T0263107

Acute-on-Chronic Liver Failure

Editor

NIKOLAOS T. PYRSOPOULOS

CLINICS IN LIVER DISEASE

www.liver.theclinics.com

Consulting Editor
NORMAN GITLIN

August 2023 • Volume 27 • Number 3

ELSEVIER

1600 John F. Kennedy Boulevard • Suite 1800 • Philadelphia, Pennsylvania, 19103-2899

http://www.theclinics.com

CLINICS IN LIVER DISEASE Volume 27, Number 3
August 2023 ISSN 1089-3261, ISBN-13: 978-0-323-94033-7

Editor: Kerry Holland
Developmental Editor: Ann Gielou M. Posedio

Clinics in Liver Disease (ISSN 1089-3261) is published quarterly by Elsevier Inc., 360 Park Avenue South, New York, NY 10010-1710. Months of issue are February, May, August, and November. Business and Editorial Offices: 1600 John F. Kennedy Blvd., Ste. 1800, Philadelphia, PA 19103-2899. Customer Service Office: 3251 Riverport Lane, Maryland Heights, MO 63043. Periodicals postage paid at New York, NY and additional mailing offices. Subscription prices are $339.00 per year (U.S. individuals), $100.00 per year (U.S. student/resident), $674.00 per year (U.S. institutions), $434.00 per year (international individuals), $200.00 per year (international student/resident), $837.00 per year (international instituitions), $393.00 per year (Canadian individuals), $100.00 per year (Canadian student/resident), and $837.00 per year (Canadian institutions). Foreign air speed delivery is included in all *Clinics* subscription prices. All prices are subject to change without notice. **POSTMASTER:** Send address changes to *Clinics in Liver Disease*, Elsevier Health Sciences Division, Subscription Customer Service, 3251 Riverport Lane, Maryland Heights, MO 63043. **Customer Service: Telephone: 1-800-654-2452 (U.S. and Canada); 314-447-8871 (outside U.S. and Canada). Fax: 314-447-8029. E-mail: journalscustomer service-usa@elsevier.com (for print support); journalsonlinesupport-usa@elsevier.com (for online support).**

Reprints. For copies of 100 or more of articles in this publication, please contact the Commercial Reprints Department, Elsevier Inc., 360 Park Avenue South, New York, NY 10010-1710. Tel.: 212-633-3874; Fax: 212-633-3820; E-mail: reprints@elsevier.com.

Clinics in Liver Disease is covered in *MEDLINE/PubMed (Index Medicus)*, Science Citation Index Expanded, Journal Citation Reports/Science Edition, and Current Contents/Clinical Medicine.

Contributors

CONSULTING EDITOR

NORMAN GITLIN, MD, FRCP (LONDON), FRCPE (EDINBURGH), FAASLD, FACP, FACG
Head of Hepatology, Southern California Liver Centers, San Clemente, California, USA

EDITOR

NIKOLAOS T. PYRSOPOULOS, MD, PhD, MBA
Professor of Medicine, Division of Gastroenterology and Hepatology, Department of Medicine, Rutgers New Jersey Medical School, Newark, New Jersey, USA

AUTHORS

KAMAL AMER, MD
Division of Gastroenterology and Hepatology, Department of Medicine, Rutgers New Jersey Medical School, Newark, New Jersey, USA

ARPIT AMIN, MD
Division of Transplant and HPB Surgery, Department of Surgery, Rutgers New Jersey Medical School, Newark, New Jersey, USA

PAOLO ANGELI, MD, PhD
Department of Medicine (DIMED), Unit of Internal Medicine and Hepatology (UIMH), University of Padova, Padova, Italy

BRYAN D. BADAL, MD
Division of Gastroenterology, Hepatology and Nutrition, Virginia Commonwealth University, Central Virginia Veterans Healthcare System, Richmond, Virginia, USA

JASMOHAN S. BAJAJ, MD
Division of Gastroenterology, Hepatology and Nutrition, Virginia Commonwealth University, Central Virginia Veterans Healthcare System, Richmond, Virginia, USA

CAMERON BEECH, MD
Department of Pathology, ARUP Laboratories, University of Utah, Salt Lake City, Utah, USA

KALYAN RAM BHAMIDIMARRI, MD, MPH, FACG, FAASLD
Division of Digestive Health and Liver Diseases, University of Miami Miller School of Medicine, Miami, Florida, USA

TALAL KHUSHID BHATTI, MD
Shaheed Zulfiqar Ali Bhutto Medical University, Islamabad, Pakistan

MADELYN J. BLAKE
Department of Medicine, University of Minnesota Medical School, Minneapolis, Minnesota, USA

ROBERT S. BROWN JR. MD, MPH
Chief, Division of Gastroenterology and Hepatology, Weill Cornell Medicine, New York, New York, USA

NAGA CHALASANI, MD
David W. Crabb Professor of Gastroenterology and Hepatology, Professor of Medicine, Vice President for Academic Affairs, Gastroenterology and Hepatology, Indiana University School of Medicine, Indiana University Health, Indianapolis, Indiana, USA

MICHAEL P. CURRY, MD
Director of Hepatology, Professor of Medicine, Beth Israel Deaconess Medical Center, Harvard Medical School, Boston, Massachusetts, USA

SUZANNE A. ELSHAFEY, MD, MPH
Fellow, Division of Gastroenterology and Hepatology, Weill Cornell Medicine, New York, New York, USA

BEN FLIKSHTEYN, MD
Division of Gastroenterology and Hepatology, Department of Medicine, Rutgers New Jersey Medical School, Newark, New Jersey, USA

MARWAN GHABRIL, MD
Professor of Medicine, Gastroenterology and Hepatology, Indiana University School of Medicine, Indiana University Health, Indianapolis, Indiana, USA

DANIELA GOYES, MD
Department of Medicine, Loyola Medicine, MacNeal Hospital, Berwyn, Illinois, USA

JAMES V. GUARRERA, MD, FACS
Professor of Surgery, Chief of Transplant and HPB Surgery, Division of Transplant and HPB Surgery, Department of Surgery, Rutgers New Jersey Medical School, Newark, New Jersey, USA

SIMONE INCICCO, MD
Department of Medicine (DIMED), Unit of Internal Medicine and Hepatology (UIMH), University of Padova, Padova, Italy

CAMILLE A. KEZER, MD
Division of Gastroenterology and Hepatology, Mayo Clinic, Rochester, Minnesota, USA

ANAND V. KULKARNI, MD
Department of Hepatology, Cluster M, Asian Institute of Gastroenterology, Hyderabad, India

PAUL Y. KWO, MD
Professor of Medicine, Director of Hepatology, Stanford University School of Medicine, Palo Alto, California, USA

VIVEK LINGIAH, MD
Division of Gastroenterology and Hepatology, Department of Medicine, Rutgers New Jersey Medical School, Newark, New Jersey, USA

CHEN LIU, MD, PhD
Department of Pathology, Yale School of Medicine, New Haven, Connecticut, USA

KERI E. LUNSFORD, MD, PhD
Department of Surgery, Division of Liver Transplant and HPB Surgery, Rutgers New Jersey Medical School, Newark, New Jersey, USA

JIAYI MA, MD
Gastroenterology and Hepatology, Indiana University School of Medicine, Indianapolis, Indiana, USA

PAUL MARTIN, MD, FRCP, FRCPI
Professor of Medicine, Chief, Division of Digestive Health and Liver Diseases, University of Miami Miller School of Medicine, Miami, Florida, USA

MUMTAZ NIAZI, MD
Division of Gastroenterology and Hepatology, Department of Medicine, Rutgers New Jersey Medical School, Newark, New Jersey, USA

GUERGANA G. PANAYOTOVA, MD
Division of Transplant and HPB Surgery, Department of Surgery, Rutgers New Jersey Medical School, Newark, New Jersey, USA

SALVATORE PIANO, MD, PhD
Department of Medicine (DIMED), Unit of Internal Medicine and Hepatology (UIMH), University of Padova, Padova, Italy

NIKOLAOS T. PYRSOPOULOS, MD, PhD, MBA
Professor of Medicine, Division of Gastroenterology and Hepatology, Department of Medicine, Rutgers New Jersey Medical School, Newark, New Jersey, USA

K. RAJENDER REDDY, MD
Founders Professor of Medicine, Division of Gastroenterology and Hepatology, University of Pennsylvania, Philadelphia, Pennsylvania, USA

RAQUEL OLIVO SALCEDO, MD
Assistant Professor of Medicine, Division of Gastroenterology and Hepatology, Rutgers New Jersey Medical School, Newark, New Jersey, USA

ANDREW R. SCHEINBERG, MD
Division of Digestive Health and Liver Diseases, University of Miami Miller School of Medicine, Miami, Florida, USA

VIJAY H. SHAH, MD
Division of Gastroenterology and Hepatology, Mayo Clinic, Rochester, Minnesota, USA

DOUGLAS A. SIMONETTO, MD
Division of Gastroenterology and Hepatology, Mayo Clinic, Rochester, Minnesota, USA

ASHWANI K. SINGAL, MD, MS
Chief of Clinical Research, Avera Transplant Institute, Professor of Medicine, University of South Dakota Sanford School of Medicine, Sioux Falls, South Dakota, USA

CLIFFORD J. STEER, MD
Departments of Medicine, and Genetics, Cell Biology and Development, University of Minnesota Medical School, Minneapolis, Minnesota, USA

ZAID H. TAFESH, MD, MSc
Assistant Professor of Medicine, Division of Gastroenterology and Hepatology, Department of Medicine, Rutgers New Jersey Medical School, Newark, New Jersey, USA

HIRSH D. TRIVEDI, MD
Faculty Physician, Transplant Hepatology, Karsh Division of Gastroenterology and Hepatology, Cedars-Sinai Medical Center, Los Angeles, California, USA

ALI WAKIL, MD
Division of Gastroenterology and Hepatology, Department of Medicine, Rutgers New Jersey Medical School, Newark, New Jersey, USA

FLORENCE WONG, MBBS, MD, FRACP, FRCPC, FAASLD
Department of Medicine, Division of Gastroenterology and Hepatology, University Health Network, University of Toronto, Toronto, Ontario, Canada

XUCHEN ZHANG, MD, PhD
Department of Pathology, Yale School of Medicine, New Haven, Connecticut, USA

Contents

advances have been made in our understanding of the mechanisms underlying regeneration following loss of hepatic mass. Liver regeneration in acute liver failure possesses several classic pathways, while also exhibiting unique differences in key processes such as the roles of differentiated cells and stem cell analogs. Here we summarize these unique differences and new molecular mechanisms involving the gut–liver axis, immunomodulation, and microRNAs with an emphasis on applications to the patient population through stem cell therapies and prognostication.

Acute-on-chronic liver failure (ACLF) is a potentially reversible syndrome that develops in patients with cirrhosis or with underlying chronic liver disease (CLD) and is characterized by acute decompensation, organ failure, and high short-term mortality. Hepatitis A and hepatitis E are major causes of ACLF. Hepatitis B may also cause ACLF through a flare of hepatitis B, acute infection, or reactivation. Besides supportive care, nucleoside/nucleotide analog therapy should also be initiated in this setting. Nonhepatotropic viruses may rarely also cause ACLF with the severe acute respiratory syndrome coronavirus 2 virus recently being identified with poorer outcomes in those with underlying CLD.

Drug-induced liver injury (DILI) is a global problem related to prescription and over-the-counter medications as well as herbal and dietary supplements. It can lead to liver failure with the risk of death and need for liver transplantation. Acute-on-chronic liver failure (ACLF) may be precipitated by DILI and is associated with a high risk of mortality. This review addresses the challenges in defining the diagnostic criteria of drug-induced ACLF (DI-ACLF). The studies characterizing DI-ACLF and its outcomes are summarized, highlighting geographic differences in underlying liver disease and implicated agents, as are future directions in the field.

Vascular, autoimmune hepatitis, and malignant causes of acute-on-chronic liver failure are rare but important to consider and investigate in patients with underlying liver disease who present with acute deterioration and other more common etiologies have been excluded. Vascular processes including Budd–Chiari syndrome and portal vein thrombosis require imaging for diagnosis and anticoagulation is the mainstay of therapy. Patients may require advanced interventional therapy including transjugular intrahepatic portosystemic shunt or consideration of liver transplantation. Autoimmune hepatitis is a complex disease entity that requires a high degree of clinical suspicion and can present heterogeneously.

Acute-on-Chronic liver failure (ACLF) is a unique disease process associated with significant short-term mortality wherein patients with either chronic liver disease or cirrhosis suffer rapid decompensation in hepatic function accompanied by extrahepatic organ failures. Alcohol-associated hepatitis (AH) is a common precipitant of ACLF and has been shown to uniquely affect the pathophysiology of systemic and hepatic immune responses in patients with ACLF. Treatment of AH-associated ACLF includes supportive measures as well as treatment directed at AH; however, AH-directed therapies unfortunately remain limited and are of suboptimal efficacy.

Acute-on-chronic liver failure (ACLF) is characterized by abrupt decompensation in a patient with chronic liver disease with extrahepatic organ dysfunction and is implicated in an increased risk of mortality. ACLF may be present in approximately 20% to 40% of hospitalized cirrhosis. There are several diagnostic scoring systems for ACLF; one defined by the North American Consortium for Study of End-stage Liver Disease is the presence of acutely decompensated cirrhosis complicated by failure of two or more organ systems: circulatory, renal, neurological, coagulopathy, and/or pulmonary.

Acute-on-chronic liver failure (ACLF) is a clinical syndrome characterized by severe hepatic dysfunction leading to multiorgan failure in patients with end-stage liver disease. ACLF is a challenging clinical syndrome with a rapid clinical course and high short-term mortality. There is no single uniform definition of ACLF or consensus in predicting ACLF-related outcomes, which makes comparing studies difficult and standardizing management protocols challenging. This review aims to provide insights into the common prognostic models that define and grade ACLF.

Acute-on-chronic liver failure (ACLF) is characterized by the presence of chronic liver disease and extrahepatic organ failure and is associated with a high rate of short-term mortality. International societies have sought to define the criteria for ACLF and differ on definitions. Encephalopathy is an important organ failure in ACLF cases and is included as a marker of ACLF across society definitions. Both brain failure and ACLF commonly occur in the presence of a triggering event and in the setting of the large amount of inflammation that ensues. The presence of encephalopathy as a part of ACLF not only increases the chances of mortality but also provides unique challenges in that the patient will be limited in conversations around major decisions such as need for advanced level of care, liver transplant, or even end-of-life decisions. Many decisions need to be made quickly and occur in parallel in the care of patients with encephalopathy and ACLF and include stabilizing the patient, identifying precipitants or alternative diagnoses, and medical management. Infections has emerged as a major trigger for both ACLF and encephalopathy, and special attention should be given to identifying and treating infections as they occur.

Owing to inherent limitations of static cold storage, marginal liver grafts from donors after circulatory death and extended criteria donors after brain death are prone to be discarded secondary to the increased risk of severe early allograft dysfunction and ischemic cholangiopathy. Marginal liver grafts resuscitated with hypothermic machine perfusion and normothermic machine perfusion demonstrate lower degree of ischemia-reperfusion injury and have decreased risk of severe early allograft dysfunction and ischemic cholangiopathy. Marginal grafts preserved by ex vivo machine perfusion technology can be used to rescue patients with acute-on-chronic liver failure who are underserved by the current deceased donor liver allocation system.

Acute-on-chronic liver failure (ACLF) results from an acute decompensation of cirrhosis due to exogenous insult. The condition is characterized by a severe systemic inflammatory response, inappropriate compensatory anti-inflammatory response, multisystem extrahepatic organ failure, and high short-term mortality. Here, the authors evaluate the current status of potential treatments for ACLF and assess their efficacy and therapeutic potential.

CLINICS IN LIVER DISEASE

SERIES OF RELATED INTEREST

Gastroenterology Clinics of North America
https://www.gastro.theclinics.com

THE CLINICS ARE AVAILABLE ONLINE!
Access your subscription at:
www.theclinics.com

Preface

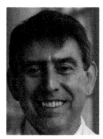

Nikolaos T. Pyrsopoulos, MD, PhD, MBA
Editor

Acute-on-Chronic Liver Failure (ACLF) is a syndrome defined as rapid decompensation of liver function and organ failure on a patient suffering from chronic liver disease with potentially lethal complications. Managing a patient with ACLF is extremely challenging requiring a "team approach" composed by an army of highly specialized and dedicated clinicians and researchers. We are excited, as several causes inducing liver disease can now be controlled, viral in particular, but the way we treat late stages of ACLF still remains the same: Liver Transplantation. The major preexisting chronic liver disease is alcohol-associated and fatty liver; we have seen a significant decline in Hepatitis C–related cause. Regarding the health care cost per patient in comparison to the most common causes of hospitalization, it is noteworthy to mention that ACLF is much higher. A number of trials utilizing new compounds or even noncellular and cellular-assisted devices have been conducted, but the survival benefit has not been proven or it is equivocal.

This issue of *Clinics in Liver Disease* is focused on Acute-on-Chronic Liver Failure and provides an explicit comprehensive approach emphasizing the multidisciplinary to epidemiologic aspects, pathophysiology of the diseases and syndromes in a state-of-the-art review of the literature, diagnostic modalities, clinical manifestations, management, and potential future directions.

An outstanding international panel of clinicians and researchers who defined this field has provided a thorough review of the current literature along with their experience in a superior academic way. This issue of the *Clinics in Liver Disease* Acute-on-Chronic

Clin Liver Dis 27 (2023) xiii–xiv
https://doi.org/10.1016/j.cld.2023.03.001
1089-3261/23/© 2023 Published by Elsevier Inc.

liver.theclinics.com

Liver Failure provides exceptional insight into the multidisciplinary approach these patients should have.

Nikolaos T. Pyrsopoulos, MD, PhD, MBA
Division of Gastroenterology and Hepatology
Department of Medicine
Rutgers New Jersey Medical School
185 South Orange Avenue, MSB H, Room - 536
Newark, NJ 07101-1709, USA

E-mail address:
pyrsopni@njms.rutgers.edu

Classification and Epidemiologic Aspects of Acute-on-Chronic Liver Failure

Zaid H. Tafesh, MD, MSc[a], Raquel Olivo Salcedo, MD[b],
Nikolaos T. Pyrsopoulos, MD, PhD, MBA[c],*

KEYWORDS

- Acute on chronic liver failure • Definition • Classification • Epidemiology • Triggers

KEY POINTS

- Acute-on-chronic liver failure (ACLF) has several definitions including those presented by North American Consortium for Study of End-stage Liver Disease, Asian Pacific Association for the Study of the Liver, and European Association for the Study of the Liver-Chronic Liver Failure.
- ACLF is an entity associated with a high risk of mortality in a short period of time.
- Both the cause of the chronic liver disease and the instigating factor for ACLF formulate the epidemiology of this disorder.

DEFINITION AND CLASSIFICATION OF ACUTE ON CHRONIC LIVER FAILURE
Introduction

Acute liver failure and acute decompensation of cirrhosis are both well-defined entities that may be indications for advanced liver care and potential liver transplantation. Some of the major differences between these two conditions include the absence of preexisting liver disease and the high rate of short-term mortality (measured in weeks) among patients with acute liver failure.[1] Although the rate of short-term mortality among patients with newly decompensated cirrhosis is lower than in fulminant liver failure, the presence of complications of portal hypertension continue to be associated with a reduction in transplant-free survival.[2] Acute-on-chronic liver failure (ACLF) is recognized as a separate disorder combining features commonly associated with acute liver failure and decompensated cirrhosis. It is defined in such a way to allow for the identification of patients with underlying chronic liver disease who carry

[a] Division of Gastroenterology and Hepatology, Rutgers New Jersey Medical School, 185 South Orange Avenue, MSB H Room-534, Newark, NJ 07103, USA; [b] Division of Gastroenterology and Hepatology, Rutgers New Jersey Medical School, 185 South Orange Avenue, MSB H Room-532, Newark, NJ 07103, USA; [c] Division of Gastroenterology and Hepatology, Rutgers New Jersey Medical School, 185 South Orange Avenue, MSB H Room-536, Newark, NJ 07103, USA
* Corresponding author. 185 South Orange Avenue, MSB H Room - 536, Newark, NJ 07101-1709.
E-mail address: pyrsopni@njms.rutgers.edu

Clin Liver Dis 27 (2023) 553–562
https://doi.org/10.1016/j.cld.2023.03.002
1089-3261/23/© 2023 Elsevier Inc. All rights reserved.
liver.theclinics.com

an elevated rate of short-term mortality. Hepatic failure and other associated extrahepatic organ failures, often triggered by events such as gastrointestinal bleeding or infection (among others) severe as the primary hallmarks of this condition.[2–4] Despite increased global recognition among clinicians in recent years,[5] ACLF continues to be a challenge to accurately define. Various international liver societies have proposed unique definitions with overlapping elements, but differ in key components (Table 1). This is in part likely related to different methodologies in the formulation of ACLF databases with different inclusion and exclusion criteria. Moreover, regional differences in liver disease prevalence and incidence by etiology is likely taken into consideration when developing each society's specific ACLF definition.

The most used definitions of ACLF are derived by the North American Consortium for Study of End-stage Liver Disease (NACSELD), the European Association for the Study of the chronic liver failure (CLIF) Acute-on-Chronic Liver Failure in Cirrhosis (CANONIC) study, and the Asian Pacific Association for the Study of the Liver (APASL). Despite the variations in the way hepatic and extrahepatic organ failures are used to classify the syndrome, the EASL-CLIF definition is very specific in its parameters, whereas the NACSELD definition is more broad and simple, and the APASL define ACLF based on intrahepatic triggers.[6] In addition, epidemiologic similarities and differences in chronic liver disease and cirrhosis within each of these different regions as well as variations in the triggers leading to ACLF have resulted in diverse cohorts used to define ACLF globally. In this article, the authors present the differences and similarities that characterize the three most cited positions on ACLF definition, classification, and epidemiologic considerations.

DEFINITION AND CLASSIFICATION OF ACUTE-ON-CHRONIC LIVER FAILURE
North America

Defining the syndrome
The NACSELD developed a definition for ACLF among a cohort of hospitalized infected patients with cirrhosis. In 2014, the NACSELD published prospective, multicenter data on patients with cirrhosis admitted with infections and described their survival at 30 days. They found that the outcomes among this patient population were directly related to the number of organ failures identified during their hospitalization. Four organ systems were used and assessed in this definition: circulatory, respiratory, renal, and cerebral. Circulatory failure was defined as mean arterial pressure less than 60 mm Hg; respiratory failure was present when the patient required any type of mechanical ventilation; the use of hemodialysis defined renal failure and cerebral failure was included when the patient had hepatic encephalopathy of grade III or IV based on the West Haven criteria.[3] The investigator found that 30-day survival was significantly reduced in patients meeting criteria for ≥ 2 organ failures, thus serving as the benchmark used to define infection-related ACLF (I-ACLF).[3,6]

This definition may seem overly simplistic owed to the fact that it does not provide detailed parameters when describing most organ failures (such as renal or respiratory), which is in contrast to the European definition of ACLF using the chronic liver failure-Sequential Organ Failure Assessment (CLIF-SOFA) criteria.[2] In addition, the NACSELD criteria do not include hepatic-related organ failure such as evaluation of bilirubin or INR—both variables are included in the CLIF-SOFA criteria.[2] However, the investigators justify this with the fact that they were prioritizing formulating "simple clinical criteria" that could be used at the bedside to make accurate and rapid decisions. Nevertheless, the NACSELD criteria provide a significant prognostic value that has been validated in both hospitalized infected and noninfected patients since

Table 1
Comparing definitions and classification of acute on chronic liver failure

	North American Consortium for the Study of End-Stage Liver Disease[3]	European Association for the Study of the Liver Chronic Liver Failure Consortium[2]	Asian Pacific Association for the Study of the Liver ACLF Research Consortium[4]
Patients included	Acutely decompensated cirrhosis with or without prior decompensation	Acutely decompensated cirrhosis with or without prior decompensation	Cirrhosis or other chronic liver disease without previous decompensation
Definition	Presence of two or more organ Failures	ACLF Grade 1: • Single kidney failure • Single circulatory, respiratory or liver failure + Cr 1.5 mg/dL – 1.9 mg/dL or grade I or II hepatic encephalopathy • Single cerebral failure + Cr 1.5 mg/dL – 1.9 mg/dL ACLF Grade 2: two organ failures ACLF Grade 3: three or more organ failures	"Acute hepatic insult" in a patient with underlying chronic liver disease presenting with jaundice (serum bilirubin[3] 5 mg/dL) and coagulopathy (INR[3] 1.5) and resulting in the development of ascites and/or encephalopathy within a 4-wk time frame
Organ Failures	1. Circulatory: MAP < 60 mm Hg 2. Respiratory: Mechanical ventilation 3. Renal: Dialysis 4. Cerebral: Grade III or IV hepatic encephalopathy	1. Circulatory: use of vasopressors 2. Respiratory: PaO2/FiO2 ≤ 200 or SpO2/FiO2 ≤ 214 3. Renal: Creatinine ≥ 2 mg/dL or RRT 4. Cerebral: Grade III or IV hepatic encephalopathy 5. Liver: Total bilirubin ≥ 12 mg/dL 6. INR ≥ 2.5	Liver failure only. Extrahepatic organ failures are considered consequences of ACLF
Triggers	Primarily infection	Intrahepatic and extrahepatic including infection, gastrointestinal bleeding, alcohol and so forth	Only intrahepatic such as HBV reactivation, alcohol, and so forth
Strengths	• Simple and easy to use at the bedside • Externally validated including in noninfected patients • Carries significant prognostic value	• Allows for accurate definition of ACLF • Recognize significance of early renal dysfunction • Carries significant prognostic value	• Includes patients with chronic liver disease but who do not have cirrhosis • Allows for earlier identification of ACLF

Abbreviations: ACLF, acute on chronic liver failure; HBV, hepatitis B virus; MAP, mean arterial pressure; RRT, renal replacement therapy.

their publication in 2014.[7] Ultimately, the NACSELD-ACLF score performed well in predicting 30-day survival in infected and noninfected patients with cirrhosis.[7] Moreover, Rosenblatt and colleagues externally validated the NACSELD-ACLF score by examining data from the Nationwide Inpatient Sample from 2005 to 2014. This cohort was thought to be more representative as it included hospitals from all over the United States. The results of the study revealed that patients with ACLF as defined by NACSELD had a 52% inpatient mortality rate, as compared with a 6% mortality rate among those who did not meet the definition of ACLF.[8] Therefore, the NACSELD-ACLF score is a validated, reliable, and simple tool to assess prognosis in patients admitted with decompensated cirrhosis.

Categorization of acute-on-chronic liver failure by grade
In the original NACSELD cohort, the presence of any organ failure carried an increased risk of mortality, whereas the combination of two or more organ system failures was associated with a significant decrease in overall survival.[3] The presence of a single organ failure (renal, respiratory, circulatory, or cerebral) carried a morality of 28% at 30 days. This increased to 49% when two organ system failures were identified, and to 77% when all four organ systems failed. Based on this reported mortality data, the NACSELD-ACLF score is considered positive if there are two or more organ system failures with no further grading system provided. Similar findings were observed in the subsequent validation cohort of noninfected patients with cirrhosis with a 59% survival rate in patients with a positive NACSELD-ACLF score, compared with a 93% rate of survival in patients not meeting the NACSELD-ACLF criteria.[7]

Epidemiologic considerations in North America
In the NACSELD cohort, the most common underlying etiologies for cirrhosis were hepatitis C and hepatitis C with concomitant alcohol use (24% and 27%, respectively), reflecting the epidemiology of cirrhosis in North America at the beginning of the 2010s. In terms of precipitating events, infection was the universal trigger among the entire cohort.[3] By definition, the initial score developed by the NACSELD—the I-ACLF—only took into account patients with cirrhosis admitted with infection. Although the fact that only infected patients were included can be seen as a significant limitation, it can also provide valuable insight about infections as a trigger for ACLF. In general, infections have been sighted as the most recognized trigger for liver decompensation among patients with cirrhosis globally.[2,6] Urinary tract infections were the most common infection (28%), followed by spontaneous bacterial peritonitis (22%), and bacteremia (13%). In contrast to older studies, the predominant bacterial isolates were gram-positive organisms, with a notably high prevalence of fungal infections as well. Nosocomial infections were identified in 15% of the study cohort. Finally, the most common gender was male with a median age of 55 years.[3,6] In both subsequent validation studies of the NACSELD-ACLF definition, the most common etiology of underlying liver disease included hepatitis C virus (HCV) and alcohol-related liver disease, and again, the most common gender remained as male within a similar age group.[7]

Asia-Pacific Region

Defining the syndrome
The APASL has since 2004 developed a consensus working group aimed at formulating regional definitions and guidelines for the management of ACLF.[4] When compared with North America and Europe, major differences still exist in the way ACLF is both defined and classified in the Asia-Pacific region. Detailed justification for these differences is provided in the APASLs most up to date consensus statement on ACLF that was published in 2019.

ACLF is defined by the presence of an "acute hepatic insult" in a patient with underlying chronic liver disease presenting with jaundice (serum bilirubin $\geq$ 5 mg/dL) and coagulopathy (international normalized ratio [INR] $\geq$ 1.5) and resulting in the development of ascites and/or encephalopathy within a 4-week time frame.[4] Moreover, the definition specifies that this disease entity is coupled with a high 28-day mortality. ACLF was defined this way by the APASL with the aim of describing a clinical syndrome that was distinct from that of a patient with decompensated cirrhosis with gradual or sudden deterioration or acute liver failure where no preexisting liver condition is present.

Conceptually, in the Asia-Pacific region, ACLF is seen as an index presentation and is defined in a way as to allow for early detection of the condition with increasing potential for reversibility. In fact, of patients with ACLF among this cohort who achieved reversal of the syndrome at 90 days (ie, resolution of coagulopathy followed by improvement in jaundice), around two-thirds maintained stability at 1 year of follow-up.[4] Therefore, patients with prior decompensation and those presenting with extrahepatic organ dysfunction are excluded from this definition, which is in contrast from the way ACLF is defined in North America and Europe.[2,3] The acute insult precipitating ACLF must be directly hepatic, whereas extrahepatic manifestations such as sepsis are felt to be consequences of ACLF rather than potential precipitants. In addition, ACLF is not reserved only for patients with underlying cirrhosis and can include any patient with underlying chronic liver disease without cirrhosis. Although this may raise the concern that ACLF may overlap with the mere progression toward cirrhosis and related decompensating events such as ascites, the expectation of a high 28-day mortality remains a distinguishing feature of ACLF.[9] In fact, a threshold of at least 33% mortality at 4 weeks was used to identify patients with ACLF since 2014, with updated data identifying a mortality rate at 4 weeks of nearly 40% among subjects enrolled in the APASL-ACLF Research Consortium (AARC).[4] In addition, patients must meet laboratory criteria that indicate liver failure (jaundice and coagulopathy) before developing jaundice and encephalopathy,[10] which further clarifies differences between ACLF and decompensated cirrhosis.

Categorization of acute hepatic insults

The APASL further classifies ACLF based on the defined types of hepatic insults. Acute events can be defined as hepatotropic infections (viral and nonviral), drug-induced liver injury, autoimmune hepatitis flare, acute variceal bleeding, and vascular liver diseases.[4] Although generally each of these direct hepatic insults is often classified as diseases of the liver or a related complication, when associated with ACLF, they manifest in a much more aggressive manner with a poorer prognosis. Practically, when coupled with ACLF, these causes of hepatic injury are unique disease entities, a point stressed by experts in the Asia-Pacific region.

Although hepatotropic viral infections are well-defined acute precipitants of ACLF, with viral hepatitis B constituting the majority of reported cases, other less common nonviral hepatotropic infections of the liver are included in the definition of an acute event leading to ACLF. Despite knowledge that preexisting liver disease is a known risk factor for drug-induced liver injury,[11] hepatotoxicity related to drugs is less documented in the West. In contrast, drug-induced liver injury-related ACLF is a well-documented entity in Asia[12] and categorized as a separately within the spectrum of ACLF by the APASL.[4] On the other hand, because of the stringent ACLF definition aimed at excluding decompensating events of cirrhosis or subsequent consequences of ACLF, variceal bleeding is not universally accepted in the Asia-Pacific society as trigger for ACLF. However, the consensus among experts was that variceal bleeding could be considered as an acute episode leading to ACLF if such an event lead to coagulopathy and jaundice as outlined in the APASL definition for the syndrome, in light of the fact that gastrointestinal hemorrhage can lead to ischemic liver injury.[4]

Categorization of acute-on-chronic liver failure by grade

The AARC-ACLF grade is a point-based system that includes total bilirubin, hepatic encephalopathy grade, PT-INR, lactate and creatinine.[4] Patients with ACLF are divided into grade I, II, and III depending on the severity of their presentation. This score was derived using a 480-patient cohort and validated amongst 922 individuals with ACLF enrolled in the AARC.[13] In the derivation and validation cohorts, the area under the receiver operating characteristics curve (AUROC) of the AARC-ACLF score was 0.8 and 0.78, respectively. Patient mortality incrementally worsened with increased ACLF grade, with reported cumulative 28-day mortality of 12.7% with grade I ACLF and 85.9% in patients with grade III ACLF. Moreover, AARC-ACLF score at baseline was predictive of death from ACLF, with a score of greater than 10 at baseline detecting those at highest risk.[13]

Epidemiologic considerations in the Asia-Pacific region

Unfortunately, data on epidemiology in ACLF are inconsistent and sparse, likely owed to inconsistent global and intraregional definitions for the syndrome. In Asia, although the APASL consensus definition for ACLF is the most accepted definition, country-specific variations continue to exist,[14,15] complicating the ability to report epidemiological data with adequate accuracy. Precipitating events leading to ACLF serve as the primary drivers of epidemiology and provide insight into the distribution of ACLF in the Asia-Pacific region. Unfortunately, large ACLF registries are lacking in Asia, and the most epidemiologic data are based on patients treated within tertiary care centers.[10]

Although intraregional differences in the most predominant triggers for ACLF within Asia exists, acute viral hepatitis, primarily hepatitis B virus (HBV) reactivation remains one of the most common identified causes of this condition.[4,16] The reported rate of ACLF in the setting of HBV reactivation in Asia varies considerably. In one Indian study of 151 patients with HBV reactivation, over 40% of patients developed ACLF.[10] In contrast, among 110 hepatitis B e-antigen seropositive patients in Taiwan, an acute exacerbation of HBV resulted in liver decompensation in only 5% of patients.[17] This large discrepancy in the risk of ACLF secondary to HBV reactivation may be related to the baseline severity of the underlying liver disease. In particular, the patients with low ACLF risk within the Taiwan study did not have underlying cirrhosis. The only identified predictor of liver decompensation within this cohort was HBV DNA level.[17] The high incidence of HBV-related ACLF within the Asia-Pacific region is consistent across definitions for ACLF. A study from China that used the European definition for ACLF identified that 35.8% of cases were related to an HBV flare. Other viral etiologies such as superimposed hepatitis A and E constituted only 6.4% of ACLF precipitating events. Overall, patients with intrahepatic insults resulting in ACLF overwhelmingly (>90%) carried a diagnosis of chronic hepatitis B-related cirrhosis.[16] Although this study only reported a small amount of hepatitis A and E-related cases, there has been variability in the prevalence particularly of hepatitis E, with higher prevalence noted in India.[18] A study from China exploring the outcomes among patients with chronic hepatitis B with hepatitis A and E superinfections noted poorer outcomes among those with hepatitis E, with a mortality rate of 33.8% versus 1.9%.[19]

The rapid increase in harmful alcohol consumption within the Asia-Pacific region has resulted in a rise in the prevalence of acute alcohol-associated hepatitis cases and consequent ACLF in the region. In fact, some data have suggested that alcohol, rather than viral hepatitis, has become the most common hepatic insult triggering ACLF in the region, with the prevalence of alcohol-related liver disease doubling in some Asian countries.[10,20] In one study using the APASL-ACLF definition, 47% of ACLF cases were linked to alcohol use versus 25% related to viral hepatitis.[21] Patients suffering from alcohol-related ACLF tended to be younger and faced increased morbidity and mortality owed to the risk of developing rapid multisystem organ failures.[10]

Within the AARC database, drugs as a trigger for ACLF have been reported in 10% of participants. Among studies throughout Asia, 1.8% to 5.7% of ACLF-related events are linked to drugs.[4] The most cited culprits are antituberculosis drugs in India and herbal alternative medicines in China.[18,22]

The underlying liver disease in patients with ACLF within the Asia-Pacific region is most commonly hepatitis B. However, other etiologies of liver disease including alcohol-related liver disease and cryptogenic cirrhosis have been well-documented.[16]

Europe

Defining the syndrome

The EASL-CLIF Consortium has proposed an alternative definition for ACLF. This definition assesses organ failures in patients with acutely decompensated cirrhosis, taking into consideration the hepatic, circulatory, renal, brain, respiratory, and coagulation functions.[23] Similar to ACLF as defined by the APASL, the EASL-CLIF definition aims to identify patients with a high risk for short-term mortality. The European definition of ACLF was first formulated in 2013 based on the initial findings of the CANONIC study. The premise of the study was that patients with cirrhosis who were admitted with an acute decompensation of their underlying liver disease were at high risk for mortality when associated organ failures developed. The study included 1343 patients who were hospitalized throughout 29 liver units in Europe with acute decompensation. The aim was to identify those patients with a high 28-day mortality estimated at greater than 15%.[2] Among this cohort, patients with presented with ACLF had the highest mortality at 33.9%, whereas those who developed ACLF had only a slightly lower mortality rate at 29.7%. What was most striking was that despite some patients developing acute decompensation of cirrhosis, those who did not meet ACLF criteria had a mortality rate of only 1.9%, a vast difference from their ACLF inflicted counterparts. As expected, the presence of kidney failure or kidney dysfunction along with "non-kidney" organ failure was linked to a high 28-day mortality. Of note, the cohort included both patients with and without prior acute decompensation,[24] and notably, those with prior acute decompensation had a more favorable prognosis.

The EASL-CLIF definition of ACLF is based on identifying the presence of one of the six listed organ failures using the CLIF-C score and is graded based on the increasing severity of ACLF and therefore increasing risk for mortality. Within the CANONIC study, a high 28-day mortality was noted among patients with two or more organ failures, the presence of kidney failure alone, or the presence of a non-kidney organ failure with evidence of kidney dysfunction with or without mild to moderate hepatic encephalopathy. These findings formed the basis of the EASL-CLIF ACLF grading system.

Categorization of acute-on-chronic liver failure by grade

ACLF is divided into three different grades based on the number of organ failures present. ACLF grade 1 includes patients with non-kidney organ failure if renal dysfunction and/or hepatic encephalopathy (grade 1 or 2) is present, kidney failure alone, or brain failure with the presence of kidney dysfunction. ACLF grade 2 is defined by the presence of two organ failures, whereas ACLF grade 3, which carries the highest rate of mortality, is defined by the presence of three organ failures.[24] ACLF grades 1, 2, and 3 were associated within the CANONIC study with 28-day mortality rates of 22.1%, 32%, and 76.7%, respectively.[2]

Epidemiologic considerations in Europe

Given the differences in how ACLF is defined in Europe, particularly with the inclusion of patients with cirrhosis and acute decompensation (including those with a prior history of decompensation) and the identification of both intrahepatic and extrahepatic precipitants, epidemiologically, certain precipitants of ACLF have been identified in the original CANONIC cohort that are not reported in Asian cohorts. Compared with hospitalized patients with cirrhosis and acute decompensations without ACLF, those with ACLF were often younger and primarily male. Although most of the ACLF precipitating events could not be identified (43.6%), up to 13.5% of patients had more than one potential triggering event. Most commonly, bacterial infections (32.6%) precipitated ACLF, followed by active alcoholism (24.5%) and gastrointestinal bleeding (13.2%). In patients with ACLF grade 3, bacterial infections and alcohol as a precipitating event was even more common, noted in 44.7% and 40.4% of patients, respectively. The overwhelming etiology of cirrhosis was related to alcohol use (60.3% of all ACLF grades), followed by hepatitis C and hepatitis C plus alcohol.[2]

A systematic review and meta-analysis by Mezzano and colleagues[5] explored the global burden of ACLF based on 30 cohort studies using the ACLD-EASL-CLIF criteria. Among hospitalized patients with cirrhosis and decompensation, the reported prevalence of ACLF was as high as 35% with an associated 90-day mortality of 58%, underscoring the importance of identifying patients with ACLF and the prognostic value of the EASL-CLIF criteria. Interestingly, the highest prevalence of ACLF was in South Asia (65%) and globally, alcohol was the most common etiology of underlying liver disease, estimated at 45% of patients with ACLF. The most common trigger was infections, consistent with the findings of the CANONIC study.

SUMMARY

ACLF has proven to be both challenging to define and inconsistently described among various global populations with underlying chronic liver disease. However, despite variabilities in cohorts from which this condition has been described, universally, the aim is to identify a group of patients with underlying chronic liver disease with the potential to develop multisystem organ failure and face an exceedingly higher rate of short-term mortality. The three major definitions of ACLF carry significant prognostic value which can aide the practicing clinician. Although the EASL-CLIF definition allows for the most detailed description of ACLF, the North American definition provides an equally valuable simpler definition that may be easier to recall at the patient bedside. The APASL-ACLF definition on the other hand allows for earlier recognition of ACLF and the potential for more timely interventions to prevent further decompensation and the risk of death.

CLINICS CARE POINTS

- Patients with underlying chronic liver disease (primarily cirrhosis) who are hospitalized with acute decompensation of their liver disease should be evaluated for the presence of acute-on-chronic liver failure (ACLF) by one or more of the available definitions for the syndrome to help identify those at increased risk for short-term mortality.

- When possible, the trigger for ACLF should be promptly identified, with the understanding that a large portion of cases of ACLF present with an unidentifiable trigger.
- With a rapid increase in alcohol related liver disease globally, the presence of ACLF in hospitalized patients with alcohol-associated hepatitis should be recognized to help in identifying patients at risk of death without liver transplantation (if they are considered eligible candidates).

DISCLOSURE

The authors have nothing to declare related to the content of this article.

REFERENCES

1. European Association for the Study of the Liver. Electronic address eee, Clinical Practice Guidelines Panel, Wendon J, et al. EASL Clinical Practical Guidelines on the management of acute (fulminant) liver failure. J Hepatol 2017;66(5):1047–81.
2. Moreau R, Jalan R, Gines P, et al. Acute-on-chronic liver failure is a distinct syndrome that develops in patients with acute decompensation of cirrhosis. Gastroenterology 2013;144(7):1426–37, 1437 e1-9.
3. Bajaj JS, O'Leary JG, Reddy KR, et al. Survival in infection-related acute-on-chronic liver failure is defined by extrahepatic organ failures. Hepatology 2014; 60(1):250–6.
4. Sarin SK, Choudhury A, Sharma MK, et al. Acute-on-chronic liver failure: consensus recommendations of the Asian Pacific association for the study of the liver (APASL): an update. Hepatol Int 2019;13(4):353–90.
5. Mezzano G, Juanola A, Cardenas A, et al. Global burden of disease: acute-on-chronic liver failure, a systematic review and meta-analysis. Gut 2022;71(1): 148–55.
6. Bajaj JS, Moreau R, Kamath PS, et al. Acute-on-Chronic liver failure: getting ready for prime time? Hepatology 2018;68(4):1621–32.
7. O'Leary JG, Reddy KR, Garcia-Tsao G, et al. NACSELD acute-on-chronic liver failure (NACSELD-ACLF) score predicts 30-day survival in hospitalized patients with cirrhosis. Hepatology 2018;67(6):2367–74.
8. Rosenblatt R, Shen N, Tafesh Z, et al. The North American consortium for the study of end-stage liver disease-acute-on-chronic liver failure score accurately predicts survival: an external validation using a national cohort. Liver Transplant 2020;26(2):187–95.
9. Sarin SK, Kedarisetty CK, Abbas Z, et al. Acute-on-chronic liver failure: consensus recommendations of the Asian Pacific association for the study of the liver (APASL) 2014. Hepatol Int 2014;8(4):453–71.
10. Jindal A, Sarin SK. Epidemiology of liver failure in Asia-Pacific region. Liver Int 2022;42(9):2093–109.
11. Lo Re V 3rd, Carbonari DM, Lewis JD, et al. Oral azole antifungal medications and risk of acute liver injury, overall and by chronic liver disease status. Am J Med 2016;129(3):283–291 e5.
12. Duseja A, Chawla YK, Dhiman RK, et al. Non-hepatic insults are common acute precipitants in patients with acute on chronic liver failure (ACLF). Dig Dis Sci 2010;55(11):3188–92.
13. Choudhury A, Jindal A, Maiwall R, et al. Liver failure determines the outcome in patients of acute-on-chronic liver failure (ACLF): comparison of APASL ACLF

research consortium (AARC) and CLIF-SOFA models. Hepatol Int 2017;11(5):
461–71.

14. Liver F. Artificial liver group CSolDCMA, severe liver D, artificial liver group
CSoHCMA. [Diagnostic and treatment guidelines for liver failure (2012 version)].
Zhonghua Gan Zang Bing Za Zhi 2013;21(3):177–83.

15. Mochida S, Nakayama N, Ido A, et al. Proposed diagnostic criteria for acute-on-
chronic liver failure in Japan. Hepatol Res 2018;48(4):219–24.

16. Shi Y, Yang Y, Hu Y, et al. Acute-on-chronic liver failure precipitated by hepatic
injury is distinct from that precipitated by extrahepatic insults. Hepatology
2015;62(1):232–42.

17. Jeng WJ, Sheen IS, Liaw YF. Hepatitis B virus DNA level predicts hepatic decompensation in patients with acute exacerbation of chronic hepatitis B. Clin Gastroenterol Hepatol 2010;8(6):541–5.

18. Shalimar, Saraswat V, Singh SP, et al. Acute-on-chronic liver failure in India: the
Indian national association for study of the liver consortium experience.
J Gastroenterol Hepatol 2016;31(10):1742–9.

19. Zhang X, Ke W, Xie J, et al. Comparison of effects of hepatitis E or A viral superinfection in patients with chronic hepatitis B. Hepatol Int 2010;4(3):615–20.

20. Lee SS, Byoun YS, Jeong SH, et al. Type and cause of liver disease in Korea:
single-center experience, 2005-2010. Clin Mol Hepatol 2012;18(3):309–15.

21. Hernaez R, Sola E, Moreau R, et al. Acute-on-chronic liver failure: an update. Gut
2017;66(3):541–53.

22. Qin G, Shao JG, Zhu YC, et al. Population-representative incidence of acute-on-
chronic liver failure: a prospective cross-sectional study. J Clin Gastroenterol
2016;50(8):670–5.

23. Arroyo V, Moreau R, Jalan R. Acute-on-Chronic liver failure. N Engl J Med 2020;
382(22):2137–45.

24. Zaccherini G, Weiss E, Moreau R. Acute-on-chronic liver failure: definitions, pathophysiology and principles of treatment. JHEP Rep 2021;3(1):100176.

Mechanisms of Disease and Multisystemic Involvement

Kamal Amer, MD[a], Ben Flikshteyn, MD[a], Vivek Lingiah, MD[a], Zaid Tafesh, MD, MSc[b], Nikolaos T. Pyrsopoulos, MD, PhD, MBA[c],*

KEYWORDS

- Acute-on-chronic liver failure • Apoptosis • Hepatocytes • Multiorgan

KEY POINTS

- Liver failure in ACLF involves complex cellular signaling resulting from both apoptosis and hepatic necrosis.
- Immune system activation plays a vital role in the pathophysiology of ACLF and includes activation by PAMPs and DAMPs.
- Multiple pathophysiologic mechanisms have been proposed to be involved in the developed of hepatic encephalopathy in patients with ACLF.
- ACLF-related acute kidney failure is often multifactorial, triggered by events just as hypotension, immune activation by DAMPs/PAMPs, SIRS, and acute tubular necrosis.

INTRODUCTION

Acute-on-chronic liver failure (ACLF) represents a syndrome of multiorgan system dysfunction associated with underlying chronic liver disease. Patients with ACLF present with acute deterioration of their liver function and associated organ failures secondary to several potential triggers. Given the complexity of this syndrome, the variable presentations associated with ACLF, and the exhaustive list of potential triggers, the exact mechanism of ACLF is not fully understood. This article describes the proposed pathophysiologic mechanisms believed to be contributing and driving ACLF.

LIVER

There are 2 main categories of pathologic changes that can lead to liver failure: acute, severe liver necrosis and chronic, progressive damage to hepatocytes. In the case of

[a] Division of Gastroenterology and Hepatology, Department of Medicine, Rutgers University, 185 South Orange Avenue, MSB H Room - 538, Newark, NJ 07101-1709, USA; [b] Division of Gastroenterology and Hepatology, Department of Medicine, Rutgers University, 185 South Orange Avenue, MSB H Room - 53, Newark, NJ 07101-1709, USA; [c] Division of Gastroenterology and Hepatology, Department of Medicine, Rutgers University, 185 South Orange Avenue, MSB H Room - 536, Newark, NJ 07101-1709, USA
* Corresponding author.
E-mail address: pyrsopni@njms.rutgers.edu

Clin Liver Dis 27 (2023) 563–579
https://doi.org/10.1016/j.cld.2023.03.003
1089-3261/23/© 2023 Elsevier Inc. All rights reserved.

liver.theclinics.com

liver failure, a severe and sudden injury to hepatocytes results in competition between cell death and regeneration. The injured hepatocytes release inflammatory cytokines, which attract inflammatory cells and consequently inhibit the process of cell division. Hepatocyte damage causes increased waste product accumulation leading to a systemic inflammatory response. The ultimate result of this cascade of events is impairment in hepatocyte regeneration.

Both apoptosis and hepatic necrosis are implicated in the pathophysiology of liver failure. Apoptosis, or programmed cell death, is a complex process that involves multiple signaling pathways.[1] The severity of apoptosis in the liver can vary based on the trigger that ultimately results in cell death.[2] Apoptosis is often a silent process, resulting in minimal hepatic inflammation. In contrast, necrosis results in a rapid and severe inflammatory response in which the depletion of ATP leads to cell edema causing hepatocyte rupture.[3] Cell death can be caused by various interconnected processes such as caspases, oxidative stress and antioxidants, transcription factors, cytokines, and kinases.[2,4] The type and duration of cellular injury determines whether cell death will occur through apoptosis or necrosis.

Necrosis involves a series of events including oxidative stress, depletion of ATP, and loss of membrane integrity that collectively result in the initiation of an inflammatory immune response. Mitochondrial depolarization, breakdown of lysosomes, and rapid ion changes contribute to a cycle of volume shifts, cell edema, and the formation of blebs (small bulges on the surface of cells) that ultimately triggers cell death. Other notable features of necrosis include significant energy loss, the production of reactive oxygen species (ROS), and the activation of nonapoptotic proteases. In addition, there is a significant increase in cytosolic calcium levels during necrosis, which leads to an overload of calcium in the mitochondria, stopping ATP production. The interplay between calcium shifts, ATP loss, and oxidative stress results in extensive hepatocyte death, with the release of intracellular contents from the ruptured hepatocytes causing downstream secondary inflammation.[5–8]

Apoptosis is a common theme in most cases of hepatocyte injury. Factors such as viruses and hepatotoxins can prompt apoptosis through ligands and receptors on the cell membrane. Two pathways identified in hepatic failure include the extrinsic pathway and the intrinsic pathway. The extrinsic pathway involves the direct activation of caspases through the interaction of apoptosis-causing factors and their respective ligands.[9] For example, binding of tumor necrosis factor alpha (TNF-α) and Fas ligand (FasL) to their respective transmembrane proteins (TNF-R1 and Fas) results in the activation of caspase-8, caspase-3, and DNA fragmentation.[10,11] The intrinsic pathway involves the activation of caspases through mitochondrial signals. Mitochondrial damage, caused by excess ROS, leads to the release of cytochrome c and activation of caspase-9, which in turn activates caspase-3 and triggers apoptosis.[12] Both apoptosis and necrosis often occur simultaneously in the setting of liver failure. This pathway overlap is described as necroapoptosis.

Activation of cellular receptors involved in apoptosis can result in liver failure, which has been described in animal models[9,13] and patients with viral hepatitis C.[14] Nearly all cases of acute-on-chronic liver disease involve apoptosis, which can affect hepatic regeneration and fibrosis, and consequently result in the development of hepatic cirrhosis. Liver failure can result from hepatocyte loss surpassing the liver's ability to regenerate. The loss of hepatocytes leads to a decline in liver function, disruption of intrahepatic metabolism, and extrahepatic organ dysfunction. Hepatocyte death through necrosis increases systemic inflammation and reduces the liver's ability to clear circulating cytokines. The combined effects of these processes cause severe liver injury, which can have serious consequences and a poor prognosis.

ACLF is typically characterized by coagulopathy and hyperbilirubinemia. The mechanism of liver failure is determined by the type of liver injury. For example, alcohol-related ACLF may involve apoptosis, whereas flare-ups of hepatitis B-related ACLF may cause massive hepatic necrosis. Injured hepatocytes have a reduced ability to secrete bile salts, and inflammation resulting from tissue damage or pathogens can lead to decreased bile transporters in hepatocytes, resulting in cholestasis.[15]

IMMUNE SYSTEM

The liver plays a key role in cellular and innate immunity and contains immune cells and cytokines that can mediate immune responses. Bacterial by-products enter the portal circulation and are processed within the liver. Activation of the immune system plays a crucial role in the development of ACLF. Both the body's inflammatory response and its compensatory anti-inflammatory response are more pronounced in people with cirrhosis and especially pronounced in those with ACLF. Dysbiosis (imbalance in the gut microbiome) and increased gut permeability that allows for antigens to translocate through the gut lining are associated with increased levels of endotoxins in the blood in patients with cirrhosis and ACLF. The presence of chronic liver disease and cirrhosis impairs the body's innate immunity by reducing the function of pattern recognition receptors and other proteins that help destroy bacteria, thereby decreasing the body's defense mechanisms against infections.

Both the innate and adaptive immune systems play complementary roles in the process of ACLF. The innate immune system is activated by pathogen-associated molecular patterns (PAMPs) or damage-associated molecular patterns (DAMPs), which are signals released as a result of cellular damage. Different triggers for ACLF can result in variable signaling of the innate immune system. Sterile inflammation triggered by DAMPs can results from triggers such as alcohol, surgery, or acetaminophen exposure. PAMPs, on the other hand, can cause an inflammatory response commonly seen in the setting of sepsis. Immune cells express Toll-like receptors (TLRs) that recognize both PAMPs and DAMPs. These TLRs play a role in detecting foreign substances and activating intracellular defense mechanisms. This activation of inflammatory cascades often leads cellular damage that overwhelms regeneration and consequently results in hepatic failure.[16]

There is significant overlap in symptoms associated with ACLF and severe sepsis or systemic inflammatory response syndrome (SIRS) with multiorgan failure (**Box 1**).[17–20] Like sepsis, immune paralysis has been demonstrated in liver failure. The impact of SIRS on the outcome of liver failure has been well studied and is linked to multiorgan failure and increased mortality (**Fig. 1**).[18–20] SIRS is caused by the release of proinflammatory cytokines like TNF-α, interleukin (IL)-1, and IL-6.[21] In parallel, there is a compensatory anti-inflammatory response syndrome (CARS) that

---

Box 1
Systemic inflammatory response syndrome, defined by meeting 2 or more of the following criteria

- Temperature greater than 38°C or less than 36°C
- Heart rate more than 90 beats per minute
- Respiratory rate more than 20 breaths per minute or $Paco_2$ less than 32 mm Hg
- White blood cell count greater than 12,000/mm^3 or less than 4000/mm^3 or less than 10% immature neutrophils

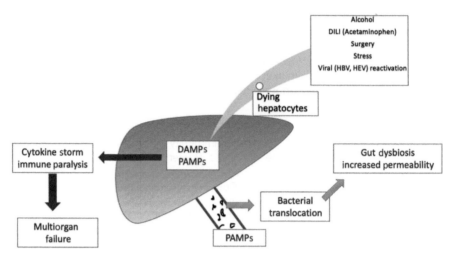

Fig. 1. In the pathogenesis of immune activation in ACLF, several factors can contribute to immune activation. Dysbiosis in the gut and increased gut permeability can lead to increased rates of bacterial translocation and endotoxemia, activating the immune system through PAMPs. In addition, various "sterile" inflammatory pathways such as alcohol use, surgery, acetaminophen toxicity, and viral hepatitis reactivation can cause hepatocyte necrosis and the release of DAMPs, leading to immune activation. This immune activation, in the form of a cytokine storm, can eventually lead to immune paralysis and multiorgan failure, increasing the risk of bacterial infection. DILI, drug induced liver injury; HBV, hepatitis B Virus; HEV, hepatitis E Virus.

involves the release of anti-inflammatory cytokines including IL-4, IL-10, and transforming growth factor-β, which helps reduce the systemic impact of SIRS. However, prolonged CARS has been shown to lead to sepsis and thus may not be beneficial and result in increased rates of mortality. Despite having a strong inflammatory immune response, patients with ACLF are more prone to infections and have high morbidity and mortality.[22–24] The relationship between SIRS and high susceptibility to infection in patients with liver failure may be due to immune dysregulation caused by the inflammatory response.[25]

Monocytes and macrophages/Kupffer cells play key roles in innate and adaptive immune responses. Their activation leads to the production of cytokines, which can enhance both proinflammatory and anti-inflammatory responses and stimulate T-cell activation. There are several changes in monocyte function and secretion in ACLF, such as increased levels of IL-6 and C-reactive protein (CRP). In liver failure, there is a decrease in TNF-α secretion accompanied by an increase in the level of anti-inflammatory/immunosuppressive cytokine IL-10 and a decrease in HLA-DR expression, leading to impaired monocyte antigen presentation.[26–29]

The liver is the primary site of fibronectin and complement synthesis. Fibronectin is a glycoprotein involved in opsonization, a process that helps clear pathogens through Kupffer cells and the reticuloendothelial system. Decreased levels of fibronectin have been seen in patients with ACLF, and this has been associated with increased mortality.[30] In addition to reducing complement levels, particularly C3 and C5, liver failure also leads to qualitative changes in both the classical and alternative pathways of complement activation, resulting in impaired opsonization.[31]

Neutrophils are an essential part of the innate immune system. Research suggests that neutrophils in cirrhosis have high resting ROS production but impaired neutrophil-endothelial adhesion and neutrophil chemotaxis.[29] Neutrophil dysfunction in cirrhosis may be reversible. Granulocyte colony-stimulating factor, an immunomodulatory glycoprotein that promotes neutrophil cell growth, differentiation, and function, has been shown in small studies to improve survival in ACLF. This benefit is likely due to liver regeneration, improved immune response, and the reversal of significant immune dysfunction through improved neutrophil activity, which helps prevent sepsis and reduce mortality.[32]

Although the immune mechanisms triggering and resulting in liver failure are variable and complex, the imbalance between proinflammatory and anti-inflammatory processes within the liver ultimately determines whether liver failure or hepatic regeneration occurs. Massive hepatocyte necrosis leads to the release of proinflammatory and anti-inflammatory cytokines that results in immune dysregulation. This immune dysregulation in ACLF leads to poor outcomes in patients with chronic liver disease who ultimately develop multiorgan failure because of increased systemic inflammation.

BRAIN

Neurological deterioration is a major feature commonly seen in ACLF. The onset of hepatic encephalopathy (HE) can be sudden, starting with mild confusion or agitation and potentially progressing to delirium, seizures, and coma, which is associated with reduced survival (**Table 1**).[33,34]

HE, which is associated with worse outcomes in cases of ACLF,[35] is caused by hyperammonemia, systemic inflammation, and problems with cerebral blood flow. The development of HE in cases of ACLF is influenced by ammonia. In astrocytes, ammonia is converted to glutamine, which can cause osmotic stress within the cell or lead to ammonia production in the mitochondria, resulting in oxidative stress.[35,36] Hyperammonemia has been significantly associated with HE in patients with ACLF. Higher ammonia levels are correlated with a greater severity of HE, whereas a reduction in serum ammonia levels is associated with improvement in HE symptoms.[37]

Cerebral edema can be caused by hyperammonemia and systemic inflammation due to a hepatic insult. There seems to be an additive relationship between ammonia and inflammation in the development of this condition, as observed in murine models of ACLF wherein rats with cirrhosis given endotoxin had similar results as patients with ACLF who developed cerebral edema.[36]

Patients with cirrhosis are more prone to infection, which is a common trigger for HE.[38] Shawcross and colleagues[38] studied 100 patients with cirrhosis admitted for grade 3 to 4 HE and found that 46% had positive blood cultures and 22% had SIRS. SIRS was significantly more common in patients with grade 4 HE compared with those with grade 3 HE.[38] In addition to systemic inflammation, neuroinflammation caused by the release of TNF-α and IL-6 from microglial cells may also contribute to the neuropsychological damage caused by elevated ammonia levels.[35]

Table 1	
West Haven criteria grades of severity of hepatic encephalopathy and the associated signs and symptoms[33]	
Grade	**Signs/Symptoms**
1	Mild lack of awareness, shortened attention span, sleep disturbance
2	Lethargy, minimal disorientation for time/place, asterixis
3	Stuporous, incoherent speech, sleeping but wakes with stimulation
4	Comatose

Although cerebral blood flow is generally reduced in cirrhosis, there is evidence that it may be increased in ACLF. The effect of this alteration in cerebral blood flow has been demonstrated by assessing the outcomes related to placement of a transjugular intrahepatic portosystemic shunt (TIPS) in patients with cirrhosis. TIPS has been demonstrated to cause endotoxemia and consequently, increased levels of nitric oxide. This cascade of events is associated with endothelial dysfunction and results in increased cerebral blood flow.[36,37] The result is an increased risk for HE, a well-documented risk after TIPS. Cerebral oxygenation, as measured by jugular venous O_2 (JVO$_2$, which is thought to indicate cerebral oxygen use and be linked to changes in cerebral blood flow), has also been studied. Sawhney and colleagues[37] found that abnormal baseline JVO$_2$ was significantly associated with both the presence and severity of HE and slower recovery from HE.

ACLF is characterized by less frequent instances of increased intracranial pressure and deaths caused by cerebral edema compared with acute liver failure. Studies have shown that overt cerebral edema occurs in approximately 5% of patients with ACLF. The low occurrence of death from cerebral herniation may be due to cerebral atrophy or decreased cerebral perfusion.[35]

In acute liver failure, it is widely accepted that cerebral edema is caused by the production of glutamine in astrocytes, leading to cytotoxic edema. However, there is controversy surrounding the cause of cerebral edema in ACLF. In chronic liver failure, the process of glutamine production in astrocytes occurs more slowly, providing the brain with enough time to shift other organic osmolytes like myoinositol and choline to compensate for imbalances caused by increased intra-astrocyte glutamine.[39,40]

There have been several MRI studies aimed at understanding fluid shifts within the brain. Mean diffusivity (MD) is a measure of the movement of water through cell membranes. Kale and colleagues[41] found that increased MD in patients with chronic liver failure was associated with interstitial edema, in contrast to controls. Nath and colleagues[39] compared MD in patients with ACLF with those with chronic liver failure and found that both MD and CS (spherical isotropy) were significantly increased in patients with chronic liver failure, but MD was nonsignificantly decreased and CS was significantly increased in patients with ACLF. The researchers suggested that the increase in CS was due to increased extracellular fluid. In patients with chronic liver failure, both CS and MD were increased, leading to interstitial edema (likely due to the decreased expression of glial fibrillary acid protein in astrocytes). In patients with ACLF, the initial precipitating event is thought to cause a decrease in MD (associated with intracellular, cytotoxic edema) and an increase in CS resulting in increased extracellular and interstitial edema. Nath and colleagues[39] concluded that both interstitial and cytotoxic edema were present in ACLF, but that interstitial edema was more predominant due to the nonsignificant change in MD.

Gupta and colleagues[42] studied cerebral edema in patients with ACLF using MRI. The investigators divided the patients into 2 groups: one with cerebral failure (all grades 3 of ACLF) and a second group without cerebral failure. Cerebral failure included all patients with grades 3 and 4 HE. The investigators found that patients with ACLF had evidence of cerebral edema on MRI, as measured by MD scores, which increased in severity with higher grades of ACLF. Levels of IL-6 were also significantly elevated in grade 3 ACLF compared with controls. All patients with grade 3 ACLF had similar degrees of disease severity. The increased MD scores with increasing severity of ACLF suggested that ACLF is more likely associated with vasogenic/interstitial edema, rather than cytotoxic edema. This association is thought to be due to blood-brain barrier dysfunction and neuroinflammation caused by SIRS and cytokine release in ACLF, which correlates with the increased IL-6 levels seen in more severe

ACLF and higher MD values. These findings suggest that higher IL-6 levels are related to higher levels of cerebral edema.[42]

In acute liver failure (ALF) and ACLF, the release of DAMPs from damaged hepatocytes leads to the production and release of proinflammatory cytokines from the portal circulation into the systemic circulation.[43,44] This production and release causes a decrease in systemic vascular resistance and hypotension resulting in a decrease in cerebral perfusion pressure (CPP).[43] Despite the reduced CPP, cerebral blood flow may significantly increase due to impaired autoregulation and a drastic reduction in cerebrovascular resistance (CVR); this leads to an increased delivery of potentially harmful substances, such as ammonia and cytokines, to the brain.[45]

SIRS associated with ACLF causes the release of proinflammatory cytokines such as TNF-alpha, IL-1, IL-6, IL-8, and IL-12.[46] Previous research has linked SIRS to the development of conditions such as HE, increased intracranial pressure, and multiorgan dysfunction syndrome.[47,48] Cytokine production and release also occurs locally in the brain by activated microglia,[49] a type of immune cell found in the brain that can respond to tissue damage, local vascular compromise, and reduction in oxygenated blood flow. In a study using mouse models of acute liver failure, researchers observed increased levels of cytokines in the brain and increased expression of the genes that encode these cytokines, suggesting that they were being produced within the brain.[49,50]

The severity of HE can vary, and mild forms (grades 1–2) are less likely to be accompanied by cerebral edema. Severe HE (grades 3–4) is more commonly associated with cerebral edema, which occurs in 50% to 80% of cases of acute liver failure.[51,52] The exact cause of cerebral edema is not well understood, but there are 2 main theories: vasogenic edema, in which the blood-brain barrier is damaged and fluid and solutes accumulate outside of the brain cells, and cytotoxic edema, in which the blood-brain barrier remains intact but brain cells swell due to an accumulation of intracellular fluid.[53]

Astrocytes, the primary type of brain cell that swells in cases of ALF and ACLF, make up about one-third of the brain's volume.[54,55] In patients with ACLF, MRI scans have shown a decrease in extracellular space, indicating an accumulation of intracellular fluid.[56] Although the exact cause of astrocyte swelling is not fully understood, there is evidence that ammonia plays a significant role. Ammonia is produced in the digestive system by the enzyme glutaminase and by certain types of bacteria, and it is carried to the liver through the hepatic portal circulation, where it is primarily processed through the urea cycle.[46] This pathway is disrupted in ALF and ACLF due to liver cell damage, resulting in elevated ammonia levels in the blood.[53] High levels of ammonia in the blood have been linked to increased uptake of ammonia in the brain, development of cerebral edema, and herniation.[57] Similar findings have been observed in children with urea cycle disorders, suggesting that hyperammonemia alone may cause brain edema.[58] In the brain, astrocytes are responsible for detoxifying ammonia through the use of an enzyme called glutamine synthetase, which converts ammonia and glutamate into the amino acid glutamine. Previous research has found elevated levels of glutamine in the brain tissues of patients with ALF, leading to the hypothesis that high ammonia levels increase the production and accumulation of glutamine in astrocytes, causing them to swell.[53]

The osmotic gliopathy hypothesis suggests that high levels of the amino acid glutamate can lead to increased cellular fluid retention and result in cellular edema. This theory has been supported by the use of methionine-S-sulfoximine, a substance that reduces glutamate levels and reduces swelling in normal and abnormal brain cells in both living and laboratory environments.[53] An alternate version of this theory proposes that in cases of ALF and ACLF, there may be abnormal activity in a protein called SNAT5, which helps to remove glutamate from cells. This abnormal activity leads to increased intracellular glutamine, a decrease in the pool of releasable glutamate, resulting in a decline in glutamatergic neurotransmission with extreme neuroinhibition, leading to decreased brain activity.[49,59]

The "Trojan horse" hypothesis is an alternative theory that aims to explain the roles of ammonia and glutamine in astrocyte swelling. According to this theory, excess glutamine produced within astrocytes is transported into the mitochondria, where it is converted into glutamate and ammonia by an enzyme called phosphate-activated glutaminase (PAG). Glutamine acts as the Trojan horse, carrying ammonia into the mitochondria. The accumulation of ammonia leads to oxidative stress, astrocyte swelling, and ultimately, cell degeneration.[60]

Ammonia has been linked to the development of cerebral changes secondary to oxidative and nitrosative stress. Prior studies have demonstrated an increase in lipid peroxidation in mice with hyperammonemia.[61] Furthermore, hyperammonemia has been shown to produce free radicals in the brain and to decrease the activity of antioxidant enzymes, leading to the increased production of superoxide.[62] Astrocyte swelling, which can occur both in living organisms and in cell cultures, has been linked to oxidative stress. Antioxidants like superoxide dismutase, catalase, and vitamin E[63] have been found to reduce astrocyte swelling caused by ammonia. Nitrosative stress has also been shown to contribute to ammonia-induced brain disorders. The inhibition of nitric oxide synthase with nitroarginine has been found to significantly reduce death in hyperammonemic mice, and ammonia infusions have been observed to increase nitric oxide levels in animals with portosystemic shunts.[53]

The induction of the mitochondrial permeability transition (MPT) can be caused by either the release of cytokines or the presence of oxidative/nitrosative stress. This calcium-dependent process exposes the inner mitochondrial membrane's permeability transition pore, leading to increased ion and solute permeability and a drop in the potential of the inner mitochondrial membrane; this results in impaired oxidative phosphorylation and reduced ATP production and can also generate secondary oxidative stress and free radicals, creating a cycle of damage.[34,53] MPT inhibitors like cyclosporine and trifluoperazine have been shown to prevent astrocyte swelling in culture, whereas compounds like magnesium, pyruvate, and L-histidine can variably inhibit ammonia-induced astrocyte swelling.[34] It is not yet fully understood how MPT induction contributes to brain edema, but it is known to play a role in the development of this condition. One possibility is that MPT induction leads to the production of free radicals and oxidative stress. Another possibility is that decreases in oxidative phosphorylation and ATP generation caused by MPT induction lead to energy failure and dysfunction of ion transporters that regulate cell volume. The agent 6-diazo-5-oxo-L-norleucine, which blocks PAG, can prevent the production of free radicals, MPT induction, and astrocyte swelling.[53] It is possible that MPT induction may occur as a result of ammonia entering the mitochondria through the Trojan Horse mechanism.

The Na/K/Cl cotransporter-1 has also been identified as a factor in astrocyte swelling. Ammonia exposure leads to the overactivation of this channel due to increased oxidation/nitration, causing an influx of ions into the cell and resulting in cellular edema, according to research by Jayakumar and colleagues.[64] The ATP-dependent, nonselective cation channel (NCCa-ATP channel) may also contribute to astrocyte swelling. The same research group found that the NCCa-ATP channel was significantly more active in ammonia-exposed astrocytes, as indicated by elevated levels of the channel's regulatory protein, sulfonylurea receptor 1 protein

(SUR1). Higher SUR1 levels were associated with astrocyte swelling, and activation of SUR1 was only seen in situations with low ATP levels.[65]

KIDNEY

Acute kidney injury (AKI) is a common manifestation of ALF and ACLF.[66]

The European Association for the Study of the Liver-Chronic Liver Failure (EASL-CLIF) consortium defines kidney dysfunction as creatinine levels between 1.5 and 1.9 mg/dL and kidney failure as creatinine levels greater than 2 mg/dL or requirement of renal replacement therapy.[66] Studies have demonstrated rates of AKI in ACLF ranging from 22.8% to 51%, which is even higher than the prevalence in hospitalized patients with cirrhosis.[67,68]

The pathogenesis of AKI is variable as summarized in the following discussion (**Box 2**). Prerenal azotemia can be secondary to systemic vasodilation and volume loss in the setting of vomiting, gastrointestinal bleeding, or aggressive lactulose therapy.[69] Renal failure in ACLF is hypothesized to mimic hepatorenal syndrome with splanchnic and systemic vasodilatation resulting in decreased effective circulatory volume. In turn, decreased renal perfusion stimulates the sympathetic nervous system, release of antidiuretic hormone, and the renin-angiotensin-aldosterone system. These systems fail to normalize renal perfusion and ironically worsen kidney injury.[70,71]

SIRS and sepsis also contribute to ACLF-related AKI.[72] SIRS is a result of a systemic inflammatory cascade propelled by cytokine release. Patients with ACLF have elevated cytokine levels irrespective of the presence of sepsis. The sources of these cytokines include hepatocyte breakdown in hepatic necrosis, endotoxemia, and impaired hepatic cytokine metabolism.[73–75] Increased circulating TNF-α, IL-1, IL-6, and others induce renal parenchymal inflammation and tubule apoptosis.[76,77] Renal cell and hepatocyte necrosis release DAMPs, which activate the renal innate immune system. DAMPs function as ligands for TLRs, especially TLR-4, triggering inflammation. Inflammation affecting the renal system is exacerbated in the setting of infection, with release of PAMPs.[76] Patients with ACLF have elevated levels of various inflammatory cytokines and markers of oxidative stress like human nonmercaptalbumin 2.[78] Furthermore, the degree of elevation correlated with the severity of ACLF. In this study,

---

Box 2
Causes of acute kidney injury in acute and acute-on-chronic liver failure

Hypotension
- Prerenal azotemia
- GI losses (GI bleeding, vomiting, diarrhea from increased lactulose)
- Volume reduction/poor volume resuscitation

DAMPs/PAMPs
- Cyclophilin A
- HMBG1
- Bacterial sepsis

SIRS/cytokines
- TNF-α, IL-1, and IL-6

ATN
- Ischemic
- Toxic (acetaminophen, amanita poisoning, trimethoprim-sulfamethoxazole, and so on)

Renal hypoperfusion

ATN, acute tubular necrosis; GI, gastrointestinal.

AKI was associated with elevated IL-6, IL-8, and human nonmercaptalbumin 2 but not with plasma renin activity. This association implies direct renal consequences of systemic inflammation independent of hemodynamics.[78] Murine studies in which mice with cirrhosis were given lipopolysaccharide (LPS) demonstrated a correlation with renal tubular injury and increased renal expression of TLR-4 and caspase-3. Inflammatory cytokines and LPS spur tubular damage via caspase-mediated pathways; this may help explain the observation that rifaximin and norfloxacin given for spontaneous bacterial peritonitis (SBP) prophylaxis apparently decrease the incidence of AKI.[79]

There are interesting differences between the causes of AKI in patients with cirrhosis versus ACLF, despite the presence of underlying chronic liver disease in ACLF. The most common causes of AKI in cirrhosis range from prerenal azotemia and hepatorenal syndrome (HRS) (functional) to acute tubular necrosis (ATN) (structural).[80] In decompensated cirrhosis, functional and structural AKI comprised two-thirds and one-third of cases, respectively. This observation is in contrast to ACLF as demonstrated in a study by Maiwall and colleagues[81] evaluating the presence and cause of AKI in hospitalized patients with ACLF versus patient with acutely decompensated cirrhosis (ADC). Both groups had similar rates of AKI, but patients with ACLF were less likely to respond to volume resuscitation (21 vs 34%, $P = .02$) and had significantly higher prevalence of structural AKI (32 vs 18%, $P = .013$). Patients with ACLF had higher model for end stage liver disease (MELD) and child-turcotte-pugh (CTP) scores, bilirubin levels, and inflammatory markers. Granular casts were more common in urine microscopy for patients with ACLF, representing the structural damage to the renal tubules.[81] The increased prevalence of structural kidney disease in ACLF versus ADC was reproduced in a study by Jiang and colleagues[82] via biomarkers of tubule injury. In this same study, ACLF-related AKI was significantly less likely to respond to terlipressin than ADC-related AKI (32.6 vs 57.9%, $P = .018$). This observation reinforces the notion that functional causes of AKI related to splanchnic vasodilatation were not the major driver of renal injury in ACLD.[82] In fact, resolution of HRS-AKI with albumin and splanchnic vasoconstriction fails in up to 40% of patients, implicating other pathophysiologic processes underlying tubular injury.[79]

Maiwall's group[81] also examined postmortem kidney biopsies in patients with ACLF and ADC. Patients with ACLF were more likely to have bile pigment nephropathy and correlating elevations in serum bilirubin levels, which were a significant predictor on multivariate analysis. This process is referred to as cholemic nephrosis and has been shown to correlate with renal damage on histology in animal studies.[83] Bile acids can lead to both direct nephrotoxicity and tubular obstruction. Another study of patients with cirrhosis revealed tubular bile casts on 11 of 13 kidney biopsies in the setting of HRS-AKI.[80]

Because of the increased bleeding risks in patients with cirrhosis due to underlying coagulopathy, kidney biopsy is rarely performed to diagnose structural disease. Trawale and colleagues[84] performed kidney biopsies on 65 patients with cirrhosis and AKI defined by serum creatinine greater than 1.5 mg/dL. Eighteen of these patients had less than 0.5 mg/d of proteinuria and no hematuria but still had signs of glomerular injury as well as both acute and chronic tubulointerstitial lesions. This finding implies that even patients thought to have functional kidney disease based on presentation and laboratory studies may have undiagnosed structural kidney disease.[84]

HEMOSTASIS

Normal hemostasis involves 3 individual phases. Primary hemostasis is the process by which activated platelets seal a breach in the integrity of the vascular endothelium.

Secondary hemostasis involves coagulation, fibrin mesh formation, and clot stabilization. Ultimately, fibrinolysis can occur during which the clot/fibrin mesh is dissolved (**Table 2**).[85]

Most of the plasma proteins involved in each stage of hemostasis are synthesized within the liver. As a result, liver failure is associated with significant disturbances in hemostasis including thrombocytopenia, platelet dysfunction, and imbalance of prothrombotic and antithrombotic factors related to synthetic dysfunction and portal hypertension. Aside from factor VIII, produced in the endothelium, procoagulant factors are observed to have decreased plasma concentrations in the setting of liver failure; this is also true of anticoagulant proteins like antithrombin and proteins C and S.[85]

Primary hemostasis is characterized by platelet adhesion and aggregation at the site of endothelial injury. Thrombopoietin (TPO) is the primary regulator of protein synthesis and is synthesized in the liver. TPO levels in chronic liver disease are variable and may be low, high, or normal.[86,87] Thrombocytopenia in liver failure is likely multifactorial with contributions from splenic sequestration from hypersplenism as well as decreased production secondary to bone marrow toxicity from agents such as alcohol. In addition, the parallels drawn between ACLF and SIRS with multiorgan failure extend to hemostasis. A recent study of patients with ACLF demonstrated a correlation between the presence of SIRS and development of thrombocytopenia, and furthermore between the presence of thrombocytopenia and multiorgan system failure. The investigators hypothesized that SIRS-induced activation of platelets yielded microparticles that resulted in clearance of platelet remnants leading to thrombocytopenia. Patients with ACLF have elevated levels of von Willebrand factor (vWF), which may encourage platelet adhesion in spite of thrombocytopenia.[88] Elevated vWF levels have also been noted in cirrhosis and are a known predictor of decompensation and mortality, as well as organ failure.[89,90]

Secondary hemostasis is also disrupted. ACLF is associated with significant dysregulation in the production of procoagulant factors II, V, VII, IX, X, and XI. Because of the rapid reduction in procoagulant factor production and the short half-life of these factors, the onset of coagulopathy can be rapid. This rapid onset of coagulopathy manifests as elevations in prothrombin time (PT) and international normalized ratio (INR). However, INR is an imperfect measure in patients with cirrhosis because it is calibrated for the general population. Furthermore, this coagulopathy is not consistently shown to predict bleeding complications during hospitalization.[91] In a study of 169 patients with ADC, the degree of inflammation, as assessed by the CRP and severity of underlying disease, was a predictor of both progression to ACLF and bleeding complications.[92] ACLF is characterized by systemic inflammation, which

Table 2	
Phases of hemostasis and abnormalities seen in liver failure	
Phases of Hemostasis	**Abnormalities**
Platelets/primary hemostasis	• Thrombocytopenia • Elevated level of vWF
Coagulation/secondary hemostasis	• Elevated level of factor 8 • Decreased level of procoagulant and anticoagulant proteins
Fibrin dissolution	• Decreased level of plasminogen • Decreased level of antiplasmin • Increased level of plasminogen activator inhibitor-1

Abbreviation: vWF, von Willebrand factor.

may actually drive hemostasis-related complications with a more causative relationship than biochemical coagulopathy.

Fibrinolysis is an important component of hemostasis that describes the breakdown of the fibrin clot. The liver is the principal site of production and clearance of fibrinolytic proteins including plasminogen, fibrinogen, and thrombin activatable fibrinolysis inhibitor (TAFI). It is speculated that impaired fibrinolysis in ACLF plays a pivotal role in the development of multiorgan dysfunction by promoting microvascular fibrin deposition.[93]

Although all patients with ACLF have coagulopathy, PT/INR is a poor measure of hemostasis. In fact, even more broad assays are unable to consistently predict bleeding. Laboratory values are not necessarily associated with bleeding diathesis. Hemostasis in this setting is more aptly described as a rebalancing of procoagulant and anticoagulant factors. Relative risks of bleeding and clotting are further modulated by coexisting conditions like sepsis and AKI.

SUMMARY

A dysregulated inflammatory immune response triggered by severe liver injury leads to multiorgan failure. The pathophysiologic mechanisms associated with ACLF are often related to the type of injury, the type of underlying liver disease, and the host's ability of balance between inflammatory mechanisms leading to cellular regeneration and death. As the collective understanding of mechanisms of ACLF improves, so too may the available treatments and related survival outcomes.

REFERENCES

1. Neuman MG, Cameron RG, Haber JA, et al. Inducers of cyto- chrome P450 2E1 enhance methotrexate-induced hepatocytotoxicity. Clin Biochem 1999;32: 519–36.
2. Wang K. Molecular mechanisms of hepatic apoptosis. Cell Death Dis 2014;5: e996.
3. Kaplowitz N. Mechanisms of liver cell injury. J Hepatol 2000;32:39–47.
4. Riordan SM, Williams R. Mechanisms of hepatocyte injury, multiorgan failure, and prognostic criteria in acute liver failure. Semin Liver Dis 2003;23:203–16.
5. Jaeschke H, Lemasters JJ. Apoptosis versus oncotic necrosis in hepatic ischemia/reperfusion injury. Gastroenterology 2003;125:1246–57.
6. Bantel H, Schulze-Osthoff K. Mechanisms of cell death in acute liver failure. Front Physiol 2012;3:79.
7. Wang K. Molecular mechanisms of liver injury: apoptosis or necrosis. Exp Toxicol Pathol 2014;66:351–6.
8. Trump BF, Berezesky IK, Chang SH, et al. The pathways of cell death: oncosis, apoptosis, and necrosis. Toxicol Pathol 1997;25:82–8.
9. Ogasawara J, Watanabe-Fukunaga R, Adachi M, et al. Lethal effect of the anti-Fas antibody in mice. Nature 1993;364:806–9.
10. Bertin J, Armstrong RC, Ottilie S, et al. Death effector domain-containing herpesvirus and poxvirus proteins inhibit both Fas- and TNFR1-induced apoptosis. Proc Natl Acad Sci U S A 1997;94:1172–6.
11. Yoon JH, Gores GJ. Death receptor-mediated apoptosis and the liver. J Hepatol 2002;37(3):400–10.
12. Wang K, Lin B. Pathophysiological significance of hepatic apoptosis. ISRN Hepatol 2013;2013:1–14.

13. Leist M, Gantner F, Bohlinger I, et al. Tumor necrosis factor- induced hepatocyte apoptosis precedes liver failure in experimental murine shock models. Am J Pathol 1995;146(5):1220.
14. Volkmann X, Fischer U, Bahr MJ, et al. Increased hepatotoxicity of tumor necrosis factor- related apoptosis-inducing ligand in diseased human liver. Hepatology 2007;46:1498–508.
15. Weichselbaum L, Gustot T. The organs in acute-on-chronic liver failure. Semin Liver Dis 2016;36(2):174–80.
16. Chung RT, Stravitz RT, Fontana RJ, et al. Pathogenesis of liver injury in acute liver failure. Gastroenterology 2012;143:e1–7.
17. Bone RC, Balk RA, Cerra FB, et al. Definitions for sepsis and organ failure and guidelines for the use of innovative therapies in sepsis. Chest 1992;101(6):1644–55.
18. Wasmuth HE, Kunz D, Yagmur E, et al. Patients with acute on chronic liver failure display "sepsis-like" immune paralysis. J Hepatol 2005;42:195–201.
19. Rolando N, Wade J, Davalos M, et al. The systemic inflammatory response syndrome in acute liver failure. Hepatology 2000;32(4I):734–9.
20. Katoonizadeh A, Laleman W, Verslype C, et al. Early features of acute-on-chronic alcoholic liver failure: a prospective cohort study. Gut 2010;59:1561–9.
21. Shubin NJ, Monaghan SF, Ayala A. Anti-inflammatory mechanisms of sepsis. Contrib Microbiol 2011;17:108–24.
22. Linderoth G, Jepsen P, Schønheyder HC, et al. Short-term prognosis of community-acquired bacteremia in patients with liver cirrhosis or alcoholism: a population-based cohort study. Alcohol Clin Exp Res 2006;30:636–41.
23. Fernández J, Acevedo J, Wiest R, et al. Bacterial and fungal infections in acute-on-chronic liver failure: prevalence, characteristics and impact on prognosis. Gut 2017;67:1870–80.
24. Vaquero J, Polson J, Chung C, et al. Infection and the progression of hepatic encephalopathy in acute liver failure. Gastroenterology 2003;125:755–64.
25. Jalan R, Mookerjee RP, Gines P, et al. Acute-on chronic liver failure. J Hepatol 2012;57:1336–48.
26. Izumi S, Hughes RD, Langley PG, et al. Extent of the acute phase response in fulminant hepatic failure. Gut 1994;35:982–6.
27. Wigmore SJ, Walsh TS, Lee A, et al. Pro-inflammatory cytokine release and mediation of the acute phase protein response in fulminant hepatic failure. Intensive Care Med 1998;24:224–9.
28. Antoniades CG, Berry PA, Wendon JA, et al. The importance of immune dysfunction in determining outcome in acute liver failure. J Hepatol 2008;49:845–61.
29. Irvine KM, Ratnasekera I, Powell EE, et al. Causes and consequences of innate immune dysfunction in cirrhosis. Front Immunol 2019;10. https://doi.org/10.3389/fimmu.2019.00293.
30. Acharya SK, Dasarathy S, Irshad M. Prospective study of plasma fibronectin in fulminant hepatitis: association with infection and mortality. J Hepatol 1995;23:8–13.
31. Wyke RJ, Rajkovic I, Eddleston ALWF, et al. Defective opsonisation and complement deficiency in serum from patients with fulminant hepatic failure. Gut 1980;21:643–9.
32. Chavez-Tapia NC, Mendiola-Pastrana I, Ornelas-Arroyo VJ, et al. Granulocyte-colony stimulating factor for acute-on-chronic liver failure: systematic review and meta-analysis. Ann Hepatol 2015;14:631–41.

33. Vilstrup H, Amodio P, Bajaj J, et al. Hepatic encephalopathy in chronic liver disease: 2014 practice guideline by the American association for the study of liver diseases and the European association for the study of the liver. Hepatology 2014;60(2):715–35.

34. Rama Rao KV, Jayakumar AR, Norenberg MD. Brain edema in acute liver failure: mechanisms and concepts. Metab Brain Dis 2014;29(4):927–36.

35. Romero-Gómez M, Montagnese S, Jalan R. Hepatic encephalopathy in patients with acute decompensation of cirrhosis and acute-on-chronic liver failure. J Hepatol 2015;62(2):437–47.

36. Lee GH. Hepatic encephalopathy in acute-on-chronic liver failure. Hepatol Int 2015;9(4):520–6.

37. Sawhney R, Holland-Fischer P, Rosselli M, et al. Role of ammonia, inflammation, and cerebral oxygenation in brain dysfunction of acute-on-chronic liver failure patients. Liver Transpl 2016;22(6):732–42.

38. Shawcross DL, Sharifi Y, Canavan JB, et al. Infection and systemic inflammation, not ammonia, are associated with grade 3/4 hepatic encephalopathy, but not mortality in cirrhosis. J Hepatol 2011;54(4):640–9.

39. Nath K, Saraswat VA, Krishna YR, et al. Quantification of cerebral edema on diffusion tensor imaging in acute-on-chronic liver failure. NMR Biomed 2008;21(7): 713–22.

40. Rai R, Ahuja CK, Agrawal S, et al. Reversal of low-grade cerebral edema after lactulose/rifaximin therapy in patients with cirrhosis and minimal hepatic encephalopathy. Clin Transl Gastroenterol 2015;6(9):e111–8.

41. Kale RA, Gupta RK, Saraswat VA, et al. Demonstration of interstitial cerebral edema with diffusion tensor MR imaging in type C hepatic encephalopathy. Hepatology 2006;43(4):698–706.

42. Gupta T, Dhiman RK, Ahuja CK, et al. Characterization of cerebral edema in acute-on-chronic liver failure. J Clin Exp Hepatol 2017;7(3):190–7.

43. Bernal W, Lee WM, Wendon J, et al. Acute liver failure: a curable disease by 2024? J Hepatol 2015;62(S1):S112–20.

44. Anand AC, Singh P. Neurological recovery after recovery from acute liver failure: is it complete? J Clin Exp Hepatol 2019;9(1):99–108.

45. Larsen FS, Wendon J. Prevention and management of brain edema in acute liver failure. Liver Transpl 2008;14:S90–6.

46. Aldridge DR, Tranah EJ, Shawcross DL. Pathogenesis of hepatic encephalopathy: role of ammonia and systemic inflammation. J Clin Exp Hepatol 2015; 5(S1):S7–20.

47. Rolando N. The systemic inflammatory response syndrome in acute liver failure. Hepatology 2000;32(4):734–9.

48. Miyake Y, Yasunaka T, Ikeda F, et al. Sirs score reflects clinical features of non-acetaminophen-related acute liver failure with hepatic coma. Intern Med 2012; 51(8):823–8.

49. Butterworth RF. Pathogenesis of hepatic encephalopathy and brain edema in acute liver failure. J Clin Exp Hepatol 2015;5(S1):S96–103.

50. Jiang W, Desjardins P, Butterworth RF. Cerebral inflammation contributes to encephalopathy and brain edema in acute liver failure: protective effect of minocycline. J Neurochem 2009;109(2):485–93.

51. Leventhal TM, Liu KD. What a nephrologist needs to know about acute liver failure. Adv Chronic Kidney Dis 2015;22(5):376–81.

52. Paschoal Junior FM, Nogueira RDC, Oliveira MDL, et al. Cerebral hemodynamic and metabolic changes in fulminant hepatic failure. Arq Neuropsiquiatr 2017; 75(7):470–6.
53. Scott TR, Kronsten VT, Hughes RD, et al. Pathophysiology of cerebral oedema in acute liver failure. World J Gastroenterol 2013;19(48):9240–55.
54. Traber PG, Canto MD, Ganger DR, et al. Electron microscopic evaluation of brain edema in rabbits with galactosamine-induced fulminant hepatic failure: ultrastructure and integrity of the blood-brain barrier. Hepatology 1987;7(6):1272–7.
55. Kato M, Hughes RD, Keays RT, et al. Electron microscopic study of brain capillaries in cerebral edema from fulminant hepatic failure. Hepatology 1992;15(6): 1060–6.
56. Chavarria L, Alonso J, Rovira A, et al. Neuroimaging in acute liver failure. Neurochem Int 2011;59(8):1175–80.
57. Clemmesen JO, Larsen FS, Kondrup J, et al. Cerebral herniation in patients with acute liver failure is correlated with arterial ammonia concentration. Hepatology 1999;29(3):648–53.
58. Kendall BE, Kingsley DPE, Leonard JV, et al. Neurological features and computed tomography of the brain in children with ornithine carbamoyl transferase deficiency. J Neurol Neurosurg Psychiatry 1983;46(1):28–34.
59. Desjardins P, Du T, Jiang W, et al. Pathogenesis of hepatic encephalopathy and brain edema in acute liver failure: role of glutamine redefined. Neurochem Int 2012;60(7):690–6.
60. Albrecht J, Norenberg MD. Glutamine: a Trojan horse in ammonia neurotoxicity. Hepatology 2006;44(4):788–94.
61. O'Connor JE, Costell M. New roles of carnitine metabolism in ammonia cytotoxicity. Adv Exp Med Biol 1990;272(1):183–95.
62. Kosenko E, Kaminsky Y, Kaminsky A, et al. Superoxide production and antioxidant enzymes in ammonia intoxication in rats. Free Radic Res 1997;27(6):637–44.
63. Jayakumar AR, Panickar KS, Murthy CRK, et al. Oxidative stress and mitogen-activated protein kinase phosphorylation mediate ammonia-induced cell swelling and glutamate uptake inhibition in cultured astrocytes – Jayakumar et al. 26(18):4774. J Neurosci 2006;26(18):4774–84.
64. Jayakumar AR, Liu M, Moriyama M, et al. Na-K-Cl cotransporter-1 in the mechanism of ammonia-induced astrocyte swelling. J Biol Chem 2008;283(49): 33874–82.
65. Jayakumar A, Valdes V, Tong XY, et al. Sulfonylurea receptor 1 contributes to the astrocyte swelling and brain edema in acute liver failure. Transl Stroke Res 2014; 5:28–37.
66. Betrosian A-P, Agarwal B, Douzinas EE. Acute renal dysfunction in liver diseases. World J Gastroenterol 2007;13(42):5552–9.
67. Cardoso FS, Marcelino P, Bagulho L, et al. Acute liver failure: an up-to-date approach. J Crit Care 2017;39:25–30.
68. Mazer M, Perrone J. Acetaminophen-induced nephrotoxicity: pathophysiology, clinical manifestations, and management. J Med Toxicol 2008;4(1):2–6.
69. Karvellas CJ, Stravitz RT. 20 - acute liver failure. 7th edition. Elsevier; 2017. https://doi.org/10.1016/B978-0-323-37591-7.00020-3.
70. Moore K. Renal failure in acute liver failure. Eur J Gastroenterol Hepatol 1999;11: 967–75.
71. Wong F. Recent advances in our understanding of hepatorenal syndrome. Nat Rev Gastroenterol Hepatol 2012;9(7):382–91.

72. Mindikoglu AL, Pappas SC. New developments in hepatorenal syndrome. Clin Gastroenterol Hepatol 2018;16(2):162–77.
73. Bone R. Toward a theory regarding the pathogenesis of the systemic inflammatory response syndrome: what we do and do not know about cytokine regulation. Crit Care Med 1996;24:163–72.
74. Boermeester MA, Houdijk APJ, Meyer S, et al. Liver failure induces a systemic inflammatory response: prevention by recombinant n-terminal bactericidal/permeability-increasing protein. Am J Pathol 1995;147(5):1428–40.
75. Donnelly MC, Hayes PC, Simpson KJ. Role of inflammation and infection in the pathogenesis of human acute liver failure: clinical implications for monitoring and therapy. World J Gastroenterol 2016;22(26):5958–70.
76. Moore JK, Love E, Craig DG, et al. Acute kidney injury in acute liver failure: a review. Expert Rev Gastroenterol Hepatol 2013;7(8):701–12.
77. Wan L, Bagshaw SM, Langenberg C, et al. Pathophysiology of septic acute kidney injury: what do we really know? Crit Care Med 2008;36(4):198–203.
78. Claria J, Stauber RE, Coenraad MJ, et al. Systemic inflammation in decompensated cirrhosis: characterization and role in acute-on-chronic liver failure. Hepatology 2016;64(4):1249–64.
79. Davenport A, Sheikh MF, Lamb E, et al. Acute kidney injury in acute-on- chronic liver failure: where does hepatorenal syndrome fit? Kidney Int 2017;92(5):1058–70.
80. Van Slambrouck CM, Salem F, Meehan SM, et al. Bile cast nephropathy is a common pathologic finding for kidney injury associated with severe liver dysfunction. Kidney Int 2013;84(1):192–7.
81. Maiwall R, Kumar S, Chandel SS, et al. AKI in patients with acute on chronic liver failure is different from acute decompensation of cirrhosis. Hepatol Int 2015;9(4):627–39.
82. Jiang QQ, Han MF, Ma K, et al. Acute kidney injury in acute-on-chronic liver failure is different from in decompensated cirrhosis. World J Gastroenterol 2018;24(21):2300–10.
83. Fickert P, Krones E, Pollheimer MJ, et al. Bile acids trigger cholemic nephropathy in common bile-duct-ligated mice. Hepatology 2013;58(6):2056–69.
84. Trawalé JM, Paradis V, Rautou PE, et al. The spectrum of renal lesions in patients with cirrhosis: a clinicopathological study. Liver Int 2010;30(5):725–32.
85. Northup PG, Caldwell SH. Coagulation in liver disease: a guide for the clinician. Clin Gastroenterol Hepatol 2013;11:1064–74.
86. Temel T, Cansu DU, Temel HE, et al. Serum thrombopoietin levels and its relationship with thrombocytopenia in patients with cirrhosis. Hepat Mon 2014;14:e18556.
87. Peck-Radosavljevic M, Zacherl J, Meng YG, et al. Is inadequate thrombopoietin production a major cause of thrombocytopenia in cirrhosis of the liver. J Hepatol 1997;27:127–31.
88. Hugenholtz GCG, Adelmeijer J, Meijers JCM, et al. An unbalance between von Willebrand factor and ADAMTS13 in acute liver failure: implications for hemostasis and clinical outcome. Hepatology 2013;58:752–61.
89. Kalambokis GN, Oikonomou A, Christou L, et al. von Willebrand factor and procoagulant imbalance predict outcome in patients with cirrhosis and thrombocytopenia. J Hepatol 2016;65(5):921–8.
90. Prasanna KS, Goel A, Amirtharaj GJ, et al. Plasma von Willebrand factor levels predict in-hospital survival in patients with acute-on-chronic liver failure. Indian J Gastroenterol 2016;35(6):432–40.

91. Campello E, Zanetto A, Bulato C, et al. Coagulopathy is not predictive of bleeding in patients with acute decompensation of cirrhosis and acute-on-chronic liver failure. Liver Int 2021;41(10):2455–66.

92. Zanetto A, Pelizzaro F, Campello E, et al. Severity of systemic inflammation is the main predictor of ACLF and bleeding in individuals with acutely decompensated cirrhosis. J Hepatol 2023;78(2):301–11.

93. Blasi A, Patel VC, Adelmeiier J, et al. Mixed fibrinolytic phenotypes in decompensated cirrhosis and acute-on-chronic liver failure with hypofibrinolysis in those with complications and poor survival. Hepatology 2020;71(4):1381–90.

Pathology of Acute and Acute-on-Chronic Liver Failure

Cameron Beech, MD[a], Chen Liu, MD, PhD[b,*],
Xuchen Zhang, MD, PhD[b,*]

KEYWORDS

- Liver failure • Acute liver failure • Acute-on-chronic liver failure • Pathology

KEY POINTS

- The precise diagnosis of acute and acute-on-chronic liver failure requires a combination of clinical, laboratory, and histologic correlation.
- Histopathology can provide insights into the etiology of acute and acute-on-chronic liver failure as well as the presence of underlying chronic liver disease.
- Unlike acute liver failure, an understanding of the pathologic features of acute-on-chronic liver disease is still in its infancy, and further study is necessary to characterize this complex and heterogeneous entity.

INTRODUCTION

Liver failure can develop either as acute liver failure (ALF) in the absence of any preexisting liver disease or acute-on-chronic liver failure (ACLF) in a patient with underlying chronic liver disease or cirrhosis. Workup for liver transplant for patients with ALF should be initiated immediately. Although liver transplantation is considered an option in patients with ACLF, transplant candidacy is not evaluated immediately, but efforts are directed at identifying and treating the precipitating factors and reversing hepatic and extrahepatic organ failures.[1] Although the diagnosis and management of ALF and ACLF are mainly based on clinical features, a timely liver biopsy evaluation may help to distinguish acute and chronic liver disease, recognize the precipitating factors, provide prognostic information based on pathologic changes, and help decision-making to proceed with liver transplantation.[2,3] The pathologic features of ALF and its etiologies have been well characterized.[4,5] However, the pathologic features of the relatively newly defined ACLF have not been well described. In this review, the

a Department of Pathology, ARUP Laboratories, University of Utah, Salt Lake City, UT 84112, USA; b Department of Pathology, Yale School of Medicine, New Haven, CT 06520-8023, USA
* Corresponding authors.
E-mail addresses: chen.liu@yale.edu (C.L.); xuchen.zhang@yale.edu (X.Z.)

Clin Liver Dis 27 (2023) 581–593
https://doi.org/10.1016/j.cld.2023.03.004
1089-3261/23/© 2023 Elsevier Inc. All rights reserved.

pathologic features and diagnostic implications in both ALF and ACLF will be discussed.

ACUTE LIVER FAILURE
Definition and Classification of Acute Liver Failure

ALF, also termed as fulminant hepatitis or fulminant liver failure, is a severe form of hepatocyte injury, which clinically is usually unexpected and abrupt in onset, frequently affecting healthy individuals without preexisting liver disease, and is characterized by the development of encephalopathy and/or coagulopathy.[6] Clinical definitions for ALF also commonly include subclassifications based on the time from onset of symptoms to the onset of hepatic encephalopathy and/or coagulopathy.[7] The O'Grady system subclassified ALF into hyperacute, acute, and subacute liver failure.[7] Hyperacute liver failure occurs very rapidly, usually less than 1 week (often with hours) from symptoms onset. This is in contrast to acute and subacute liver failure, which is predominantly immune-mediated injury, occurring approximately 1 to 4 weeks and 5 to 12 weeks from the time of clinical presentation, respectively. The Bernuau system subclassified ALF into fulminant (<2 weeks) and subfulminant (2–12 weeks) liver failure.[8] The Japanese system divided ALF into fulminant hepatitis, which was further divided into acute (<10 days) and subacute (10 days to 8 weeks) types, and late-onset (8–24 weeks) liver failure.[9] These classification schemes may help to define the etiology and pathologic changes and predict prognosis. For example, ALF with a hyperacute or fulminant presentation is commonly related to acetaminophen toxicity, a viral infection, or ischemic/hypoxic injury to the liver presenting predominantly with zone 3 necrosis, and patients generally have a better survival. Whereas ALF with acute or subfulminant presentation is often related to idiosyncratic drug-induced liver injury (DILI), Wilson's disease, or autoimmune hepatitis (AIH), demonstrating diffuse, panlobular/panacinar hepatitis, and patients often have a worse outcome. Furthermore, when ALF presents beyond 8 weeks (subacute or late-onset), the liver often shows regenerative changes in the background of necrosis with irregular nodular appearance, which may mimic liver cirrhosis. The admixture of confluent necrosis with these regenerative nodules in such livers is termed as submassive necrosis, although the presence of submassive necrosis has been suggested to be a feature distinguishing hepatitis B virus-associated ACLF from cirrhotic patients with acute decompensation.[10]

Pathology of Acute Liver Failure

The pathologic changes of ALF fall into two main patterns, either marked inflammation often with necrosis or extensive bland necrosis with very little inflammation. With time, these two patterns converge, leading to a nonspecific pattern characterized by bile ductular proliferation, hepatocyte regeneration, liver parenchymal collapse, and chronic inflammation, referred to as subacute or submassive necrosis. Generally, the pathologic changes are closely associated with etiologies leading to ALF. The etiology of ALF is the most important determinant to predict prognosis and provides a guide to potential targeted treatments. The etiology of ALF varies around the world. Based on the two largest series,[11,12] the most common causes of ALF in developed countries include acetaminophen or non-acetaminophen DILIs, ischemic/hypoxic injury, AIH, and hepatitis B virus (HBV). This differs from developing countries where the most prevalent causes include viral hepatitis A (HAV), HBV, and E (HEV).[6] Other etiologies (malignant infiltration of the liver (lymphoma/leukemia, carcinoma), mushroom poisoning (Amanita spp), heat shock, heat stroke, Reye's syndrome, hemophagocytic lymphohistiocytosis, Wilson's disease, acute fatty liver of pregnancy,

Table 1
Etiology and clinical presentation of acute liver failure

Etiologies	Clinical Presentation
Drugs/Toxins	
Acetaminophen (paracetamol)	Hyperacute/fulminant
Non-acetaminophen drugs/toxins	Acute/subacute/subfulminant
Viral infections	
Hepatotropic (hepatitis A, B, and E)	Hyperacute/acute/fulminant
Other viruses (CMV, HSV, adenovirus, VZV, parvovirus B19, dengue, and yellow fever)	Hyperacute/acute/fulminant
Autoimmune hepatitis	Hyperacute/acute/fulminant and subacute/subfulminant
Ischemia/hypoxia Budd–Chiari syndrome, heart failure, sinusoidal obstruction syndrome, hypovolemic/hypotensive/septic shock	Acute/fulminant and subacute/subfulminant
Genetic/metabolic diseases Wilson's disease, acute fatty liver of pregnancy, mitochondrial diseases, galactosemia, tyrosinemia type 1	Acute/fulminant and subacute/subfulminant
Miscellaneous Malignant infiltration of the liver (lymphoma/leukemia, carcinoma), mushroom poisoning (amanita spp), heat shock, hemophagocytic lymphohistiocytosis, heat stroke, Reye's syndrome	Acute/fulminant and subacute/subfulminant
Indeterminate/unknown	Hyperacute/Acute/fulminant and subacute/subfulminant

Abbreviations: CMV, cytomegalovirus; HSV, herpes simplex virus; VZV, varicella-zoster virus.

mitochondrial diseases, galactosemia, tyrosinemia, and α1-antitrypsin deficiency) (**Table 1**), although rare, may also cause ALF, and should be kept in mind. Approximately 6% of patients with ALF have an indeterminate cause for liver failure.[13]

DILI is a challenging area of liver pathology, given the wide spectrum of histologic changes that can occur. In the non-ALF setting, DILI can have a variety of patterns including portal and/or lobular hepatitis, cholestatic pattern with bile duct injury and chronic cholestasis, steatosis and steatohepatitis, granulomatous hepatitis, and vascular injury patterns.[14] However, in the ALF setting, the pathologic patterns of injury of DILI are mainly limited to three histologic patterns including necrosis predominant hepatocellular injury, an inflammatory predominant pattern of injury (acute hepatitis), and microvesicular steatosis[15] (**Table 2**).

Acetaminophen is the most common drug to cause necrosis predominant hepatocellular injury. Acetaminophen toxicity represents a leading cause of DILI in the United States, making up for nearly half of the cases of drug-induced ALF.[16,17] The drug undergoes glutathione-dependent conjugation to water soluble metabolites in the liver. With higher doses of acetaminophen, glutathione is depleted, enabling metabolism of the drug to toxic intermediates. The histologic pattern characteristically seen with acetaminophen toxicity includes a necrosis predominant acute hepatitis, dominated

Table 2
Pathologic patterns of drug-induced liver injury

Pattern of Injury	Drugs	Differential Diagnosis
Inflammatory predominant with variable degree of necrosis	Antimicrobial (eg, isoniazid, trimethoprim-sulfamethoxazole, albendazole, zidovudine), NSAIDs, chemotherapeutic agents (eg, cyclophosphamide, vincristine), lipid lowering drugs (eg, statins), hypoglycemic drugs (eg, sulfonylureas)	Autoimmune hepatitis, acute viral hepatitis, Wilson disease
Necrosis predominant with scant inflammation	Halothane, acetaminophen, cocaine, industrial toxins	Budd–Chiari syndrome, mushroom poisoning, non-hepatotropic viral infection, ischemia
Microvesicular steatosis	Tetracycline, valproic acid, zidovudine	Mitochondria disease, alcoholic injury, fatty liver disease of pregnancy

by confluent necrosis without significant inflammation. The necrosis often begins at the centrizonal region (**Fig. 1**A, B), however, can expand to bridging necrosis, panacinar necrosis and even massive necrosis (**Fig. 1**C) if severe toxicity is present. Grossly, the liver with massive necrosis is reduced in weight and has a wrinkled capsule due to extensive necrosis of liver parenchyma (**Fig. 1**D). It is important to note that this pattern; however, it is not necessarily unique to acetaminophen as other drugs such as halothane, organic compounds such as carbon tetrachloride, and cocaine have described to be associated with this pattern.[18]

Non-acetaminophen drug-induced ALF is uncommon, which often presents as an inflammatory predominant pattern of injury (acute hepatitis). Histologically, the liver shows lobular and portal inflammation, hepatocyte ballooning, acidophilic bodies (apoptosis), spotty necrosis, cholestasis, and lobular disarray (**Fig. 2**A, B). Severe and confluent necrosis, characterized by bridging hepatic necrosis (**Fig. 2**C), multilobular necrosis, panacinar necrosis (**Fig. 2**D), and even massive necrosis, may occur in some cases. The degree of necrosis is associated with severe or fatal hepatic injury.[15] Of note, these histologic changes are not specific for any particular drug and can be seen in acute viral hepatitis, such as HAV, HBV, and HEV. Therefore, a thorough clinical history investigation of medication use, including herbal remedies, nutritional supplements, over-the-counter medications, and their chronology of administration is essential in the diagnosis of drug-induced ALF. Furthermore, serologic test for HAV, HBV, and HEV plays an important role in establishing or excluding viral hepatitis-caused ALF.

Ischemic/hypoxic injury to the liver, also known as ischemic hepatitis or shock liver, leads to hypoxic injury and can be characterized by a sudden increase in transaminase level, consistent with marked hepatic necrosis and injury. Most cases of ischemic hepatitis occur in the setting of systemic hypoperfusion caused by various shock conditions (septic, cardiogenic, obstructive, hypovolemic, neurogenic, or anaphylactic). The characteristic pathologic pattern of injury is centrilobular (zone 3) hepatocyte necrosis with congestion, as the centrilobular hepatocytes are more susceptible to ischemic/hypoxic injury. Oftentimes there is no lobular or portal

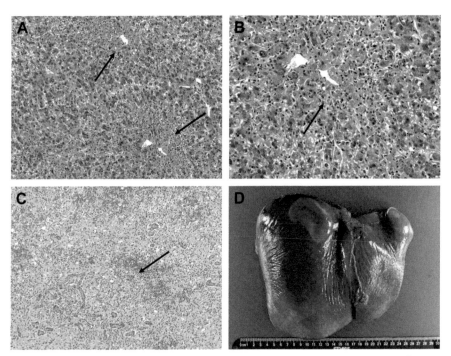

Fig. 1. Acetaminophen-induced acute liver failure. (A) Lower power examination showing centrilobular necrosis without significant inflammation (*arrows*) (H&E, X100). (B) Higher power examination showing centrilobular necrosis without significant inflammation (*arrow*) (H&E, X200). (C) Lower power examination showing panacinar necrosis without significant inflammation (*arrows*) (H&E, X100). (D) Explanted liver specimen showing the liver with a wrinkled capsule due to extensive necrosis of liver parenchyma.

inflammation. This histologic finding can be identical to acetaminophen toxicity and thus histologic discrimination between these two etiologies often cannot be made, and clinical correlation is the key.[19]

AIH can have a range of histologic appearances, depending on the severity and when the biopsy was taken in the natural history of the patient's disease. Among these patterns is a fulminant hepatitis pattern resembling acute hepatitis of other etiologies, such as viral hepatitis or DILI. In this setting, AIH can present as chronic AIH with acute exacerbation, chronic AIH with superimposed viral, toxic, or DILI, or as acute onset "de novo" AIH.[20] In contrast to classic histologic changes of AIH with features of chronic hepatitis, acute onset fulminant AIH is characterized by more diffuse lobular necroinflammation with a marked plasma cell infiltrate. Furthermore, unlike other patterns of AIH, the fulminant pattern of AIH shows marked hepatocellular necrosis which starts with pericentral hepatocytes (zone 3) (**Fig. 3**A) and can expand in severity to be bridging necrosis, panacinar necrosis, and even massive necrosis (**Fig. 3**B–D).[21–24] If the biopsy was taken after ALF began to resolve, other histologic findings could be encountered including parenchymal collapse, ductular proliferation and nodular hyperplasia of hepatocytes may be seen as the liver attempts to regenerate after injury. It is important to note that the diagnosis of AIH in this setting should be based on the presence of compatible clinical and serologic findings as well as the exclusion of other etiologies including DILI and viral hepatitis. A liver biopsy plays an important role in

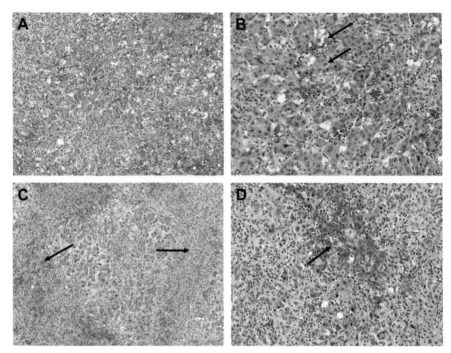

Fig. 2. Drug-induced acute liver failure. (*A*) Lower power examination showing acute hepatitis (H&E, X100). (*B*) Higher power examination showing acute hepatitis characterized by lobular inflammation, hepatocyte ballooning, acidophilic bodies (*arrow*), cholestasis, and lobular disarray (H&E, X200). (*C*) Lower power examination showing bridging necrosis (*arrows*) (H&E, X100). (*D*) Higher power examination showing acute hepatitis with lobular necrosis (*arrow*) (H&E, X200).

excluding other etiologies of acute hepatitis and helping to establish a diagnosis of acute onset fulminant AIH.

Viral hepatitis, although primarily due to hepatotropic viral infections (A, B, C, D, and E), can also occur from non-hepatotropic viruses including Epstein–Barr virus, herpes simplex virus (HSV), varicella zoster virus, parvoviruses, and cytomegalovirus (CMV), and adenovirus. However, ALF in the setting of viral hepatitis usually is related to hepatotropic viral infections, although non-hepatotropic viral infections have been occasionally implicated in ALF, particularly in immunosuppressed patients.[13,25,26] The morphologic features of acute viral hepatitis are not particularly unique among the different viruses, characterized by a lobular inflammation composed predominantly of a lymphocytic inflammatory infiltrate with variable portal inflammation and hepatocellular injury including hepatocyte ballooning and vacuolation. Occasional cholestasis can be identified in the acute viral infection setting, which may invoke consideration for a biliary disorder or DILI. With progression toward ALF, severe hepatocellular injury leading to panacinar necrosis can be identified. Occasionally, viral cytopathic changes in intact hepatocytes and non-zonal necrosis can be seen in the setting of CMV, HSV (**Fig. 4**A–D), or adenovirus, however, even in the absence of these morphologic findings, a high degree of suspicion for infection should be considered and a low threshold for ordering immunostains is warranted.

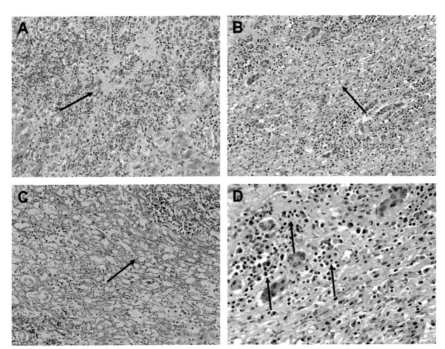

Fig. 3. Autoimmune hepatitis-induced acute liver failure. (*A*) Lower power examination showing autoimmune hepatitis with central necrosis and lymphoplasmacytic inflammation (*arrow*) (H&E, X100). (*B*) Lower power examination showing autoimmune hepatitis with panacinar necrosis with collapsed liver parenchyma (*arrow*) (H&E, X100). (*C*) Reticulin stain highlighting the collapsed necrotic liver parenchyma (*arrow*) (reticulin stain, 100X). (*D*) Higher power examination showing residual portal tract and necrotic parenchyma with lymphoplasmacytic infiltrate (*arrow*) (H&E, X200).

ACUTE-ON-CHRONIC LIVER FAILURE
Definition and Classification of Acute-on-Chronic Liver Failure

ACLF is a clinical syndrome of sudden hepatic decompensation observed in patients with preexisting chronic liver disease with or without cirrhosis that is associated with one or more extrahepatic organ failures and high mortality within 3 months, in the absence of treatment of the underlying liver disease, liver support, or liver transplantation.[27] One of the challenges in evaluating pathologic changes of ACLF is that there are different definitions used in different parts of the world. In Asia, the Asian Pacific Association for the Study of the Liver (APASL) defines ACLF as "an acute hepatic insult manifesting as jaundice and coagulopathy complicated within 4 weeks by clinical ascites and/or hepatic encephalopathy in a patient with previously diagnosed or undiagnosed chronic liver disease/cirrhosis and is associated with a high 28-day mortality."[28] However, in the West, the North American Consortium for the Study of End-Stage Liver Disease and the European Association for the Study of the Liver-Chronic Liver Failure consortium define ACLF as a syndrome that develops in patients with cirrhosis and is characterized by acute decompensation, organ failure, and high short-term mortality.[29–31] Because of the varying definition of ACLF, many studies have differed in their inclusion criteria, making generalizability of the pathologic findings of such studies limited.

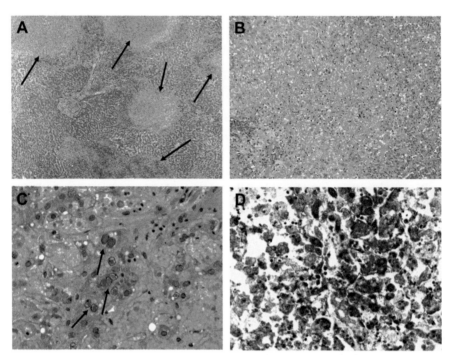

Fig. 4. Herpes simplex virus-induced acute liver failure. (*A*) Lower power examination showing non-zonal necrosis of liver parenchyma (*arrow*) (H&E, X40). (*B*) Higher power examination showing liver parenchyma necrosis with necrotic debris without significant inflammation (H&E, X200). (*C*) Higher power examination showing hepatocyte nuclear viral inclusion with clear halo (*arrow*) (H&E, X400). (*D*) Immunohistochemistry showing nuclear and cytoplasmic herpes simplex virus (Immunohistochemical stain, X400).

Pathology of Acute-on-Chronic Liver Failure

Although ACLF remains a diagnosis defined by clinical criteria, liver histology can be helpful in situations where the etiology of the acute decompensation is unclear or to distinguish ACLF from ALF in patients without a history of chronic liver disease. The etiology of ACLF would be related to a precipitating event in the context of a preexisting liver condition. Viral hepatitis, alcohol, or combination of both are the predominant causes of underlying preexisting chronic liver disease in ACLF in the world. As to the precipitating event, it can be hepatic or extrahepatic.[32] Hepatic precipitating events include excessive alcohol intake, DILI, viral hepatitis, ischemic/hypoxic injury, or liver surgeries including transjugular intrahepatic portosystemic shunt placement. Extrahepatic precipitating events mainly are bacterial infections and major surgery. However, the etiology causing underlying chronic liver disease/cirrhosis and the precipitating event to trigger ACLF vary according to geographical areas. Although reactivation of chronic HBV, acute HAV or HEV superimposed infection, acute alcoholic hepatitis, and acute bacterial infection are the most common precipitating events of ACLF in Asia[33]; active alcoholism and bacterial infections are most frequent in the west.[30] The differences in etiology and in precipitating events can give rise to different pathologic changes. The published studies surrounding the histologic features of ACLF are limited. Many studies examining ACLF lack a standardized control group matched for fibrosis, etiology or precipitating event of liver disease, and some studies have

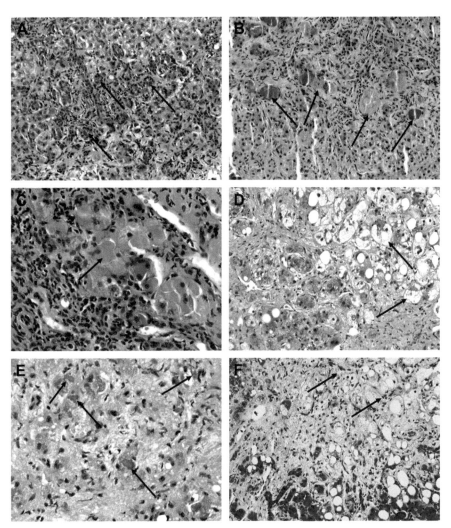

Fig. 5. Alcoholic steatohepatitis-associated acute-on-chronic liver failure. (*A*) Prominent bile ductular proliferation (*arrow*) (H&E, X100). (*B*) Ductular bile plugs/ductular bilirubinostasis (*arrow*) (H&E, X200). (*C*) Hepatocytes with eosinophilic degeneration (*arrow*) (H&E, X200). (*D*) Hepatocytes with ballooning degeneration (*arrow*) (H&E, X200). (*E*) Hepatocytes with Mallory–Denk bodies (*arrow*) (H&E, X200). (*F*) Pericellular fibrosis (*arrow*) (Trichrome-Masson, X200).

used compensated chronic liver disease with varying levels of fibrosis as a control group rather than patients with decompensated chronic liver disease without organ failure. Despite these significant limitations, several histologic features have been described, some of which may have clinical utility.

Histologic features of ACLF have been characterized into two different pathologic pattern groups, which have previously been shown to have two distinct clinical outcomes. Pattern I pathologic features include marked ductular proliferation, coarse inspissated ductular bile plugs, eosinophilic degeneration of hepatocytes, foci of confluent necrosis/bridging necrosis, higher apoptosis, pericellular fibrosis,

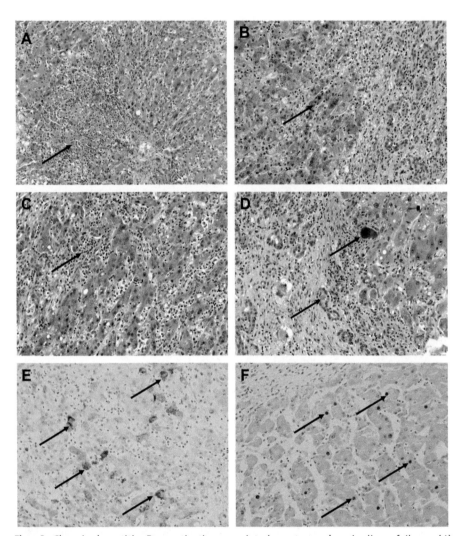

Fig. 6. Chronic hepatitis B reactivation-associated acute-on-chronic liver failure. (*A*) Confluent necrosis (*arrow*) (H&E, X100). (*B*) Ductular proliferation and lobular hepatocytic and canalicular cholestasis (*arrow*) (H&E, X200). (*C*) Dense lobular inflammatory infiltrate (*arrow*) (H&E, X200). (*D*) Ductular bile plugs/ductular bilirubinostasis (*arrow*) (H&E, X200). (*E*) Immunohistochemistry showing cytoplasmic hepatitis B surface antigen in hepatocytes (*arrow*) (Immunohistochemical stain, X200). (*F*) Immunohistochemistry showing nuclear hepatitis B core antigen in hepatocytes (*arrow*) (Immunohistochemical stain, X200).

Mallory–Denk body, and higher stage of fibrosis (**Fig. 5**A–F). Pattern II pathologic features demonstrate prominent hepatocyte ballooning with lesser parenchymal involvement by fibrosis and necrosis,[34–36] although earlier studies showed that patients with pattern I pathologic features in liver biopsies had decreased short-term survival, comparing to patients with pattern II pathologic features.[34,35] However, a recent study attempting to correlate these histologic patterns with survival have found no differences.[36] On multivariate analysis, dense lobular necroinflammatory activity, characterized by the presence of necrosis and a dense lobular inflammatory infiltrate (**Fig. 6**A–F), was independently associated with increased 28-day mortality in ACLF patients.[36] Similar results have been found in other studies examining patients with hepatitis B virus cirrhosis, whose presence of submassive hepatic necrosis within the explanted liver after liver transplantation, correlated with clinical measures of liver injury and ACLF severity and helped distinguish from patients with acute decompensation in the setting of cirrhosis.[10] A prospective study by Katoonizadeh and colleagues assessed clinical and pathologic features of ACLF (using the APASL definition) versus decompensated cirrhosis in patients with alcoholic cirrhosis. They found that during the first 6 months since presentation with their acute exacerbation, ACLF patients had a worse transplant-free survival, however, the difference in survival attenuated once they survived after a year. Also, the presence of ductular bilirubinostasis and cholangiolitis, characterized by the presence of bile plugs in dilated ductules and inflammatory cells involving the bile duct epithelium, corresponded with earlier markers of sepsis and multiorgan failure in patients with ACLF.[37] Given the challenges listed previously for studying ACLF, the histologic findings represent a heterogenous pattern of histologic changes. Further investigation with standardized definitions of ALCF, taking into account the etiology of the patient's chronic liver disease as well their precipitating events is necessary to further characterize the histologic features surrounding this complex entity.

SUMMARY

The pathologist's role in the diagnostic interpretation of ALF and ACLF is crucial for disease management. The histopathologic features of ALF have been well described and biopsy interpretation may help to further guide patient care. ACLF remains a life-threatening syndrome with a high mortality, which is clinically and pathophysiologically distinct from ALF. As the definition of ACLF is further refined over time, further study regarding the pathologic features of this entity may help to guide further biomarker development and aid in stratifying which therapeutic route is most appropriate for each individual patient.

CLINICS CARE POINTS

- ALF represents a severe form of hepatocyte injury caused by various etiologies, including infectious, autoimmune, drug/toxin, and ischemia-related factors, among others.
- Definitions of ACLF vary in their requirements, including the presence or absence of established cirrhosis, as well as the presence or absence of organ failure(s).
- Patients with ALF and ACLF can have overlapping clinical presentations, and a liver biopsy may help to aid in establishing the presence of chronic liver disease as well as suggest possible etiologies for acute liver injury.

DISCLOSURE

The authors have nothing to disclose.

REFERENCES

1. Garcia-Tsao G. Acute-on-Chronic liver failure: an old entity in search of clarity. Hepatol Commun 2018;2(12):1421–4.

2. van Leeuwen DJ, Alves V, Balabaud C, et al. Acute-on-chronic liver failure 2018: a need for (urgent) liver biopsy? Expert Rev Gastroenterol Hepatol 2018;12(6): 565–73.

3. Flamm SL, Yang YX, Singh S, et al. American gastroenterological association institute guidelines for the diagnosis and management of acute liver failure. Gastroenterology 2017;152(3):644–7.

4. Lefkowitch JH. The pathology of acute liver failure. Adv Anat Pathol 2016;23(3): 144–58.

5. Fyfe B, Zaldana F, Liu C. The pathology of acute liver failure. Clin Liver Dis 2018; 22(2):257–68.

6. Bernal W, Wendon J. Acute liver failure. N Engl J Med 2013;369(26):2525–34.

7. O'Grady JG, Schalm SW, Williams R. Acute liver failure: redefining the syndromes. Lancet 1993;342(8866):273–5.

8. Bernuau J, Rueff B, Benhamou JP. Fulminant and subfulminant liver failure: definitions and causes. Semin Liver Dis 1986;6(2):97–106.

9. Mochida S, Nakayama N, Matsui A, et al. Re-evaluation of the Guideline published by the Acute Liver Failure Study Group of Japan in 1996 to determine the indications of liver transplantation in patients with fulminant hepatitis. Hepatol Res 2008;38(10):970–9.

10. Li H, Xia Q, Zeng B, et al. Submassive hepatic necrosis distinguishes HBV-associated acute on chronic liver failure from cirrhotic patients with acute decompensation. J Hepatol 2015;63(1):50–9.

11. Bernal W, Hyyrylainen A, Gera A, et al. Lessons from look-back in acute liver failure? A single centre experience of 3300 patients. J Hepatol 2013;59(1):74–80.

12. Reuben A, Tillman H, Fontana RJ, et al. Outcomes in adults with acute liver failure between 1998 and 2013 an observational cohort study. Ann Intern Med 2016; 164(11):724–+.

13. Ganger DR, Rule J, Rakela J, et al. Acute liver failure of indeterminate etiology: a comprehensive systematic approach by an expert committee to establish causality. Am J Gastroenterol 2018;113(9):1319.

14. Zhang X, Ouyang J, Thung SN. Histopathologic manifestations of drug-induced hepatotoxicity. Clin Liver Dis 2013;17(4):547–64, vii-viii.

15. Kleiner DE, Chalasani NP, Lee WM, et al. Hepatic histological findings in suspected drug-induced liver injury: systematic evaluation and clinical associations. Hepatology 2014;59(2):661–70.

16. Reuben A, Koch DG, Lee WM. Acute Liver Failure Study G. Drug-induced acute liver failure: results of a U.S. multicenter, prospective study. Hepatology 2010; 52(6):2065–76.

17. Larson AM, Polson J, Fontana RJ, et al. Acetaminophen-induced acute liver failure: results of a United States multicenter, prospective study. Hepatology 2005; 42(6):1364–72.

18. Ramachandran R, Kakar S. Histological patterns in drug-induced liver disease. J Clin Pathol 2009;62(6):481–92.

19. Tapper EB, Sengupta N, Bonder A. The incidence and outcomes of ischemic hepatitis: a systematic review with meta-analysis. Am J Med 2015;128(12): 1314–21.

20. Zhang X, Jain D. The many faces and pathologic diagnostic challenges of autoimmune hepatitis. Hum Pathol 2022;132:114–25.

21. Kessler WR, Cummings OW, Eckert G, et al. Fulminant hepatic failure as the initial presentation of acute autoimmune hepatitis. Clin Gastroenterol H 2004;2(7): 625–31.

22. Stravitz RT, Lefkowitch JH, Fontana RJ, et al. Autoimmune acute liver failure: proposed clinical and histological criteria. Hepatology 2011;53(2):517–26.
23. Singh R, Nair S, Farr G, et al. Acute autoimmune hepatitis presenting with centrizonal liver disease: case report and review of the literature. Am J Gastroenterol 2002;97(10):2670–3.
24. Fujiwara K, Fukuda Y, Yokosuka O. Precise histological evaluation of liver biopsy specimen is indispensable for diagnosis and treatment of acute-onset autoimmune hepatitis. J Gastroenterol 2008;43(12):951–8.
25. Onda Y, Kanda J, Sakamoto S, et al. Detection of adenovirus hepatitis and acute liver failure in allogeneic hematopoietic stem cell transplant patients. Transpl Infect Dis 2021;23(2):e13496.
26. Riediger C, Sauer P, Matevossian E, et al. Herpes simplex virus sepsis and acute liver failure. Clin Transplant 2009;23(Suppl 21):37–41.
27. Bajaj JS, O'Leary JG, Lai JC, et al. Acute-on-Chronic liver failure clinical guidelines. Am J Gastroenterol 2022;117(2):225–52.
28. Sarin SK, Choudhury A, Sharma MK, et al. Acute-on-chronic liver failure: consensus recommendations of the Asian Pacific association for the study of the liver (APASL): an update. Hepatol Int 2019;13(4):353–90.
29. Bajaj JS, O'Leary JG, Reddy KR, et al. Survival in infection-related acute-on-chronic liver failure is defined by extrahepatic organ failures. Hepatology 2014; 60(1):250–6.
30. Moreau R, Jalan R, Gines P, et al. Acute-on-Chronic liver failure is a distinct syndrome that develops in patients with acute decompensation of cirrhosis. Gastroenterology 2013;144(7):1426. U1189.
31. Jalan R, Saliba F, Pavesi M, et al. Development and validation of a prognostic score to predict mortality in patients with acute-on-chronic liver failure. J Hepatol 2014;61(5):1038–47.
32. Shi Y, Yang Y, Hu Y, et al. Acute-on-chronic liver failure precipitated by hepatic injury is distinct from that precipitated by extrahepatic insults. Hepatology 2015;62(1):232–42.
33. Zhang Q, Li Y, Han T, et al. Comparison of current diagnostic criteria for acute-on-chronic liver failure. PLoS One 2015;10(3):e0122158.
34. Rastogi A, Kumar A, Sakhuja P, et al. Liver histology as predictor of outcome in patients with acute-on-chronic liver failure (ACLF). Virchows Arch 2011;459(2): 121–7.
35. Jain R, Jha AA, Jha G. Clinical and histological markers of poor prognosis in acute on chronic liver failure (ACLF) - an Indian perspective. Int J Sci Res 2018;7(2):388–90.
36. Baloda V, Anand A, Yadav R, et al. Histologic changes in core-needle liver biopsies from patients with acute-on-chronic liver failure and independent histologic predictors of 28-day mortality. Arch Pathol Lab Med 2022;146(7):846–54.
37. Katoonizadeh A, Laleman W, Verslype C, et al. Early features of acute-on-chronic alcoholic liver failure: a prospective cohort study. Gut 2010;59(11):1561–9.

Liver Regeneration in Acute on Chronic Liver Failure

Madelyn J. Blake[a],*, Clifford J. Steer, MD[a,b]

KEYWORDS

- Acute liver failure • Acute on chronic liver failure • Cytokines • Growth factors
- Homeostasis • microRNAs • Partial hepatectomy • Regeneration

KEY POINTS

- Liver regeneration is a tightly regulated process of coordinated cytokines, growth factors, inflammation, and cell fate.
- Emerging pathophysiologic mechanisms of this process or processes include the gut-liver axis, microRNAs, the Hippo-YAP pathway, and stem cell function.
- Promising therapeutics include immunomodulation, microRNA technology, and stem cell therapy.

INTRODUCTION

The study of liver regeneration has advanced rapidly in recent decades from the earliest model of liver injury and regeneration, the two-thirds (~70%) partial hepatectomy (PHx), in 1931 to the recent discovery of liver progenitor cells (LPCs).[1,2] Furthermore, a more robust understanding of the temporal course associated with liver disease has also been established with chronic liver disease, acute liver failure (ALF) and acute-on-chronic liver failure (ACLF).

The overarching goal of this review is to detail acute liver injury and corresponding liver regeneration in the setting of ischemic, surgical, and infectious insults in addition to acute on chronic liver injury, which involves further insult in the presence of preexisting cirrhosis and chronic hepatic fibrosis. For the purposes of this review, it is necessary to underscore the importance of the PHx model to the understanding of liver disease because it has historically been the crestal model for liver injury and the basis for examining pathways of liver regeneration. The PHx model induces an

[a] Department of Medicine, University of Minnesota Medical School, 420 Delaware Street Southeast, MMC 36, Minneapolis, MN 55455, USA; [b] Department of Genetics, Cell Biology and Development, University of Minnesota Medical School, 420 Delaware Street Southeast, MMC 36, Minneapolis, MN 55455, USA
* Corresponding author.
E-mail address: blake561@umn.edu

Clin Liver Dis 27 (2023) 595–616
https://doi.org/10.1016/j.cld.2023.03.005
1089-3261/23/© 2023 Elsevier Inc. All rights reserved.

acute insult that can lead to subsequent liver failure in its host without inflicting any additional injury in remaining hepatocytes.

BACKGROUND

Homeostasis is central to the role of the liver—an organ in the body whose functions extend from detoxification and metabolism of hormones, proteins, and lipids to storage of essential nutrients and vitamins. Moreover, the liver also assists in immune regulation through the reticuloendothelial system and nutritional utilization with the synthesis of bile salts. Given the capacious nature of the liver's broad homeostatic functions, it is not surprising that the liver also possesses novel mechanisms to preserve its own homeostasis following an injury. These novel features of liver homeostasis include swift initiation of mitosis from quiescent hepatocytes with the capacity to synchronize this process among the varying hepatic cell types, as well as the impressive ability to modulate a baseline hepatic mass.

Early study using parabiotic models proposed that an extrahepatic "humoral" factor possessed an initiating role in regeneration. These studies involved induced cross circulation with a donor rat that had recently undergone PHx and a normal rat. The investigators reported a substantial increase in mitotic activity and DNA synthesis in the normal rat's hepatocytes. Moreover, the livers of the donor rats regained liver mass to preoperative weight and failed regeneration in the setting of irreversible necrosis was only observed after an immense degree of hepatic resection.[3] Subsequent studies illustrated a synchronized bout of regeneration, described as a "wave" of mitoses in the injured liver, spanning from periportal to pericentral hepatic regions. Of note, this "wave" of synchronous regeneration was found to be cell autonomous.[4] This finding was further elucidated by early xenotransplantation studies that used mouse hepatocytes that were embedded into a rat liver. The implanted mouse hepatocytes did not differ from the intrinsic temporal course of regeneration observed in the mouse liver and were impervious to the surrounding cellular milieu.[5]

Following these findings, the search for the "quintessential" mitogen, one that would modulate the initiation and coordination of liver regeneration until proper liver mass was obtained, ensued. Of course, this search has been overly fruitful in that myriad factors contributing to the process of hepatic regeneration have been identified and extensively detailed in the literature throughout recent decades. As such, it is our intent to underscore the fundamental components of the present day understanding of hepatic regeneration and its respective mechanisms with an application to ALF. Principally described will be the "classical" pathways of liver regeneration involving cytokines and growth factors before a later discussion of the contemporary study of microRNAs (miRNAs) and hepatic stem cells.

CLASSICAL PATHWAYS OF HEPATIC REGENERATION

The classical pathway of hepatic regeneration is centered on signaling cascades, both intrahepatic and extrahepatic, which occur with rapid precision on hepatocytes and the surrounding cellular environment. This process is commonly referred to as "priming and progression," due to the fact that regeneration is initially preceded by a signal to hepatocytes "priming" them for subsequent mitosis and division by prompting a deviation from G0.[6] However, this first signal is inadequate to propel the hepatocytes through cell cycle and therefore, a second signal, originating from a mitogen of extrahepatic origin, is required for cellular progression through the remainder of G1 and mitosis. This proposed mechanism will be discussed in greater detail later in this article.

INTRACELLULAR SIGNALING PATHWAYS

The investigation of molecular mechanisms underlying hepatic regeneration have required the identification of intracellular signaling pathways that produce an immediate response to insult, with a particular focus on transcription factors such as STAT3, NFκB, and β-catenin.[7,8] These factors were of interest because their main effects are posttranslational and they possess no reliance on protein synthesis, making them ideal candidates for a swift effect on cell cycle regulation and gene expression following hepatocyte injury. Of note, the Hedgehog signaling pathway is upregulated in liver regeneration despite extending far beyond liver development.[9] This section will discuss regulators of these processes in extensive detail (**Fig. 1**).

ROLE OF TUMOR-NECROSIS FACTOR ALPHA

In alignment with our discussion of immune involvement in hepatic regeneration, tumor-necrosis factor alpha (TNF)-α plays a pivotal role in this process. TNF-α is a signaling protein and proinflammatory cytokine produced by macrophages in the setting of acute inflammation. It possesses a broad spectrum of signaling events in cells and is significantly involved in hepatic regeneration after PHx as well as CCl_4-induced injuries.[10] TNF-α serum levels increased substantially following PHx and were suppressed by pretreatment of Kupffer cell depletion. During the priming phase, TNF-α acts directly on hepatocytes to enter the cell cycle for regeneration.[11] TNF-α deploys many of its effects through the binding to 2 receptor types, TNF receptor (TNFR)-1 and TNFR-2. In the setting of carbon tetrachloride (CCL_4)-induced injury, TNFR-1 knockout mice exhibited substantial deficits in cellular replication time and a delay in liver weight recovery, both of which were reversed with the administration of interleukin 6 (IL-6) treatment. This was paralleled in PHx models where TNFR-1 knockout mice demonstrated major impairments in the synthesis of transcription factors, and later recovered following treatment with IL-6.[12] Collectively, these studies illustrated that TNF-α possesses a vital role in the initiation of the "priming" cascade via TNFR-1, eventually pushing hepatocytes to proliferate.

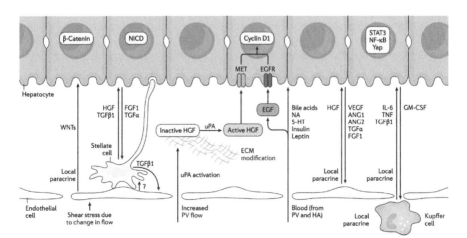

Fig. 1. Multiple signaling molecules regulate cell proliferation during liver regeneration. (*From* Michalopoulos GK, Bhushan B. Liver regeneration: biological and pathological mechanisms and implications. Nat Rev Gastroenterol Hepatol 2021;18:40-55.)

Intracellular signaling cascades initiated by TNF-α have been robustly studied, and the transcription factors NF-κB and STAT3 have been identified as maintaining vital roles in TNF-α signaling for hepatocyte proliferation. NF-κB possesses several pathways regulating the cell cycle and apoptosis, with its canonical pathway involving IKK degradation being the most pertinent to the TNF-α "priming" cascade. NF-κB is principally involved in liver development and is essential for the maintenance of hepatocyte homeostasis, including the regulation of cell survival and apoptosis.[13] When NF-κB subunit ReAl is deficient, both extensive liver degeneration and embryonic lethality have been reported.[14] It is well established that NF-κB activation within Kupffer cells is critical for hepatic regeneration in the setting of PHx and its inactivation in Kupffer cells and hepatocytes is detrimental for cellular proliferation.[15] Moreover, both NF-κB and TNF-α are integral for maintenance of the precise balance between hepatocyte regeneration and widespread necrosis after greater than the two-thirds PHx and are thought to be mediated through a combination of Myd88 and RAGE signaling.[16] Recently, NF-κB activation has been linked to long noncoding RNA molecules (lncRNAs) in a regulatory manner. lncRNAs are known regulators of the proliferation and apoptosis of hepatocytes in the process of liver fibrosis. Upregulation of NF-κB signaling is a fundamental component of the pathogenesis associated with liver fibrosis, and as such, they possess substantial promise as a novel therapeutic target.[17]

ROLE OF INTERLEUKIN 6

Interleukin 6 is a pleiotropic proinflammatory cytokine that possesses a wide variety of biological functions, including but not limited to the regulation of acute phase response, regeneration, and carcinogenesis. To perform these functions, IL-6 has 2 distinct signaling pathways, classical and trans-signaling, both of which are vital for liver regeneration. The classical IL-6 signaling pathway is characterized by IL-6 binding to its respective cell surface receptor, IL-6R (also referred to as gp-180) present on effector cells.[18] IL-6 receptors located at the cell surface membrane are characteristic of only certain cell types, of which include hepatocytes, some epithelial cells, and leukocytes. Following the binding of IL-6, the IL-6/IL-6R complex associates with a dimer of another membrane receptor, gp-130, which then results in the autophosphorylation of gp-130 and subsequent activation of its corresponding cytoplasmic tyrosine kinase, JAK1. This results in downstream activation of STAT3 and STAT1, in addition to initiation of the RAS/MAPK signaling pathway.[19] The trans-signaling pathway for IL-6 differs from the classical pathway in that it acts through a soluble IL-6R (sIL-6R). This soluble property is secondary to the cleavage of sIL-6R from the cell membrane by metalloproteinase ADAM17 before being shed into the serum and cytoplasm.[20] sIL-6R has been of particular interest as an experimental tool in liver regeneration because it allows for artificial IL-6 signal transduction in cells that do not constitutively express IL-6R. IL-6 binds to sIL-6R in a manner comparable to IL-6R and, thereafter, binds gp-130 to initiate the downstream effects of its signaling cascade. Of note, this cascade will have varied effects depending on the specific cell type, gp-130 concentrations, and sIL-6R levels in serum, establishing IL-6 as a pleiotropic cytokine.

Kupffer cells are the probable source of IL-6 in liver regeneration, as previously illustrated in knockout experiments involving macrophage-specific IL-6 and bone marrow transplants.[21] Following PHx in rats, serum levels of both TNF-α and IL-6 were found to be elevated only a few hours after the procedure and were then correlated with significant activation of downstream transcription factors STAT3 and C/EBPβ/nuclear factor-IL-6, culminating in amplified transcription of their respective genes.

Consequently, these results suggested that activation of the IL-6 signaling cascade may serve as a prominent initiating factor for G0/G1 phase transition in hepatocytes in the setting of recent PHx.[19]

The invaluable role of IL-6 in liver regeneration was illustrated in IL-6 knockout mice that exhibited ALF following PHx due to diminished levels of DNA synthesis and G1 cell cycle response. STAT3 phosphorylation was also reduced, and there was diminished expression of several cell cycle regulatory factors. Furthermore, when injected with IL-6, hepatocyte proliferation was restored in mice, and ALF was avoided, in turn cementing the importance of this pleiotropic cytokine in the process of liver regeneration.[22] Of interest, several PHx studies involving IL-6 knockout mice reported high rates of mortality and noted that outcomes were improved by subcutaneous, but not IV, injection of IL-6, in turn highlighting the requirement of sustained activity for this recapitulative effect.[23] It has been proposed that this therapeutic effect is modulated in part by preservation of Fas-mediated death in hepatocytes.

The IL-6/STAT3 pathway seems to play an important, although delicate role in liver regeneration associated with ACLF. This is centered on the fact that chronic liver injury is known to halt liver regeneration because IL-6 levels are reduced secondary to Kupffer cell damage. IFN-γ, exhibits a strong innate immune response in the setting of ACLF, and this has the downstream effect of activating the STAT1 pathway.[24] In contrast to STAT3, the STAT1 pathway is repressive and inhibits liver regeneration. As such, in liver injury models, liver regeneration is mediated through a balance of the IL-6/STAT3 and the IFN-γ/STAT1 signaling pathways.[25] The imbalance of these pathways can have deleterious effects on liver regeneration. In ACLF models, IL-22, a cytokine produced by several immune cells, was shown to upregulate the STAT3 pathway over the STAT1 pathway and subsequently enhance liver regeneration.[26] Additionally, administration of IL-22 in patients with ACLF resulted in improved regeneration and survival outcomes through reversal of the STAT1/STAT3 pathway imbalance and upregulation of several antibacterial genes associated with modulation of antiapoptotic protein BCL2. IL-22 promotes proliferation and tissue regeneration through interactions with its key cellular targets, stromal cells, and nonhematopoietic epithelial cells, and has broad therapeutic potential for ameliorating acute liver insults and ACLF.

IMMUNE REGULATION IN THE REGENERATING LIVER

The return of portal blood from the intestines to the liver establishes an intricate relationship between the gut and the liver. It is a complex balance of immune tolerance and controlled inflammation secondary to a constant onslaught of myriad toxins and microbial antigens.[27] Moreover, the gut–liver axis also fosters a reservoir of regulatory immune cells, principally Kupffer cells, which serve as resident macrophages within the liver. Kupffer cells compose a majority of macrophages found throughout all tissues and represent approximately a third of the hepatic sinusoidal cells.[28] Given their close association with portal blood, Kupffer cells are indispensable for cell signaling and possess a substantial role in the ability of the liver to regenerate.

In response to hepatocyte injury, both macrophage number and replication are upregulated, alongside increased recruitment of additional inflammatory monocytes to the liver.[29] At present, the integral role of Kupffer cells and other recruited macrophages remains unclear because several studies investigating activation and depletion report conflicting outcomes. Hepatocyte-protective effects conferred by macrophage inactivation have been reported but depletion studies have shown delayed regeneration, diminished NF-κB activation, and a significant drop in recruitment of circulating monocytes.[30,31] However, with recent advances in our understanding of the M1/M2 phenotype and macrophage polarization, a dual role for Kupffer cells has been further elucidated with likely alternation between M1/M2 during the hepatic repair process and subsequent fibrosis.

Several regenerative mediators discussed throughout this review are also indispensable signaling molecules or cytokines within the immune system. Fundamental studies involving rodent models bred to be athymic, germ-free, and lipopolysaccharide (LPS)-resistant illustrated the innate immune response in hepatic regeneration. This resistance was later linked to Toll-like receptor 4 (TLR4), a key binding protein for routine immunity, as defects in TLR4 have demonstrated intact hepatocyte regeneration.[32] Knockout models lacking signaling protein MyD88, an essential adaptor protein required for TLR-mediated signaling, however, demonstrated a significant decrease in hepatic regeneration.[33,34] Furthermore, hepatic regeneration studies involving C3 and C5 knockout mice, complement pathways involved in regeneration, also demonstrated reduced capacities for hepatic regeneration.[35] Promising results have also been observed with the drug Cenicriviroc (CVC), a C–C chemokine receptor antagonist, predominantly expressed on monocytes and various immune cells.[36] Preclinical studies involving CVC have reported significant reductions in the severity of liver fibrosis relative to placebo; and a majority of patients exhibited improvement for at least 2 years following treatment.

After PHx, serum levels of macrophage colony stimulating factor (CSF-1) increased proportionately to the quantity of tissue resected and accelerated the regenerative process.[37] ALF in the setting of acetaminophen (APAP) overdose in humans also demonstrated an altered immune response, involving a depletion of inflammatory cells recruited to the liver, increase of hepatic-derived macrophage infiltration into necrotic liver tissue, and higher concentrations of local Kupffer cells relative to normal controls. These alterations in immune function were observed secondary to elevated levels of chemokine ligands 2 and 3, IL-6 and IL-10, and transforming growth factor β1 (TGF-β1) in serum.[38] The ALF model and APAP has also shown that lower serum levels of macrophage CSF-1 were associated with a worse prognosis and therefore may predict mortality outcomes in this population.[39] Although immune-modulating therapies in ALF/ACLF and the utility of steroids to augment hepatocyte regeneration remain under investigation, these translational studies indicate that therapeutic possibilities certainly exist. Several pilot studies involving individuals with ALF/ACLF have demonstrated improved mortality in patients treated with the administration of granulocyte-colony stimulating factor (g-CSF).[40] Additionally, the emergence of improved models for the study of hepatotoxicity, such as the MPS model, allows for an earlier detection and prediction of drug-induced liver injury and work to improve patient outcomes.[41]

GROWTH FACTORS

After liver injury and the hepatocyte phase transition from G0 to G1, the importance of growth factors is augmented due to their invaluable role throughout the cellular processes involved in G1. In particular, the most pertinent growth factors and mitogens involved in G1 and liver regeneration are that of epidermal growth factor (EGF) and hepatocyte growth factor (HGF), as well as corresponding ligands.

EPIDERMAL GROWTH FACTOR AND ITS RECEPTOR

In liver regeneration, hepatocyte-derived epidermal growth factor and its receptor (EGFR) are activated by several ligands, which in turn promote cell proliferation and survival. The primary ligands of EGFR are that of amphiregulin, heparin-binding

EGF-like receptor (HB-EGFR), and TGF-α, all of which are found to be upregulated in the setting of liver injury and PHx.[42] The synthesis of these ligands occurs in various locations, which contributes to the redundancy in upregulation present in liver regeneration. The pivotal role of EGFR has been highlighted by several EGFR-knockout studies, as mice lacking EGFR survive for an average of only 8 days and possess substantial developmental impairments including those in epithelial and neural development. Moreover, conditional models involving EGFR-knockout mice have reported significant delays in liver regeneration following PHx with corresponding elevation in mortality. That increase is principally attributed to diminished hepatocyte regeneration secondary to cell cycle arrest and decreased serum concentrations of cyclin D1.[43] In addition to cyclin D1, HB-EGF is also a vital ligand involved in cell cycle regulation and progression. HB-EGF has been studied extensively in a model with varied percentages of PHx, with a focus on corresponding hepatocyte proliferation and survival. HB-EGF was undetectable following one-third PHx but was noted to exhibit an increased serum concentration in two-thirds PHx before DNA replication. Secondary to this observation, it was found that treatment of HB-EGF following one-third PHx was associated with more than a 15x increase in DNA replication, in turn cementing the indispensable roles of both HB-EGF and EGFR in hepatocyte cell cycle progression after priming by the aforementioned factors.[44] Of note, hepatocyte proliferation was suppressed following shRNA-mediated silencing of EGFR but it eventually does recover. Mesenchymal-epithelial transition factor (c-MET) signaling was temporally associated with this acute silencing of EGFR and implied a compensatory mechanism within liver regeneration. This was further elucidated in a study involving c-MET knockout mice after PHx, where canertinib-mediated inhibition of EGFR resulted in substantial impairment in liver regeneration and subsequent liver failure.[45]

Interesting findings have been reported with incremental dosing in APAP overdose with the integration of the cellular signaling cascades discussed above. At 300 mg/kg, the lower dose for the study, classical regenerative pathways performed as expected. Expression of cyclin D1 was elevated before the regenerative phase with the lower dose but exhibited complete inhibition with higher dosing, defined as 600 mg/kg. Moreover, induction of cyclin D1 expression by classical signaling molecules, such as TNF-α/NF-κB, IL-6/STAT3, was also inhibited at higher dosing despite redundancy of these pathways.[46] As such, these findings underscore the need for additional investigation of these basic pathways in acute liver injury independent of surgical models.

TGF-α and amphiregulin are synthesized by hepatocytes to serve autoendocrine roles. Surprisingly, PHx in TGF-α-knockout mice did not exhibit any abnormalities in liver regeneration, likely due to the presence of multiple redundant pathways. However, impaired amphiregulin expression resulted in impaired hepatocyte proliferation.[47,48] Salivary glands and Brunner's gland in the gut secrete EGF such that it can act in an endocrine manner. Previous studies reported impaired regeneration in the absence of EGF, with corresponding upregulation alongside administration of recombinant EGF in PHx mice.[49]

HEPATOCYTE GROWTH FACTOR

HGF, one of the earliest mitogens isolated from serum in PHx mice, plays an essential role in liver regeneration.[50] It is synthesized by mesenchymal cells within the liver, principally endothelial cells and Kupffer cells, and it is thought to function in a paracrine manner. Knockout models involving the receptor for HGF, c-MET, result in substantial liver abnormalities and failed embryonic development. Furthermore, conditional knockouts have shown diminished recovery from centrolobular lesions and increased sensitivity to Fas-induced apoptosis, likely due to direct binding and sequestration of the Fas receptor by c-MET in hepatocytes.[51] The interplay between liver sinusoidal endothelial cells (LSECs) and HGF has also been recently established as a key component in liver regeneration. LSECs have been strongly associated with the promotion of liver regeneration following PHx through the release of angiocrine factors, such as HGF, during the inductive phase of liver regeneration where hepatocytes initially proliferate.[52] Moreover, an additional study reported that a decrease in liver endothelial cells was associated with depleted hepatocyte proliferation in patients with ACLF but not patients with ALF. As such, hepatocyte replication is impaired in ACLF and is consequently associated with diminished survival outcomes.[53]

THE ROLE OF METABOLISM IN LIVER REGENERATION

The role of bile acids in liver regeneration is well documented. Early studies reported significant impairments in regeneration following PHx involving external biliary drainage as opposed to internal biliary drainage in cholestatic liver. These findings were paralleled by studies investigating CCL_4-induced injury, with the restoration of regeneration following the replacement of bile acids and alterations in FOXM1 signaling, an essential transcription factor for cell cycle progression.[54] Of note, one study involving administration of cholic acid versus a bile acid sequestrant, cholestyramine, reported that rats fed with the bile acid sequestrant exhibited a diminished bile acid pool, impaired regenerative capacity, elevated CYP7A1 expression, and decreased farnesoid X receptor (FXR) expression.[55] These findings were further supported in a corresponding clinical study using hemihepatectomy, where a significant decrease in liver volume was observed in patients possessing external biliary drainage.[56]

Nuclear receptor FXR is an invaluable receptor in bile acid signaling and its respective mechanisms. FXR is expressed in the liver and ileum in addition to several other tissues and is involved in myriad intracellular signaling pathways relating to the regulation of lipid and bile acid homeostasis.[57] FXR knockout models involving PHx and CCL_4 injury in mice have shown significant deficits in early liver regeneration, and bile acid supplementation did not recapitulate those deficits. These FXR knockout studies also established the binding of FXR to a fibroblast growth factor (FGF), and subsequent interaction with cytochrome P450 as an integral pathway in bile acid synthesis. FXR has been linked to transcription factor FOXm1B expression in hepatocytes through knockout models, and the inhibition of FOXm1b expression resulted in reduced liver regeneration.[58] A hepatic and intestine-specific FXR knockout study demonstrated that hepatocyte-derived FXR was required for the induction of FOXm1B in both PHx and CCL_4-induced injury. Enterocyte-specific FOXm1B knockout mice did not exhibit this requirement and deficits in regeneration were ameliorated with ectopic expression of FGF15 via recombinant adenovirus.[59] Additionally, FXR has been implicated in the downstream inhibition of CYP7A1, a key enzyme in bile acid synthesis, through the binding of response element mouse FGF15 in enterocytes. FGF15 is the mouse analog of human FGF19, which serves as an inhibitor of CYP7A1.[60]

Bile acids have also been implicated in the activation of constitutive androstane receptor (CAR), a key regulator for FOXO-1 and its corresponding target gene, p21, and upregulates the activity of cyclin D1, which results in augmented cell cycle progression. CAR has recently attracted substantial therapeutic interest as CAR deficiency was associated with liver failure secondary to robust loss of liver mass. Pharmacologic reactivation of CAR was shown to enhance cell cycle progression and hepatocyte survival through modulation of JNK signaling during liver regeneration, in turn cementing its importance as a potential metabolic-targeted therapy for liver disease.[61]

The interplay between the gut microbiota and maintenance of bile acid homeostasis has become an increasingly popular topic with substantial clinical implications. Acute liver injury or PHx was associated with increased bacterial translocation across the gut mucosa and exposure to microbiome byproducts.[62] The primary means by which the microbiome composition is associated with alterations in bile acid homeostasis is through changes in the synthesis of primary and secondary bile acids. The microbiome diversity is reduced in patients with cirrhosis and, therefore, is implicated in the diminished conversion of primary bile acids to secondary bile acids. Moreover, obstruction of bile acid enterohepatic circulation following PHx was associated with the inhibition of liver regeneration. These findings elucidate another potential mechanism to explain the hepatic dysfunction and corresponding risk for liver failure in individuals with ACLF.[63,64]

PLATELETS AND PLATELET-DERIVED FACTORS

Platelets and platelet-derived factors play a key role in liver regeneration following PHx. High concentrations of platelets have been found in the liver remnant after PHx in both human and murine models. Liver regeneration is also significantly delayed when platelets are depleted or functionally impaired, whereas elevated platelet levels are associated with the stimulation of liver regeneration following PHx.[65] Various clinical studies have also reported impaired survival outcomes alongside increased liver dysfunction and diminished regeneration. These findings were eventually linked to the discovery that activated platelets secrete growth factors and, therefore, possess an essential role in liver regeneration. One of the growth factors secreted by platelets is fibrinogen, which has been demonstrated to substantially increase in the liver after PHx, and the inhibition of fibrinogen deposition in the liver results in impaired hepatocyte proliferation.[66] Both human and murine PHx studies propose a unique mechanism involving the promotion of platelet accumulation by intrahepatic fibrin(ogen) deposition, which ultimately drives hepatic regeneration following PHx.[67]

PARACRINE MEDIATORS

The importance of the Wnt/β-catenin pathway applies not only to liver regeneration but also to the development and maintenance of normal physiology. When Wnt signaling is absent, β-catenin is marked and later degraded by a complex involving the tumor suppressor protein, APC. When activated, free β-catenin translocates to the nucleus and regulates target gene transcription through T-cell factor proteins. β-catenin levels are highly constrained, with a significant proportion often bound to the APC complex or E-cadherin at the cell membrane. After PHx, cytosolic β-catenin levels are elevated with a corresponding increase in the translocation of β-catenin to the nucleus.[68,69] The essential role of β-catenin in liver regeneration has been studied extensively in knockout models, which demonstrate substantial delays in hepatocyte proliferation and depleted liver mass in early regeneration. APAP overdose is also a clinically relevant model illustrating the role of β-catenin in regeneration. Of note, several murine APAP models have reported the activation of β-catenin with parallel increases in the expression of glutamine synthase and hepatocyte proliferation secondary to elevated levels of cyclin D1. Moreover, analysis of liver tissue from individuals with APAP overdose has shown an association between nuclear β-catenin localization and spontaneous liver regeneration.[70]

The Wnt/β-catenin pathway has also been linked to "metabolic zonation" in the liver during organogenesis and likely regeneration, by maintaining a balance of Wnt signaling, activation of β-catenin, and APC regulation. Hepatocytes have been shown to express a gradient between periportal and pericentral phenotypes, and their respective metabolic activities.[71,72] The close association of β-catenin with E-cadherin highlights the potential involvement of Wnt/β-catenin signaling in the architectural development involved in liver regeneration. Following PHx, the expression levels of β-catenin and E-cadherin are opposite and therefore suggest a mechanistic coordination with cell–cell adhesion.[73,74]

TRANSFORMING GROWTH FACTOR β

TGF-β plays a pivotal role in the termination of liver regeneration. Preliminary studies reported that TGF-β was associated with significant inhibition of DNA synthesis in mitogen-stimulated hepatocytes, and the decrease in this inhibition was temporally associated with the amount of time the hepatocytes were separated from the regenerating liver.[75] These findings were further supported by a corroborating study demonstrating an increase in TGF-β mRNA expression after PHx, with the highest expression occurring immediately after the initial round of hepatocyte cell division. Of note, this increase in TGF-β expression was associated with a reduction in the expression of the TGF-β receptor following liver injury.[76] TGF-β receptor knockout models highlighted the importance of the elevated TGF-β receptor expression in liver regeneration with corresponding increases in hepatocyte proliferation and liver mass. The effects of the inverse relationship between TGF-β and its receptor are thought to be mediated through inhibition of cyclin D1 and subsequent cell cycle arrest in phase G1.[77]

Beta-2 spectrin (β2SP) has been established as another essential receptor molecule in TGF-β signaling and has produced surprising results in liver regeneration models. Murine knockout models of β2SP demonstrated a significant delay in liver regeneration after PHx, as well as impaired cell cycle progression and increased DNA damage in a manner independent of p53. Collectively, these findings indicate a coordinating role for TGF-β in liver regeneration and contradict the prevailing idea that it simply serves as a terminating signal.[78]

HIPPO/YAP REGENERATION PATHWAY

The Hippo/YAP pathway serves as a key regulator of liver mass and progenitor cell determination. Yes-associated protein (YAP1) is a transcription coactivator and the primary pathway effector, with nuclear localization negatively regulated by Hippo upstream signaling. Hippo activation results in phosphorylation and subsequent activation of mammalian Sterile20-like (MST) 1 and 2, which activate large tumor suppressor kinases (LATS) 1 and 2. When Hippo is inactive, YAP can translocate to the nucleus and bind transcription factors, resulting in elevated transcription of genes pertaining to cell survival, proliferation, and growth. Phosphorylation of YAP1 by LATS prevents its nuclear translocation, in turn inhibiting its interactions with transcription factors and the Hippo/YAP pathway.[79] Transgenic models involving the induction of YAP1 with corresponding overexpression resulted in a 4-fold increase in liver size, secondary to an increase in hepatocyte number. Of note, this effect was reversible with the termination of YAP1 expression.[80] Moreover, adeno-associated virus (AAV)-mediated hepatocyte overexpression of YAP1 was associated with rapid growth of progenitor-like hepatocyte populations, and upregulated nuclear localization of YAP1 has been linked with hepatocellular carcinoma.[81] Although significant increases in YAP1 protein were observed, mRNA levels did not reflect this elevation, in turn proposing posttranslational modification or inhibition of degradation concurrent with regeneration.[82] With additional understanding of this pathway and its associated molecular mechanisms, the list of regulators has increased substantially and as such, Hippo/YAP is now considered a vital component of "hepatostat."

IDEA OF HEPATOSTAT

"Hepatostat" is a relatively new term that encompasses the homeostatic mechanisms guaranteeing appropriate liver size and architecture following injury or stress.[83] Regeneration is species-specific and follows a stereotyped time course, with complete restoration of liver mass occurring 5 to 7 days after PHx in rodents and 3 to 4 months in humans. The hepatic proliferation process does not merely consist of mitosis and cell division but rather a still incomplete understanding of cell fate and replication. It is well established that hepatocytes divide at varying rates depending on location, with periportal and zone 2 hepatocytes composing approximately 80% of all cell division, and the disparate division is impacted by nuclear ploidy.[84] Although organ size is principally confirmed by the respective number and size of its cells, this was only recently confirmed for the liver. Cell hypertrophy was found to play a substantial role in the restoration of liver mass, composing all regenerative mass following a 30% hepatectomy and an equal contribution to regenerative mass after a 70% PHx.[85,86]

THE ROLE OF microRNAs IN LIVER REGENERATION

MiRNAs are evolutionarily conserved, small noncoding RNAs that repress gene expression in a posttranscriptional manner through translational obstruction or degradation of mRNA molecules via binding of 3'-untranslated regions. MiRNAs are first transcribed by RNA polymerase as primary transcripts (pri-miRNA) and are then further modified by an endoribonuclease Dicer to become mature miRNA.[87] Various mechanisms involving miRNA rearrangements have been characterized as integral components of liver regeneration, differentiation, and hepatic carcinogenesis.[88] In postnatal Dicer knockout models, the loss of functional miRNAs resulted in elevated levels of apoptosis and cell proliferation in young mice, as well as inflammation and progressive liver damage in aged mice. These findings cemented the idea that although miRNAs are not vital to the maintenance of hepatic function by adult hepatocytes, they do possess a crucial role in the mediation of regeneration and inflammation.[89]

In several clinical studies, patients with spontaneous recovery from ALF had significantly elevated serum levels of the exosomal miRNAs, miR-122, miR-21, and miR-221, relative to nonrecovered patients.[90] It has also been reported that select regeneration-specific miRNAs are strong indicators of prognosis following liver transplantation in both acute liver injury and CLD.[91] Moreover, miR-122 was found to be elevated in both the serum and liver tissue of patients with spontaneous recovery.[92] As such, these findings have fostered widespread interest in the utility of miRNAs as a prognostic marker and therapeutic intervention for ALF.

MiR-122 is specific to the liver and is the most abundant miRNA in liver tissue, composing 70% of all cloned miRNAs.[93] As discussed previously, miR-122 has been strongly associated with improved prognosis in ALF—both clinically and in murine models.[94] In a murine APAP-induced liver injury model, miR-122 increases were noted in both a dose and duration-dependent manner.[95] MiR-122 has been suggested to play a mechanistic role in regeneration and carcinogenesis through its ability to promote hepatic differentiation and increase FoxA1 and HNF4a levels in vitro, with subsequent alterations in the balance of the transition from epithelial to mesenchymal cells and vice versa.[96]

MiR-21, another antiapoptotic miRNA, is associated with the promotion of cell proliferation following liver injury. During the initial stages of liver regeneration, the expression of miR-21 is significantly elevated. This upregulation is principally mediated by Pellino-1 and its downstream inhibition of NF-κB signaling in both PHx and in vitro models.[97] Studies involving miR-21 knockout models have also demonstrated a vital role for miR-21 in the progression through the DNA synthesis portion of the cell cycle. Impairments involving miR-21 have been associated with the pathogenesis of several forms of chronic liver disease, including that of liver fibrosis, hepatocellular carcinoma, and viral liver diseases.[98]

MiR-221 is another prominent antiapoptotic miRNA, which has been shown to confer protective effects from fas cell surface death receptor-induced ALF. In addition, it has been reported to serve as an accelerator of hepatocyte proliferation in AAV-mediated overexpression experiments with in vivo murine PHx models. MiR-221 over-expression is thought to directly target p27, p57, and Arnt mRNA, ultimately resulting in proliferation due to an increase in rapid-S phase entry in hepatocytes.[99,100]

THE ROLE OF STEM CELLS

The role of stem cells in normal liver physiology and liver regeneration following hepatectomy or injury remains somewhat unsettled. By definition, stem cells possess the ability to proliferate and differentiate into several cell lineages. It is well established that during embryonic development, the liver is constructed mainly by endodermal-derived cells, which later differentiate into the 2 primary cells of the liver, hepatocytes, and cholangiocytes.[101]

Following PHx, the regenerative process is, in part, fueled by proliferation and hypertrophy of mature hepatocytes. In several rodent bile duct ligation studies, transdifferentiation from hepatocytes to cholangiocytes seems to be fostered by the NOTCH pathway. Impairments in this pathway have been associated with repressed transdifferentiation alongside diminished YAP levels, indicating a mechanistic collaboration between the NOTCH and Hippo/YAP pathways.[102,103]

One limitation of the PHx model is that it often fails to recapitulate most liver diseases and their respective pathogenesis involving inflammatory and fibrogenic cascades, ultimately resulting in hepatocyte damage and death. Moreover, regeneration in the setting of acute liver disease and ACLF commonly requires the activation of LPCs.[104] LPCs have been strongly implicated in the maintenance of hepatic homeostasis and were recently shown to exhibit hepatocyte functions in the setting of massive hepatic necrosis.[105] The origin of these cells remains unknown but the canal of Hering has traditionally thought to be a potential source. LPCs are known by several names in the literature, such as "ductular hepatocytes" or "hepatic/liver progenitor cells" but are often referred to as "oval cells" in rat models and are reported to only occur in the damaged liver.[106] The primary protocol used for the induction of oval cells involves blocking hepatocyte proliferation via 2-AAF before PHx. Several studies using this method have demonstrated that oval cells have the potential to differentiate into both hepatocytes and cholangiocytes.[107] The 2-AAF/PHx model only works in rats, not mice, so other induction methods for hepatic injury, namely administration of a 5-diethyoxycarbonyl-1,4-dihidro-collidine-containing diet or choline-deficient ethionine-supplemented diet, have been used for murine models.[108] However, it is important to note that these models can differ significantly in the production of their respective oval cells and thus, "LPC" is a more appropriate term for the resultant cells.

When regeneration alone does not compensate for diminished metabolic function, liver transplantation is the only remaining option. Despite a recent positive trend in the rate of liver transplantation in the United States, many patients die each year waiting for a liver transplant. As such, the intersection of the field of regeneration and stem cell research has expanded rapidly to ameliorate this massive gap in human suffering. Several protocols for the differentiation of hepatic mesenchymal stem cells (MSCs) have been developed.[109] The transplantation of MSC-derived hepatocytes in CCL_4-induced murine models of liver failure has demonstrated restoration of liver function, with parallel findings being reported in drug-induced models of ALF.[110,111] Several studies have also demonstrated that small extracellular vesicles from IFN-γ-conditioned MSCs enhanced tissue repair in regeneration by inducing upregulation of anti-inflammatory macrophages and regulatory T cells.[112] Similar findings were reported with the administration of mesenchymal stromal cells, which were shown to foster liver regeneration through the inhibition of innate immune cells and activation of the adaptive immune system, namely B and T regulatory cells.[113]

Despite initial popularity surrounding hepatocyte transplantation as an alternative to liver transplantation, its expansion as a therapeutic avenue has been limited due to several factors, including poor cell engraftment in the recipient. As such, much of the focus on stem-cell therapies as an alternative to liver transplantation has been shifted to the use of human-induced pluripotent stem cells (iPSCs). In particular, the possibility of obtaining hepatocytes from iPSCs has gained a substantial amount of attention due to their ability to generate both parenchymal and nonparenchymal cells. A substantial benefit of these iPSCs is the autologous characteristic of their cell transplant, in turn diminishing the possibility of immune rejection. At present, several studies have reported exciting results with the creation and transplantation of liver organoids synthesized by iPSC-derived liver cells. One study reported that human liver organoids demonstrated a high degree of repopulation in damaged mouse livers and exhibited high levels of albumin production when examined at 90 days following transplantation. However, additional studies are needed to examine whether organoids are truly an inexhaustible source of liver cells that could meet the needs of liver bioengineering.[114]

ACUTE ON CHRONIC LIVER FAILURE

Although this discussion has predominantly focused on regeneration in the setting of acute injury in a previously functional liver, recent exploration has been centered on regeneration in ACLF, where the functionality of the liver is already compromised (**Fig. 2**). ACLF is a multifaceted condition characterized by an acute decompensation in liver function, organ failure, and high short-term mortality.[115] In addition to their impaired functional capacity, ACLF patients possess chronic inflammation secondary to substantial immune dysfunction. Although this population possesses lower serum concentrations of inflammatory markers relative to patients with sepsis, they exhibit significant depression in TNF-α production and HLA-DR expression.[116] Additionally, pervasive dysfunction is present in regulatory monocytes and macrophages as well as cytokines and cell signaling.[117] Mitochondrial dysfunction has also been frequently observed in ACLF and is implicated in the promotion of a hyperinflammatory or immunosuppressive state.[118] Of note, hepatic perfusion has been recently recognized as a valuable predictor of prognosis and mortality outcomes in critically ill patients with ACLF.[119] Hepatocyte-derived exosomes were also recently identified as prognostic markers in patients with ACLF. In particular, an exosome profile with ALB and VEGF was an accurate marker of liver regeneration and improved prognosis.[120]

Due to the complex nature of ACLF and its pathogenesis, a pivotal issue hindering robust innovation in the field is the difficulty faced when developing accurate animal models. Several strategies for the induction of ACLF in animal models have been

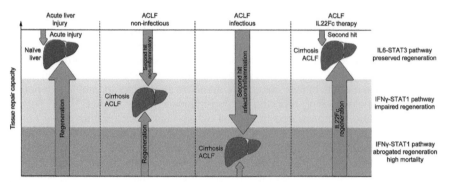

Fig. 2. Regenerative capacities in acute-on-chronic liver failure. The naïve liver has a high regenerative capacity allowing full recovery after acute liver injury. Once cirrhosis is present, the ability of hepatocytes to proliferate is impaired due to a switch from STAT3 to STAT1 pathway activation in response to injury. Additional infections in the context of ACLF abrogate regenerative capacities and lead to insufficient recovery with high mortality. Stimulation of the STAT3 pathway by IL22Fc has the potential to restore the liver's ability to regenerate in ACLF. ACLF, acute-on-chronic liver failure. (*From* Engelmann C, Mehta G, Tacke F. Regeneration in acute-on-chronic liver failure – the phantom lost its camouflage. Journal of Hepatology 2020;72:610-612.)

identified, and agents commonly selected for ACLF models include bacterial LPS, ethyl alcohol, and the combination of CCL_4 and a bacterial load.[121] CCL_4 administration is the most used model for murine liver injury when studying ACLF, with repeated administration during several weeks required for the establishment of a stable cirrhotic state. However, despite the accessibility of treatment for the study of ACLF in animal models, multiple drawbacks develop due to a limited range of animal tolerability. CCL_4-treated animals are often unstable and possess significant mortality rates during development, ultimately culminating in inconsistent outcomes and serious limitations to the applicability of results. That said, a recent study centered on improving CCL_4-based animal models for ACLF may serve as the necessary breakthrough for this concern. A 3-hit protocol consisting of chronic administration of CCL_4, acute administration of CCL_4, and consistent bacterial load in mice was shown to accurately replicate multiorgan failure, a crucial component of ACLF's pathogenesis. This novel protocol not only works to combat existing concerns with the toxin-induced model but also affords novel insight into our understanding of ACLF and regeneration.[122] In addition, promising results have been reported with an ACLF murine model composed of CCL_4 administration for 10 weeks followed by acute hepatic injury with acetaminophen (APAP) and LPS. This CCL_4/APAP/LPS model, known as CALPS, was shown to accurately mimic the pathogenesis of ACLF, including hepatocellular necrosis, impaired regeneration, portal hypertension, and multiorgan dysfunction.[123]

Unsurprisingly, depleted immune function and cytokines have a strongly negative effect on regeneration. Innovative therapies have focused on the inherent immune dysfunction associated with ACLF to enhance regenerative capacity and recovery. As discussed earlier, g-CSF therapy is one example to enhance tissue repair and alleviate inflammation following injury through mobilization of endogenous bone marrow-derived stem cells.[124] Administration of MSCs is also of significant therapeutic interest due to their ability to combat inflammation and prevent hepatic damage by inhibiting collagen synthesis and activation of hepatic stellate cells. Several ongoing clinical trials are currently investigating the use of HepaStem cells as a therapeutic avenue for ACLF. HepaStem cells are derived from human-liver MSCs and following intravenous administration, they migrate to the liver and perform various functions to mitigate fibrosis via inhibition of hepatic stellate cells and collagen secretion.[125] Pomegranate has also demonstrated immense therapeutic potential in alleviating oxidative stress and inflammation secondary to mitochondrial dysfunction. In a CCL_4-induced model of liver injury, pomegranate administration reversed the detrimental effects of the toxin by increasing anti-inflammatory serum enzymes and ROS production.[126]

SUMMARY

With the multifaceted nature of injury and recovery, the study of regeneration in ALF and ACLF will continue to evolve overtime with further identification of instigating factors and pathophysiology informing future treatments. Regenerative factors highlighted throughout this review, including that of immunomodulation and stem cell therapy, continue to exhibit significant therapeutic potential while emerging discoveries such as miRNAs and the Hippo/YAP pathway open unexplored avenues for the future of novel treatments. It is hoped that as we continue to learn more about the relationship between these elements and the host by means of the microbiome, bile homeostasis, and mechanosensing, we may be able to foster the development of innovative strategies for the prevention and regeneration of the injured liver.

CLINICS CARE POINTS

- Acute on chronic liver failure (ACLF) is a clinical syndrome of sudden hepatic decompensation in patients with pre-existing chronic liver disease. It is a serious condition with high morbidity and mortality. Given the significant heterogeneity and the multi-faceted complex nature of liver regeneration, both the etiology of liver injury and potential repair mechanisms will continue to evolve.

- Patients with ACLF have reduced hepatic reserve and chronic circulatory dysfunction. Hepatocyte death causes release of damaging molecules and incites inflammation with resultant further liver failure. Patients typically have a significantly altered immune milieu, with alterations in pro- and anti-inflammatory cytokines which can hinder liver regeneration in addition to depleted Kupffer cell populations resulting in reduced regenerative function.

- Renal failure, hepatic encephalopathy, recurrent infections and upper gastrointestinal bleeding from worsening portal hypertension are considered end- stage complications of decompensated cirrhosis and should be evaluated immediately and continuously. Gut microbiota and immune modulation are being explored as potential prognostic markers and therapeutic options.

- Clinical management of ACLF includes assessing precipitant factors that can be readily treated, including latent infections. The clinical effectiveness of liver assist devices in the context of management remains unclear, in part due to the heterogeneity of patient populations and lack of definitive data to support their use for recovery from ACLF.

- The role of liver transplantation in ACLF remains a topic of debate. While organ transplantation is potentially the only curative intervention in advanced patients, it is also associated with higher postoperative complications and longer ICU and hospital stays compared with other indications of cirrhosis. It is, however, a consideration that must be considered in maintaining survival of the patient.

DISCLOSURE

The authors declare neither competing nor commercial and/or financial conflicts of interest.

REFERENCES

1. Higgins G. Experimental pathology of the liver: restoration of the liver in the white rate following partial surgical removal. Arch Pathol 1931;12:186–202.
2. Rabinovici N, Wiener E. Liver Regeneration after partial hepatectomy in carbon tetrachloride-induced cirrhosis in the rat. Gastroenterology 1961;40:416–22.
3. Moolten FL, Bucher NL. Regeneration of rat liver: transfer of humoral agent by cross circulation. Science 1967;158:272–4.
4. Rabes HM. Kinetics of hepatocellular proliferation as a function of the microvascular structure and functional state of the liver. Ciba Found Symp 1977;31–53.
5. Weglarz TC, Sandgren EP. Timing of hepatocyte entry into DNA synthesis after partial hepatectomy is cell autonomous. Proc Natl Acad Sci U S A 2000;97:12595–600.
6. Fausto N, Laird AD, Webber EM. Liver regeneration. 2. Role of growth factors and cytokines in hepatic regeneration. FASEB J 1995;9:1527–36.
7. Cressman DE, Diamond RH, Taub R. Rapid activation of the Stat3 transcription complex in liver regeneration. Hepatology 1995;21:1443–9.
8. Cressman DE, Greenbaum LE, Haber BA, et al. Rapid activation of posthepatectomy factor/nuclear factor κB in hepatocytes, a primary response in the regenerating liver. J Biol Chem 1994;269:30429–35.
9. Sadri A-R, Jeschke MG, Amini-Nik S. Cellular and molecular cascades during liver regeneration. Surg Res Open J 2015;2:53–61.
10. Idriss HT, Naismith JH. TNF alpha and the TNF receptor superfamily: structure-function relationship(s). Microsc Res Tech 2000;50:184–95.
11. Iwai M, Cui T-X, Kitamura H, et al. Increased secretion of tumor necrosis factor and interleukin 6 from isolated, perfused liver of rats after partial hepatectomy. Cytokine 2001;13:60–4.
12. Yamada Y, Fausto N. Deficient liver regeneration after carbon tetrachloride injury in mice lacking type 1 but not type 2 tumor necrosis factor receptor. Am J Pathol 1998;152:1577–89.
13. Karin M, Lin A. NF-κB at the crossroads of life and death. Nat Immunol 2002;3:221–7.
14. Beg AA, Sha WC, Bronson RT, et al. Embryonic lethality and liver degeneration in mice lacking the RelA component of NF-κB. Nature 1995;376:167–70.
15. Fausto N, Campbell JS, Riehle KJ. Liver regeneration. Hepatology 2006;43:S45–53.
16. Zeng S, Zhang QY, Huang J, et al. Opposing roles of RAGE and Myd88 signaling in extensive liver resection. FASEB J 2012;26:882–93.
17.. Wang Z, Yang X, Gui S, et al. The roles and mechanisms of lncRNAs in liver fibrosis. Front Pharmacol 2021;12:779606.
18. Schmidt C, Bladt F, Goedecke S, et al. Scatter factor/hepatocyte growth factor is essential for liver development. Nature 1995;373:699–702.
19. Streetz KL, Luedde T, Manns MP, et al. Interleukin 6 and liver regeneration. Gut 2000;47:309–12.
20. Mackiewicz A, Schooltink H, Heinrich PC, et al. Complex of soluble human IL-6-receptor/IL-6 up-regulates expression of acute-phase proteins. J Immunol 1992;149:2021–7.
21. Aldeguer X, Debonera F, Shaked A, et al. Interleukin-6 from intrahepatic cells of bone marrow origin is required for normal murine liver regeneration. Hepatology 2002;35:40–8.

22. Cressman DE, Greenbaum LE, DeAngelis RA, et al. Liver failure and defective hepatocyte regeneration in interleukin-6-deficient mice. Science 1996;274: 1379–83.
23. Blindenbacher A, Wang X, Langer I, et al. Interleukin 6 is important for survival after partial hepatectomy in mice. Hepatology 2003;38:674–82.
24. Sun R. Gao B. Negative regulation of liver regeneration by innate immunity (natural killer cells/interferon-gamma). Gastroenterology 2004;127:1525–39.
25. Hong F, Jaruga B, Kim WH, et al. Opposing roles of STAT1 and STAT3 in T cell-mediated hepatitis: regulation by SOCS. J Clin Invest 2002;110:1503–13.
26. Xiang X, Feng D, Hwang S, et al. Interleukin-22 ameliorates acute-on-chronic liver failure by reprogramming impaired regeneration pathways in mice. J Hepatol 2020;72:736–45.
27. Balmer ML, Slack E, de Gottardi A, et al. The liver may act as a firewall mediating mutualism between the host and its gut commensal microbiota. Sci Transl Med 2014;6:237ra66.
28. Bouwens L, Baekeland M, Zanger R De, et al. Quantitation, tissue distribution and proliferation kinetics of Kupffer cells in normal rat liver. Hepatology 1986; 6:718–22.
29. Antoniades CG, Quaglia A, Taams LS, et al. Source and characterization of hepatic macrophages in acetaminophen-induced acute liver failure in humans. Hepatology 2012;56:735–46.
30. Abshagen K, Eipel C, Kalff JC, et al. Loss of NF-κB activation in Kupffer cell-depleted mice impairs liver regeneration after partial hepatectomy. Am J Physiol Gastrointest Liver Physiol 2007;292:G1570–7.
31. You Q, Holt M, Yin H, et al. Role of hepatic resident and infiltrating macrophages in liver repair after acute injury. Biochem Pharmacol 2013;86:836–43.
32. Cornell RP, Liljequist BL, Bartizal KF. Depressed liver regeneration after partial hepatectomy of germ-free, athymic and lipopolysaccharide-resistant mice. Hepatology 1990;11:916–22.
33. Poltorak A, He X, Smirnova I, et al. Defective LPS signaling in C3H/HeJ and C57BL/10ScCr mice: mutations in Tlr4 gene. Science 1998;282:2085–8.
34. Seki E, Tsutsui H, Iimuro Y, et al. Contribution of Toll-like receptor/myeloid differentiation factor 88 signaling to murine liver regeneration. Hepatology 2005;41: 443–50.
35. Markiewski MM, DeAngelis RA, Strey CW, et al. The regulation of liver cell survival by complement. J Immunol 2009;182:5412–8.
36. Torre P, Motta BM, Sciorio R, et al. Inflammation and fibrogenesis in MAFLD: role of the hepatic immune system. Front Med 2021;8:781567.
37. Sauter KA, Waddell LA, Lisowski ZM, et al. Macrophage colony-stimulating factor (CSF1) controls monocyte production and maturation and the steady-state size of the liver in pigs. Am J Physiol Gastrointest Liver Physiol 2016;311: G533–47.
38. Antoniades CG, Quaglia A, Taams LS, et al. Source and characterization of hepatic macrophages in acetaminophen-induced acute liver failure in humans. Hepatology 2021;56:735–46.
39. Stutchfield BM, Antoine DJ, Mackinnon AC, et al. CSF1 restores innate immunity after liver injury in mice and serum levels indicate outcomes of patients with acute liver failure. Gastroenterology 2015;149:1896–909.
40. Possamai LA, Thursz MR, Wendon JA, et al. Modulation of monocyte/macrophage function: a therapeutic strategy in the treatment of acute liver failure. J Hepatol 2014;61:439–45.

41. Novac O, Silva R, Young LM, et al. Human liver microphysiological system for assessing drug-induced liver toxicity in vitro. J Vis Exp 2022;179. https://doi.org/10.3791/63389.

42. Michalopoulos GK. Liver regeneration. J Cell Physiol 2007;213:286–300.

43. Natarajan A, Wagner B, Sibilia M. The EGF receptor is required for efficient liver regeneration. Proc Natl Acad Sci USA 2007;104:17081–6.

44. Mitchell C, Nivison M, Jackson LF, et al. Heparin-binding epidermal growth factor-like growth factor links hepatocyte priming with cell cycle progression during liver regeneration. J Biol Chem 2005;280:2562–8.

45. Paranjpe S, Bowen WC, Tseng GC, et al. RNA interference against hepatic epidermal growth factor receptor has suppressive effects on liver regeneration in rats. Am J Pathol 2010;176:2669–81.

46. Bhushan B, Walesky C, Manley M, et al. Pro-regenerative signaling after acetaminophen-induced acute liver injury in mice identified using a novel incremental dose model. Am J Pathol 2014;184:3013–25.

47. Berasain C, Garcia-Trevijano ER, Castillo J, et al. Amphiregulin: an early trigger of liver regeneration in mice. Gastroenterology 2005;128:424–32.

48. Russell WE, Kaufmann WK, Sitaric S, et al. Liver regeneration and hepatocarcinogenesis in transforming growth factor-α-targeted mice. Mol Carcinog 1996;15:183–9.

49. Noguchi S, Ohba Y, Oka T. Influence of epidermal growth factor on liver regeneration after partial hepatectomy in mice. J Endocrinol 1991;128:425–31.

50. Huh C-G, Factor VM, Sánchez A, et al. Hepatocyte growth factor/c-met signaling pathway is required for efficient liver regeneration and repair. Proc Natl Acad Sci USA 2004;101:4477–82.

51. Kinoshita T, Hirao S, Matsumoto K, et al. Possible endocrine control by hepatocyte growth factor of liver regeneration after partial hepatectomy. Biochem Biophys Res Commun 1991;177:330–5.

52. Li ZW, Wang L. The role of liver sinusoidal endothelial cells in liver remodeling after injury. Hepatobiliary Pancreat Dis Int 2022. https://doi.org/10.1016/j.hbpd.2022.09.007.

53. Shubham S, Kumar D, Rooge S, et al. Cellular and functional loss of liver endothelial cells correlates with poor hepatocyte regeneration in acute-on-chronic liver failure. Hepatol Int 2019;13:777–87.

54. Naugler WE. Bile acid flux is necessary for normal liver regeneration. PLoS One 2014;9:e97426.

55. Dong X, Zhao H, Ma X, et al. Reduction in bile acid pool causes delayed liver regeneration accompanied by down-regulated expression of FXR and c-Jun mRNA in rats. J Huazhong Univ Sci Technol - Med Sci 2010;30:55–60.

56. Otao R, Beppu T, Isiko T, et al. External biliary drainage and liver regeneration after major hepatectomy. Br J Surg 2012;99:1569–74.

57. Sinal CJ, Tohkin M, Miyata M, et al. Targeted disruption of the nuclear receptor FXR/BAR impairs bile acid and lipid homeostasis. Cell 2000;102:731–44.

58. Huang W, Ma K, Zhang J, et al. Nuclear receptor-dependent bile acid signaling is required for normal liver regeneration. Science 2006;312:233–6.

59. Zhang L, Wang YD, Chen WD, et al. Promotion of liver regeneration/repair by farnesoid X receptor in both liver and intestine in mice. Hepatology 2012;56:2336–43.

60. Inagaki T, Choi M, Moschetta A, et al. Fibroblast growth factor 15 functions as an enterohepatic signal to regulate bile acid homeostasis. Cell Metab 2005;2:217–25.

61. Solhi R, Lotfinia M, Gramignoli R, et al. Metabolic hallmarks of liver regeneration. Trends Endocrinol Metab 2021;32:731–45.

62. Wang XD, Soltesz V, Andersson R, et al. Bacterial translocation in acute liver failure induced by 90 per cent hepatectomy in the rat. Br J Surg 1993;80:66–71.

63. Kakiyama G, Pandak WM, Gillevet PM, et al. Modulation of the fecal bile acid profile by gut microbiota in cirrhosis. J Hepatol 2013;58:949–55.

64. Xu Z, Jiang N, Xiao Y, et al. The role of gut microbiota in liver regeneration. Front Immunol 2022;13:1003376.

65. Murata S, Ohkohchi N, Matsuo R, et al. Platelets promote liver regeneration in early period after hepatectomy in mice. World J Surg 2007;31:808–16.

66. Beier JI, Guo L, Ritzenthaler JD, et al. Fibrin-mediated integrin signaling plays a critical role in hepatic regeneration after partial hepatectomy in mice. Ann Hepatol 2016;15:762–72.

67. Groeneveld D, Pereyra D, Veldhuis Z, et al. Intrahepatic fibrin(ogen) deposition drives liver regeneration after partial hepatectomy in mice and humans. Blood 2019;133:1245–56.

68. Cadigan KM, Waterman ML. TCF/LEFs and Wnt signaling in the nucleus. Cold Spring Harb Perspect Biol 2012;4:a007906.

69. Monga SP, Mars WM, Pediaditakis P, et al. Hepatocyte growth factor induces Wnt-independent nuclear translocation of β-catenin after Met-β-catenin dissociation in hepatocytes. Cancer Res 2002;62:2064–71.

70. Apte U, Singh S, Zeng G, et al. β-catenin activation promotes liver regeneration after acetaminophen-induced injury. Am J Pathol 2009;175:1056–65.

71. Gougelet A, Torre C, Veber P, et al. T-cell factor 4 and β-catenin chromatin occupancies pattern zonal liver metabolism in mice. Hepatology 2014;59: 2344–57.

72. Leibing T, Geraud C, Augustin I, et al. Angiocrine Wnt signaling controls liver growth and metabolic maturation in mice. Hepatology 2018;68:707–22.

73. Monga SP, Pediaditakis P, Mule K, et al. Changes in WNT/β-catenin pathway during regulated growth in rat liver regeneration. Hepatology 2001;33: 1098–109.

74. Nelson WJ, Nusse R. Convergence of Wnt, β-catenin, and cadherin pathways. Science 2004;303:1483–7.

75. Nakamura T, Tomita Y, Hirai R, et al. Inhibitory effect of transforming growth factor-β on DNA synthesis of adult rat hepatocytes in primary culture. Biochem Biophys Res Commun 1985;133:1042–50.

76. Chari RS, Price DT, Sue SR, et al. Down-regulation of transforming growth factor beta receptor type I, II, and III during liver regeneration. Am J Surg 1995;169: 126–31.

77. Ko TC, Yu W, Sakai T, et al. A. TGF-β1 effects on proliferation of rat intestinal epithelial cells are due to inhibition of cyclin D1 expression. Oncogene 1998; 16:3445–54.

78. Thenappan A, Shukla V, Abdul Khalek FJ, et al. Loss of transforming growth factor β adaptor protein β-2 spectrin leads to delayed liver regeneration in mice. Hepatology 2011;53:1641–50.

79. Patel SH, Camargo FD, Yimlamai D. Hippo signaling in the liver regulates organ size, cell fate, and carcinogenesis. Gastroenterology 2017;152:533–45.

80. Camargo FD, Gokhale S, Johnnidis JB, et al. YAP1 increases organ size and expands undifferentiated progenitor cells. Curr Biol 2007;17:2054–60.

81. Zhao B, Wei X, Li W, et al. Inactivation of YAP oncoprotein by the Hippo pathway is involved in cell contact inhibition and tissue growth control. Genes Dev 2007; 21:2747–61.
82. Yimlamai D, Christodoulou C, Galli GG, et al. Hippo pathway activity influences liver cell fate. Cell 2014;157:1324–38.
83. Michalopoulos GK. Hepatostat: liver regeneration and normal liver tissue maintenance. Hepatology 2017;65:1384–92.
84. Grisham JW. A morphologic study of deoxyribonucleic acid synthesis and cell proliferation in regenerating rat liver; autoradiography with thymidine-H3. Cancer Res 1962;22:842–9.
85. Miyaoka Y, Ebato K, Kato H, et al. Hypertrophy and unconventional cell division of hepatocytes underlie liver regeneration. Curr Biol 2021;22:1166–75.
86. Abu Rmilah A, Zhou W, Nelson E, et al. Understanding the marvels behind liver regeneration. Wiley Interdiscip Rev Dev Biol 2019;8:e340.
87. Ha M, Kim VN. Regulation of microRNA biogenesis. Nat Rev Mol Cell Biol 2014; 15:509–24.
88. Chen Y, Verfaillie CM. MicroRNAs: the fine modulators of liver development and function. Liver Int 2014;34:976–90.
89. Hand NJ, Master ZR, Le Lay, et al. Hepatic function is preserved in the absence of mature microRNAs. Hepatology 2009;49:618–26.
90. Abdel Halim AS, Rudayni HA, Chaudhary AA, et al. MicroRNAs: small molecules with big impacts in liver injury. J Cell Physiol 2023;238:32–69.
91. Salehi S, Tavabie OD, Verma S, et al. Serum microRNA signatures in recovery from acute and chronic liver injury and selection for liver transplantation. Liver Transpl 2020;26:811–22.
92. John K, Hadem J, Krech T, et al. MicroRNAs play a role in spontaneous recovery from acute liver failure. Hepatology 2014;60:1346–55.
93. Bandiera S, Pfeffer S, Baumert TF, et al. miR-122–a key factor and therapeutic target in liver disease. J Hepatol 2015;62:448–57.
94. Lagos-Quintana M, Rauhut R, Yalcin A, et al. Identification of tissue-specific microRNAs from mouse. Curr Biol 2020;12:735–9.
95. Kang LI, Mars WM, Michalopoulos GK. Signals and cells involved in regulating liver regeneration. Cells 2012;12:1261–92.
96. Deng X-G, Qiu R-L, Wu Y-H, et al. Overexpression of miR-122 promotes the hepatic differentiation and maturation of mouse ESCs through a miR-122/FoxA1/ HNF4a-positive feedback loop. Liver Int 2014;34:281–95.
97. Marquez RT, Wendlandt E, Galle CS, et al. MicroRNA-21 is upregulated during the proliferative phase of liver regeneration, targets Pellino-1, and inhibits NF-κB signaling. Am J Physiol Gastrointest Liver Physiol 2010;298:G535–41.
98. Zhang T, Yang Z, Kusumanchi P, et al. Critical role of microRNA-21 in the pathogenesis of liver diseases. Front Med 2020;7:7.
99. Yuan Q, Loya K, Rani B, et al. MicroRNA-221 overexpression accelerates hepatocyte proliferation during liver regeneration. Hepatology 2013;57:299–310.
100. Sharma AD, Narain N, Handel EM, et al. MicroRNA-221 regulates FAS-induced fulminant liver failure. Hepatology 2011;53:1651–61.
101. Michalopoulos GK, Khan Z. Liver stem cells: experimental findings and implications for human liver disease. Gastroenterology 2015;149:876–82.
102. Yanger K, Zong Y, Maggs LR, et al. Robust cellular reprogramming occurs spontaneously during liver regeneration. Genes Dev 2013;27:719–24.
103. Huang R, Zhang X, Gracia-Sancho J, et al. Liver regeneration: cellular origin and molecular mechanisms. Liver Int 2022;42:1486–95.

104. Van Haele M, Snoeck J, Roskams T. Human liver regeneration: an etiology dependent process. Int J Mol Sci 2019;20:2332.

105. Lin T, Feng R, Liebe R, et al. Liver progenitor cells in massive hepatic necrosis-How can a patient survive acute liver failure? Biomolecules 2022;12:66.

106. Dollé L, Best J, Mei J, et al. The quest for liver progenitor cells: a practical point of view. J Hepatol 2010;52:117–29.

107. Evarts RP, Nagy P, Nakatsukasa H, et al. *In vivo* differentiation of rat liver oval cells into hepatocytes. Cancer Res 1989;49:1541–7.

108. Akhurst B, Croager EJ, Farley-Roche CA, et al. A modified choline-deficient, ethionine-supplemented diet protocol effectively induces oval cells in mouse liver. Hepatology 2001;34:519–22.

109. Lee C-W, Chen Y-F, Wu H-H, et al. Historical perspectives and advances in mesenchymal stem cell research for the treatment of liver diseases. Gastroenterology 2018;154:46–56.

110. Kuo TK, Hung SP, Chuang CH, et al. Stem cell therapy for liver disease: parameters governing the success of using bone marrow mesenchymal stem cells. Gastroenterology 2008;134:2111–21.

111. Tan CY, Lai RC, Wong W, et al. Mesenchymal stem cell-derived exosomes promote hepatic regeneration in drug-induced liver injury models. Stem Cell Res Ther 2014;5:76.

112. Li Y, Lu L, Cai X. Liver regeneration and cell transplantation for end-stage liver disease. Biomolecules 2021 20;11:1907.

113. Hu C, Wu Z, Li L. Mesenchymal stromal cells promote liver regeneration through regulation of immune cells. Int J Biol Sci 2020;16:893–903.

114. Papatheodoridi M, Mazza G, Pinzani M. Regenerative hepatology: in the quest for a modern prometheus? Dig Liver Dis 2020;52:1106–14.

115. Bajaj JS, O'Leary JG, Lai JC, et al. Acute-on-chronic liver failure clinical guidelines. Am J Gastroenterol 2022;117:225–52.

116. Wasmuth HE, Kunz D, Yagmur E, et al. Patients with acute on chronic liver failure display "sepsis-like" immune paralysis. J Hepatol 2005;42:195–201.

117. Bernsmeier C, Pop OT, Singanayagam A, et al. Patients with acute-on-chronic liver failure have increased numbers of regulatory immune cells expressing the receptor tyrosine kinase MERTK. Gastroenterology 2015;148:603–15.

118. Zhang IW, López-Vicario C, Duran-Güell M, et al. Mitochondrial dysfunction in advanced liver disease: emerging concepts. Front Mol Biosci 2021;8:772174.

119. Vogg J, Maier-Stocker C, Munker S, et al. Hepatic perfusion as a new predictor of prognosis and mortality in critical care patients with acute-on-chronic liver failure. Front Med 2022;9:1008450.

120. Jiao Y, Lu W, Xu P, et al. Hepatocyte-derived exosome may be as a biomarker of liver regeneration and prognostic valuation in patients with acute-on-chronic liver failure. Hepatol Int 2021;15:957–69.

121. Hassan HM, Li J. Prospect of animal models for acute-on-chronic liver failure: a mini-review. J Clin Transl Hepatol 2022;10:995–1003.

122. Huang W, Han N, Du L, et al. A narrative review of liver regeneration-from models to molecular basis. Ann Transl Med 2021;9:1705.

123. Nautiyal N, Maheshwari D, Tripathi DM, et al. Establishment of a murine model of acute-on-chronic liver failure with multi-organ dysfunction. Hepatol Int 2021;15:1389–401.

124. Jalan R. Novel approaches and therapeutics in acute-on-chronic liver failure. Liver Transpl 2016;22:14–9.

125. Khanam A, Kottilil S. Acute-on-chronic liver failure: Pathophysiological mechanisms and management. Front Med 2021;8:752875.

126. Ali H, Jahan A, Samrana S, et al. Hepatoprotective potential of pomegranate in curbing the incidence of acute liver injury by alleviating oxidative stress and inflammatory response. Front Pharmacol 2021;12:694607.

Viral Hepatitis and Acute-on-Chronic Liver Failure

Talal Khushid Bhatti, MD[a], Ashwani K. Singal, MD, MS[b], Paul Y. Kwo, MD[c],*

KEYWORDS

- Acute-on-chronic liver failure • Hepatitis A • Hepatitis B • Hepatitis C • Hepatitis D
- Hepatitis E • SARS-CoV-2 • EBV

KEY POINTS

- Hepatitis A and hepatitis E are major causes of acute-on-chronic liver failure (ACLF), particularly in India with most series having reported sporadic outbreak of hepatitis E being associated with higher rates of ACLF than hepatitis A.
- Hepatitis B may also cause ACLF through flare of hepatitis B, acute infection, or reactivation.
- Hepatitis delta and hepatitis C are rare causes of ACLF.
- Nonhepatotropic viruses may rarely also cause ACLF with the severe acute respiratory syndrome coronavirus 2 (SARS-CoV-2) virus recently being identified with poor outcomes in those with underlying chronic liver disease.
- Prevention of ACLF due to viral causes relies primarily on effective vaccination for hepatitis A, B, and E as well as vaccination for the SARS-CoV-2 virus.

BACKGROUND

Acute-on-chronic liver failure (ACLF) is a potentially reversible syndrome that develops in patients with cirrhosis or with underlying chronic liver disease (CLD) and is characterized by acute decompensation, organ failure, and high short-term mortality.[1] The precipitating causes of ACLF vary depending on the region of the world, with bacterial infections, gastrointestinal hemorrhage, and alcohol-associated liver disease comprising the majority of cases in North America and Europe, whereas exacerbation of hepatitis B and bacterial infections are the most common precipitating causes in Asia. Although the European and American definitions of ACLF factor in extrahepatic organ failure when defining ACLF and its severity, this is not a requirement of the Asian Pacific Association for the Study of the Liver (APASL) criteria.[2–4]

[a] Shaheed Zulfiqar Ali Bhutto Medical University, Islamabad, Pakistan; [b] University of SD Sanford School of Medicine, Sioux Falls, SD, USA; [c] Stanford University School of Medicine, Palo Alto, CA, USA
* Corresponding author.
E-mail address: pkwo@stanford.edu

Clin Liver Dis 27 (2023) 617–630
https://doi.org/10.1016/j.cld.2023.03.006
1089-3261/23/© 2023 Elsevier Inc. All rights reserved.

liver.theclinics.com

Organ failure develops due to a combination of tissue hypoperfusion, direct immune-mediated damage, and mitochondrial dysfunction with systemic inflammation being a hallmark of ACLF.[5] The 3 major classifications of ACLF from North America, Europe, and Asia have common features including an acute process characterized by multiple organ failures that requires treatment of the underlying liver disease, supportive care, most commonly in an intensive care unit (ICU), and the potential requirement for liver transplantation. This review will focus on viral causes contributing to ACLF including the major causes of hepatitis B and E, in addition to other hepatotropic and nonhepatotropic viruses.

Viral Hepatitis with Acute-on-Chronic Liver Failure

Hepatitis A

The hepatitis A virus (HAV) is a highly contagious picornavirus that may cause infection in individuals with cirrhosis or CLD with a potential for the development of ACLF. The global distribution and endemicity of HAV is directly proportional to socioeconomic and hygienic conditions. Globally, about 1.4 million cases of acute HAV infection occur annually with a reduction in cases noted where the HAV vaccine has been deployed.[6] Recently, mortality has increased in age groups 2 to 12 years of age and also in those aged above 35 years.[7] HAV infection is spread primarily via the fecal–oral route when an uninfected person ingests food or water contaminated with the feces of an infected person. Less common routes of transmission include oral–anal sexual contact or injection drug use with someone who is infected with HAV. Morbidity and mortality is related to age group, with subclinical infection in children aged 6 years and symptomatic presentation found more commonly in adults and the elderly.

Hepatitis A seroprevalence (Immunoglobulin G [IgG] anti-HAV) studies have demonstrated 3 zones worldwide: (1) very-high endemic zone, (2) high-to-intermediate endemic zone, and (3) low-endemic zone.

The very-high endemic zone includes countries of Southeast Asia and Sub-Saharan Africa with seroprevalence data revealing that more than 90% of children seroconvert before 10 years of age and are positive for IgG anti-HAV. The high-to-intermediate endemic zone for HAV includes developing countries of Asia, Latin America, Eastern Europe, and the Middle East. These countries have improved their sanitary conditions and HAV exposure in older children and adolescents may be symptomatic. The low-endemic zone of HAV spreads over the developed world, including Western Europe, Australia, New Zealand, Canada, the United States, Japan, Korea, and Singapore. In these countries, there is significantly less exposure to HAV infection during childhood.

HAV-related ACLF reports have originated from Asia rather than European countries and North America. One large study reported predictors of outcomes in those with Hepatitis A and E in the setting of cirrhosis from India. In this single-center study, 33 out of 121 (27%, 21 adults, 12 children) had HAV infection with dual infection in 8% compared with 80 out of 121 (61%) with Hepatitis E virus (HEV) infection. Three-month mortality rates were similar with the HAV ACLF cohort noting a 51.5% mortality rate compared with 43.8% in the HEV ACLF cohort.[8] Traditional predictors of mortality were noted including hyponatremia, as well as development of grade 3 or 4 encephalopathy. Another prospective study from India looked at 52 patients with ACLF and noted viral hepatitis representing the most common cause of ACLF in a population with underlying CLD with 8 out of 52 (15%) having acute HAV infection. Two of these individuals had dual HAV/HEV infection with outcomes worse than those with a single infection.[9] In another retrospective analysis of a hospital database, HAV infection was found to be the cause of ACLF in 7/89 (8%) cases in New Delhi.[10] Thus, in Asia, there are fewer reported cases of ACLF related to HAV infection compared with ACLF cases caused by HEV infection. There have been recent reports of HAV-related outbreaks causing ACLF in North America. A recent report from the United States, identified 20 out of 264 (8%) of individuals with acute HAV infection with underlying cirrhosis.[11] In this cohort, 6 out of 20 developed ACLF with 5 out of 6 developing advanced ACLF (grade 3), with one death and higher rates of ascites and hepatic encephalopathy compared with those with HAV infection without underlying cirrhosis. In this cohort intravenous drug use was the predominant mode of transmission.

The pathogenesis of development of ACLF in patents with HAV infection is not clear.

HAV is a noncytopathic virus that replicates in hepatocytes and generates a cytotoxic immune response in T-cells that likely increases systemic inflammation and inflammatory cytokines.[12] The common clinical presentation of ACLF in HAV infection includes jaundice, encephalopathy, and renal failure with poorer outcomes found in those with dual infections. The diagnosis of HAV infection relies on the presence of anti-IgM HAV detected at the time of clinical presentation (**Table 1**). A wide range of mortality rates have been reported with HAV-related ACLF of up to 50% with traditional factors predicting worse outcomes.[10,13] There are no specific therapies for ACLF due to HAV and the treatment remains supportive. Extrahepatic organ failures, such as circulatory failure, sepsis, or renal failure, are managed in an ICU. Patients with ACLF due to HAV infection may be considered for liver transplantation although there is no data specific to HAV-related ACLF transplant outcomes. The most effective strategy to reduce ACLF from HAV infection is prevention with improved hygiene including better management of the water supply and the preparation and cooking of food. In lower prevalence countries, without childhood exposure, more adults are vulnerable to HAV infection and they should be vaccinated. Patients with CLD should be identified and vaccinated as well, especially with the growing vulnerable populations of those with nonalcoholic fatty liver disease, alcohol-associated liver disease, in addition to those with chronic hepatitis B and C (**Table 2**).[14]

The United States (US) Advisory Committee on Immunization Practice recommends a 2-dose vaccination series of HAV or a 3-dose series of HAV/hepatitis B virus (HBV) vaccinations for all patients with CLD, including those with HBV, hepatitis C virus (HCV), cirrhosis, nonalcoholic fatty liver disease (NAFLD), alcoholic liver disease, autoimmune hepatitis, or an alanine aminotransferase greater than 2 IU/L (the upper limit of normal) (https://www.immunize.org/acip/). The WHO has recommended that HAV vaccination should be given as early as possible after CLD diagnosis for maximum efficacy.[15]

Hepatitis B Virus Infection

Chronic infection with HBV is present in approximately 272 million individuals worldwide and is a major cause of liver disease, liver cancer, and liver-related mortality.[16] The prevalence of chronic hepatitis B (CHB) varies by region and is often difficult to define due to limited surveillance. In highly endemic regions of Europe and the Americas, which have immigrants from endemic regions, a predominant cause of transmission remains perinatal infection. In low-prevalence regions, sexual transmission has historically been a major source of HBV acquisition. More recently, the implementation of widespread vaccination campaigns in some regions has dramatically reduced HBV prevalence and rates of acute HBV in children and young adults. However, due to high-risk behaviors and limited access to health services, marginalized populations such as injection drug users and incarcerated individuals continue to suffer from disproportionate rates of infection relative to the general population, with new outbreaks of HBV in those with substance use disorders in the United States culminating in a health-care crisis.[17]

Table 1
Diagnostic testing for acute-on-chronic liver failure caused by viral hepatitis

Virus	Diagnostic Testing	Comments
Hepatitis A	Anti-HAV IgM	Supportive treatment
Acute hepatitis B	IgM anti-HBc, HBsAg	COSSH criteria for ACLF caused by
Acute hepatitis B	HBV DNA	Hepatitis B includes TB ≥ 12 mg/dL,
flare	IgM anti-HBC, HBsAg	INR >1.5
HBV-reactivation	HBV PCR DNA, HBsAg	
Hepatitis C	Anti-HCV, HCV PCR RNA	Very rare with HCV infection
Hepatitis D	Anti-HDV IgM, HDV RNA	ACLF occurs with superinfection
Hepatitis E	Anti-HEV IgM	If negative and high suspicion check HEV RNA
Epstein Barr Virus	Confirm with EBV PCR	Rare cause of ACLF
Cytomegalovirus	Confirm with CMV PCR	Rare cause of ACLF
Herpes simplex virus	HSV Culture confirm with serum HSV PCR	More sensitive than culture
SARS-CoV-2	SARS-CoV-2 antigen test with confirmation with RT-PCR NAAT	Higher rates of mortality with ACLF in the setting of cirrhosis

Abbreviations: RT-PCR NAAT, reverse transcriptase -polymerase chain reaction nucleic acid amplification test.

Hepatitis B leading to acute-on-chronic liver failure

The natural history of hepatitis B is closely associated with ACLF. In many parts of the world, CHB (failure to clear hepatitis B surface antigen) is associated with CLD with cirrhosis due to unavailable antiviral therapy for the treatment of CHB.[18] Although acute hepatitis B can rarely cause acute liver failure, ACLF due to hepatitis B reactivation may occur in up to 38% of all individuals with hepatitis B.[19] Spontaneous flares of hepatitis B may occur in those who are hepatitis Be antigen positive or negative during the immune clearance phase of hepatitis B. The potential factors associated with a higher risk of ACLF and CHB are complex and include factors related to the virus itself as well as extrahepatic factors. Several studies have suggested that HBV genotype B with basal core promoter or core promoter mutations is associated with a higher risk of development of ACLF.[20] In addition, amino acid mutations in the large hepatitis B surface antigen and hepatitis B core antigen have been associated with ACLF by potentially inducing immune dysfunction.[21] A recent genome wide association study from China identified HLA-DR regions as having the strongest genetic risk for the development of ACLF and CHB carriers with s3129859*C and HLA-DRB1*12:02 alleles being the most prominent susceptible variants, and the rs3129859*C allele being associated with a higher 28-day mortality in the setting of ACLF.[22] Extrahepatic factors that contribute to ACLF in the setting of hepatitis B reactivation are related to high degrees of systemic inflammation that is a hallmark of ACLF. This inflammatory response is associated with high levels of inflammatory cytokines in contrast to the attenuated immune response observed in CHB.

In addition, the reactivation of hepatitis B due to the administration of immunosuppressive therapies may also be associated with ACLF. The proliferation of targeted immune therapies and cytotoxic therapies for oncologic and immune-mediated disorders can lead to hepatitis B reactivation in those with CHB (HBsAg positive) or in those with resolved hepatitis B (HBsAg negative, anti-HBc positive) who are receiving potent immunosuppressive agents such as anti-CD 20 antibody therapy.[23]

Table 2
Potential therapies for acute-on-chronic liver failure caused by viral hepatitis

Virus	ACLF Therapies	Specific Antiviral Therapy	Comments
Hepatitis A	Supportive care	None	None, vaccinate at risk populations, vaccination is recommended for CLD patients
Hepatitis B	Supportive care	Entecavir, tenofovir disoproxil, tenofovir alafenamide	Vaccination is recommended for all individuals aged <60 years
Hepatitis C	Supportive care	DAA therapy to treat Acute hepatitis C	
Hepatitis D	Supportive care	Ensure treatment of hepatitis B with entecavir, tenofovir disoproxil, tenofovir alafenamide	No currently approved therapies for hepatitis D, interferon contraindicated
Hepatitis E	Supportive care	Limited reports suggest ribavirin could be considered	Vaccination of at risk groups including those with chronic liver disease. Preliminary data suggest HEV vaccine safe in pregnant women
Epstein Barr Virus	Supportive care	None	Consider reduction of immunosuppressive agents if applicable
Cytomegalovirus	Supportive care	Ganciclovir, valganciclovir may be considered limited data	Consider reduction of immunosuppressive agents if applicable
Herpes Simplex Virus	Supportive care	Acyclovir should be initiated early suspected patients	HSV infection has poor prognosis in ACLF, especially pregnant women
SARS-CoV-2	Supportive care	Remdesivir, lopinavir/ritonavir, molnupiravir, monoclonal antibodies	COVID-19 infection in CLD can lead to ACLF, has poor prognosis and high mortality in cirrhosis. Vaccination in all patients with CLD is recommended

These individuals may have recrudescence from undetectable HBV to detectable HBV DNA or seroreversion with the production of surface antigen in those who previously had resolved hepatitis B. Although current practice guidance recommends that patients who were positive for hepatitis B surface antigen or who have resolved hepatitis B be treated prophylactically with nucleoside/nucleotide analogs such as entecavir or tenofovir or monitored during therapy, screening in these at-risk populations is not universal and clinicians continue to see presentations of ACLF in those with chronic or resolved hepatitis B.[23,24]

The diagnosis of ACLF due to hepatitis B is made by confirming the presence of hepatitis B surface antigen with elevated hepatitis B DNA levels in the setting of acute liver decompensation with jaundice, elevated prothrombin time and encephalopathy in the setting of known CHB or resolved hepatitis B (see **Table 1**). The search for precipitating factors include a history of exposure to immunosuppressive or chemotherapy agents and if no such exposure is found, then a hepatitis B flare may explain the presentation of ACLF. Finally, one needs to consider viral superinfection such as hepatitis A, C, D, or E that may also lead to a presentation of ACLF in a CHB-infected individual.

Although therapy for ACLF is generally supportive, there are therapies available to suppress hepatitis B viral levels. In the United States, first-line therapies to suppress hepatitis B include tenofovir disoproxil, tenofovir alafenamide, and entecavir, all of which are known to have a high barrier to hepatitis B resistance and are first-line therapies for those with CHB.[24] Therapies for hepatitis B do seem to improve outcomes in the setting of ACLF. One meta-analysis examined 3 prospective and 8 retrospective cohort studies involving 1491 patients with acute exacerbation of hepatitis B with or without ACLF.[25] These trials evaluated short-term and long-term mortality rates in those who received entecavir or lamivudine. Neither entecavir nor lamivudine improved short-term mortality in hepatitis B-related acute exacerbations with or without ACLF. However, entecavir was superior to lamivudine in long-term outcomes in those with hepatitis B-related ACLF. Caution should be used in those receiving entecavir with decompensated cirrhosis and high Model for End Stage Liver Disease (MELD) scores as there have been reports of lactic acidosis in this population although entecavir was well-tolerated in this analysis.[26] Tenofovir disoproxil and entecavir were compared in 67 patients with hepatitis B-related ACLF due to reactivation of hepatitis B genotypes B and C.[27] Patients were followed up to 3 months with the tenofovir group having significantly higher HBV DNA reduction, higher rate of HBV DNA undetectability, a lower Child Turcotte Pugh (CTP) score, and a lower MELD score at 2 weeks. The tenofovir group also had significantly higher cumulative survival rate than entecavir (21/32, 63.6% vs 22/36, 34.3%, $P < .025$) at 3 months. Significant predictors of mortality in this study included white blood cell (WBC) count and HBV DNA at 2 weeks suggesting that rapid viral suppression may be of benefit in those presenting with HBV-related ACLF. Reassuringly, no episodes of lactic acidosis were reported in either group.

Diagnostic criteria and prognostic models have been used to predict outcomes in those with hepatitis B-related ACLF, which include the Chronic Liver Failure Consortium ACLF development score (CLIF-C), Model for End-stage Liver Disease score (MELD), Model for End-stage Liver Disease sodium (MELD-Na) score, and the CTP score. Specific criteria and prediction models for hepatitis B-related ACLF have come from the Chinese group on the Study of Severe Hepatitis B (COSSH). In their original report of 271 patients with cirrhosis and hepatitis B who developed ACLF, they proposed that serum bilirubin 12 mg/dL or greater, and international normalized ratio (INR) 1.5 or greater are diagnostic indicators for ACLF in this population.[28] A prognostic score that included INR, age, bilirubin, and a newly created hepatitis B sequential organ failure assessment score (HBV SOFA) predicted 28-day mortality more accurately than the CLIF-C ACLF score, MELD score, MELD-sodium score, or the CTP score. Subsequent prognostic models have been reported including a report of 954 hospitalized patients with acute deterioration from hepatitis B-related CLD.[29] These individuals were diagnosed with HBV-ACLF by the COSSH-ACLF criteria and 6 factors accurately predicted 28-day mortality including INR, hepatic encephalopathy score, bilirubin level, urea level, neutrophil count, and age. A recently published revised prognostic score from the same group based on alanine transferase (ALT) level, total bilirubin, INR, and ferritin levels noted high-risk and low-risk groups for ACLF onset with an improved performance over 5 other predictive models (Chronic Liver Failure Consortium ACLF development score/Model for End-stage Liver Disease score/Model for End-stage Liver Disease sodium score/COSSH-ACLF score/Chronic liver failure Consortium ACLF score).[30]

The prevention of hepatitis B-related ACLF relies on multiple strategies. Vaccination and screening of those at high risk for hepatitis B ACLF will prevent ACLF-related episodes in those with CLD in addition to preventing acute infection. In the United States, hepatitis B vaccination guidance recommendations were recently broadened to include universal vaccination for those aged 19 to 59 years and in those aged 60 years or older with risk factors for HBV infection.

(www.cdc.gov/vaccines/acip/recommendations.html). Moreover, adults aged 60 years or older without risk factors may also receive the HBV vaccine. The second strategy is to educate all practitioners who prescribe immunosuppressive or immune-modulating therapies including oncologists, hematologists, rheumatologists and immune-mediated disease specialists, and gastroenterologists to screen for hepatitis B before the initiation of these therapies with HBsAg, anti-HBc total, and anti-HBs. This will allow for the successful vaccination of appropriate patients as well as the initiation of monitoring for the reactivation in those who are HBsAg positive or anti-HBc positive with the initiation of nucleoside/nucleotide therapy as required depending on the immunosuppressive, immune-modulating agent and hepatitis B status.[23,24] Finally, diagnosis and linkage to care with appropriate therapy for CHB according to societal guidance will reduce the incidence of ACLF due to hepatitis B flares.

Hepatitis D leading to acute-on-chronic liver failure

Hepatitis D virus (hepatitis Delta-HDV) was first identified in 1977 and is an RNA virus that is dependent on the HBV surface antigen for replication. The risk factors for hepatitis D infection are the same as hepatitis B and HDV can occur as an acute infection in combination with hepatitis B or as a superinfection in those who have CHB. The precise worldwide epidemiology of hepatitis D has been difficult to determine. The World Health Organization has estimated approximately 5% of individuals with HBV infection have HDV coinfection, with other estimates being higher.[31] High prevalence areas include Africa, Asia, the Middle East, Eastern Europe, and South America. Chronic hepatitis B/D infection occurs rarely in the setting of HDV/HBV coinfection, whereas superinfection is associated with high rates of chronic hepatitis D.[32] The natural history of chronic Hepatitis D infection can be quite severe with high rates of progression to cirrhosis and hepatocellular carcinoma being observed in up to 70% of individuals after 10 years.[32] ACLF from hepatitis D superinfection may present with acute hepatic decompensation although there are limited data on this subject. The diagnosis of acute hepatitis D is made by the detection of anti-HDV IgM in the setting of hepatitis B infection and chronic hepatitis D is confirmed by the presence of HDV RNA with anti-HDV IgG being present. Specific management of ACLF due to hepatitis D is similar to the approach with those with hepatitis B and ACLF. There are no specific therapies for HDV-related ACLF to reduce the hepatitis D viral level (see **Table 2**). Pegylated interferon may be used to treat hepatitis D but it is not recommended in the setting of ACLF.[24] Bulevirtide, an entry inhibitor that blocks the sodium taurocholate cotransporting polypeptide, prevents entry of HBV and HDV into hepatocytes and has been conditionally approved in Europe for the treatment of chronic hepatitis D but has not been evaluated in ACLF.[33] Effective preventative care in those with CLD can eliminate the risk of hepatitis D infection by education combined with successful vaccination against the HBV.

Hepatitis E leading to acute-on-chronic liver failure

HEV is an RNA virus that was first discovered in 1983 and is responsible for large-scale epidemics of acute viral hepatitis in low-income and middle-income countries in Central America, Asia, and Africa. The hepatitis E virus is not cytopathic, and the damage to hepatocytes is immune-mediated. There are multiple genotypes with HEV geno-types 1 and 2 most commonly associated with acute liver failure and ACLF.[34] Similarly to hepatitis A, hepatitis E causes an acute self-limited hepatitis although acute liver failure may occur in pregnant women. Hepatitis E-related ACLF is a common cause of ACLF cases in endemic areas of the world with a recent comprehensive review noting a median mortality rate of 34%.[35] Both hepatitis A and hepatitis E cause ACLF although reported series note higher rates of hepatitis E-related ACLF compared with hepatitis A. Hepatitis E transmission occurs predominantly through the fecal–oral route and in endemic areas transmission typically is through contami-nated water. In nonendemic areas of the world, transmission may occur via animal vectors most commonly via exposure to infected swine and ACLF is rare in this setting.

The majority of cases of ACLF with hepatitis E have been reported from Asia, pri-marily China and India, and these reports utilize the APASL definition of ACLF.[2] In contrast, ACLF related to hepatitis E is extremely uncommon in the western regions of the world including Europe and North America. As previously stated, hepatitis E-related ACLF is more common than hepatitis A-ACLF with an estimated 3-month mortality rate of 45% in one report from India where hepatitis E infection occurred in a broad population of individuals with CLDs including hepatitis B, alcohol-associated liver disease, hepatitis C, and nonalcoholic fatty liver disease.[8] In China, hepatitis E-related ACLF occurs predominantly in those with CHB with lower rates of hepatitis A-related ACLF in this population. Hepatitis E-related ACLF leads to higher rates of mortality and organ failure compared with those with hepatitis A-related ACLF. In one case series of 188 individuals with CHB, higher rates of ACLF caused by hep-atitis E compared with hepatitis A (136 out of 188 vs 52 out of 188) were observed dur-ing an 8-year period.[36] Hepatitis E infection was associated with greater evidence of biochemical dysfunction with higher rates of AST and ALT elevation in the hepatitis E group compared with the hepatitis A group as well as higher bilirubin levels. Hepatic complications in this cohort included higher rates of variceal bleeding, hepatic en-cephalopathy, and ascites in those with hepatitis E-related ACLF compared with hep-atitis A-related ACLF. Finally, the mortality rate was 24% (46 out of 188) in hepatitis E-infected individuals compared with only one fatality in the hepatitis A group, with the dominant cause of mortality being hepatic failure.

Similar results have been reported from India, where the outcomes of ACLF in those with acute hepatitis A and E infection in 121 patients with preexisting cirrhosis were compared. The authors also noted higher rates of ACLF due to hepatitis E as compared with hepatitis A (61.1% vs 27.2%).[8] The presentation of ACLF caused by hepatitis E in their cohort was typical for ACLF with evidence of hepatic decompensa-tion including jaundice, ascites, and hepatic encephalopathy. A 3-month mortality rate of 44.6% was observed with high rates of hepatic and extrahepatic complications including ascites, coagulopathy, renal failure, and hepatic encephalopathy. In multi-variate analysis, grades 3 and 4 hepatic encephalopathy, hyponatremia, and renal fail-ure significantly predicted 3-month mortality in this ACLF population with cirrhosis as did MELD score.

The diagnosis of hepatitis E-related ACLF is made by antibody testing, with anti-HEV IgM to document acute infection (see **Table 1**).[37] If testing is negative and the clinical suspicion remains high, especially in endemic areas, HEV RNA PCR testing may be performed to confirm the diagnosis. Test performance may be related to differing genotypes although in Asia genotypes 1 and 2 HEV are predominant. Man-agement of HEV-related ACLF is similar to that of hepatitis A with supportive care in the ICU to address hepatic and extrahepatic complications. Ribavirin has been used to treat chronic HEV infection in immunosuppressed individuals.[38] A recent pilot study reported ribavirin use in hepatitis E patients with ACLF at a dose of 200 to 600 mg/d with 100% survival.[39] Although data are limited, selected individuals with hepatitis E-related ACLF are likely candidates for liver transplantation, this option is likely limited by the regions where HEV-related ACLF occur. Prevention of hepatitis E-related ACLF relates to improving sanitation to reduce fecal–oral transmission (see **Table 2**). A single vaccine, HEV 239 vaccine, Hecolin, is available based on a genotype 1 hepatitis E strain and has been licensed in China and other parts of the world. Vaccination for those with CLD in endemic regions of the world would likely reduce the incidence and risk of ACLF development due to acute hepatitis E infection.[40] Therefore, once again, education regarding sanitation plus vaccination could be effective preventative measures against HEV infection and the complications of ACLF and hepatic and extrahepatic decompensation.

Hepatitis C leading to acute-on-chronic liver failure
Hepatitis C, first reported in 1986, is a blood-borne RNA virus that causes both acute and chronic hepatitis.[41] Cases of ACLF related to acute hepatitis C infection are uncommon, although the incidence of acute hepatitis C is increasing in many parts of the world due to the opioid epidemic. The acute hepatitis associated with hepatitis C infection (HCV) is typically subclinical with icteric hepatitis C at acute infection more often associated with the clearance of infection.[42] Unlike CHB infection, there is no clinically meaningful reactivation in chronic hepatitis C-infected individuals who receive chemotherapy leading to ACLF although flares of hepatitis may be observed in up to 23% of individuals.[43] Treatment of hepatitis C in an acute presentation is recommended with direct-acting antiviral (DAA) therapy, although there are no reports of this strategy in the setting of ACLF (AASLD-IDSA. Recommendations for testing, managing, and treating hepatitis C. http://www.hcvguidelines.org.). However, treatment with a sofosbuvir-based regimen with NS5a inhibitor could be initiated to treat acute hepatitis C infection if required in this setting.

Other nonhepatotropic viruses leading to acute-on-chronic liver failure
Many viruses including Epstein-Barr virus (EBV), cytomegalovirus (CMV), herpes simplex virus (HSV), and severe acute respiratory syndrome coronavirus 2 (SARS-CoV-2) may cause acute hepatitis, and these viruses have rarely been associated with ACLF with less severe outcomes than experienced with ACLF caused by hepatotropic viruses.[13] EBV infection is associated with a subclinical hepatitis in most cases although reports of acute liver failure have been reported. ACLF has been noted in hepatitis B-infected individuals of which a subset had CMV and EBV infection confirmed by DNA testing. In this cohort, 23% (23 out of 100) of those tested had detectable EBV DNA and 5% (5 out of 100) had CMV DNA detected.[44] Risk factors for CMV ACLF were related to low HBV DNA levels, and in EBV-related ACLF, age greater than 60 years old predicted the presence of EBV infection. The clinical presentation of ACLF in EBV-infected individuals with hepatitis B was more severe with higher CPT scores and lower albumin levels, whereas CMV-infected patients had lower ALT levels. Another report from India noted that ACLF cases related to CMV and EBV were uncommon (2 out of 89, 2%) with no cases of mortality.[10] Although not reported for ACLF, in theory, CMV therapies such as valganciclovir could be used in this setting. Fulminant hepatitis due to herpes simplex virus 1 has been reported rarely in hepatitis B-infected individuals in China, one of whom was coinfected with HIV and in another patient on long-term corticosteroid therapy.[45] These individuals were first thought to have hepatitis B reactivation and neither had mucocutaneous manifestations of herpes simplex infection. Both patients died within

24 hours of presentation with both patients showing evidence of CLD on autopsy liver pathology slides. Acyclovir therapy is utilized to treat HSV hepatitis and could be used in this population with ACLF.

The SARS-CoV-2 virus has also been associated with poor outcomes in those with advanced liver disease with 2.38 times greater mortality being reported in a large administrative database.[46] Multiple observational cohort data have reported higher mortality rates in individuals with SARS-CoV-2 infection with CLD. Those with a diagnosis of alcohol-associated liver disease, decompensated cirrhosis, and hepatocellular carcinoma were all associated with higher mortality when infected with SARS-CoV-2.[47] A single-center report in adults with SARS-CoV-2 infection and CLD noted that 32 out of 84 (38%) patients with cirrhosis developed ACLF with extrahepatic failure, respiratory failure, and renal failure being most common.[48] Those of Hispanic/Latino ethnicity were also at higher risk of in-hospital mortality. In-hospital mortality was not different between those with CLD with cirrhosis and without cirrhosis with SARS-CoV-2 infection although higher mortality rates were observed in those who developed ACLF.

A study from 13 Asian countries reported on outcomes in those with concurrent SARS-CoV-2 infection and CLD and noted a prevalence of ACLF of 11%, with increased liver-related complications in those with more advanced liver disease. Interestingly, the mortality was similar among those without cirrhosis and those with compensated cirrhosis, although the cohort with compensated cirrhosis developed more significant liver injury and liver-related complications. However, in decompensated cirrhosis, a high rate of liver injury was observed with a 43% mortality in those with cirrhosis and evidence of acute liver injury. In this cohort a CTP score of 9 or more predicted a poor outcome.[49]

Management of ACLF and those with COVID infection include supportive care directed not only toward the extrahepatic organ failures associated with ACLF but also treatment directed toward the SARS-CoV-2 virus. This would include monoclonal antibody therapies, corticosteroids, and antiviral agents. To date, remdesivir, has been associated with low rates of clinically apparent liver injury and in general may be administered to those with cirrhosis and therapies are approved although their role in the treatment of ACLF is unknown as well (see **Table 2**).[50] Vaccination against SARS-CoV-2 virus with timely boosters should be offered to all patients with CLD as vaccination has been reported to reduce mortality in those with CLD.[51]

In summary, ACLF caused by viral hepatitis is an important cause of morbidity and mortality in those with CLD. In endemic areas of the world, hepatitis E is a common viral cause leading to ACLF and is associated with high morbidity and mortality rates. Improved sanitation and vaccination (where available) against genotype 1 hepatitis E are important strategies to reduce adverse clinical outcomes. Hepatitis A infection may also lead to ACLF, and effective vaccines are available, therefore, all patients with CLD should be vaccinated for the HAV. Hepatitis B is also a common viral cause of ACLF and in those with CHB infection with ACLF, suppression of HBV DNA with nucleoside/nucleotide analog therapy with tenofovir or entecavir should be initiated in those with hepatitis B flares and/or reactivation in addition to providing supportive care for ACLF. Vaccination against hepatitis B worldwide is the strategy not only to eliminate hepatitis B but also to reduce morbidity, mortality, and the risk of developing ACLF. Practitioners who prescribe chemotherapies or immune-modulating therapies must be educated about the risks for reactivation. Hepatitis D may also cause ACLF in the setting of superinfection, although there are no specific therapies available for hepatitis D that have been tested in this setting. Again, vaccination to prevent hepatitis B infection should be the underlying strategy to reduce ACLF risk from hepatitis D.

Clinical outcomes are less severe in ACLF caused by nonhepatotropic viruses although more data are required to better define outcomes with SARS-CoV-2 infection. EBV and CMV virus may be found in those with CLD but are rare causes of ACLF and have very-low mortality rates. COVID-19 infection (SARS-CoV-2 virus) is associated with markedly worse outcomes in those with CLD, especially in those with decompensated cirrhosis. Therefore, in addition to treatment of the SARS-CoV-2 infection, vaccination against SARS-CoV-2 virus with boosters is an important strategy to reduce morbidity and mortality in this population. Prevention of ACLF due to viral hepatitis (particularly hepatitis B and hepatitis E), with screening, education, improved sanitation, and vaccination are essential tools to mitigate the occurrence and diminish the incidence of ACLF and improve overall patient survival in patients with liver disease from any etiology.

CLINICS CARE POINTS

- All patients with chronic liver disease should be vaccinated against hepatitis A and B viruses if protective antibodies are not present.
- Vaccination against Sars-CoV-2 will reduce poor outcomes in those with chronic liver disease.

POTENTIAL CONFLICTS

P.Y. Kwo: Advisory Board: Abbvie, Gilead, Antios, Aligos, Glaxo Smith Kline, Grant Support: Eiger, Janssen, Gilead, HCV Target Registries, Altimmune Consulting: Drug Farm.

REFERENCES

1. Moreau R, Jalan R, Gines P, et al. Acute-on-chronic liver failure is a distinct syndrome that develops in patients with acute decompensation of cirrhosis. Gastroenterology 2013;144:1426–37. e9.
2. Sarin SK, Kumar A, Almeida JA, et al. Acute-on-chronic liver failure: consensus recommendations of the Asian Pacific Association for the study of the liver (APASL). Hepatology International 2009;3:269–82.
3. Arroyo V, Moreau R, Jalan R. Acute-on-chronic liver failure. N Engl J Med 2020; 382:2137–45.
4. O'Leary JG, Reddy KR, Garcia-Tsao G, et al. NACSELD acute-on-chronic liver failure (NACSELD-ACLF) score predicts 30-day survival in hospitalized patients with cirrhosis. Hepatology 2018;67:2367–74.
5. Hernaez R, Solà E, Moreau R, et al. Acute-on-chronic liver failure: an update. Gut 2017;66:541.
6. Ly KN, Klevens RM. Trends in disease and complications of hepatitis A virus infection in the United States, 1999-2011: a new concern for adults. J Infect Dis 2015;212:176–82.
7. Stanaway JD, Flaxman AD, Naghavi M, et al. The global burden of viral hepatitis from 1990 to 2013: findings from the Global Burden of Disease Study 2013. Lancet 2016;388:1081–8.
8. Radha Krishna Y, Saraswat VA, Das K, et al. Clinical features and predictors of outcome in acute hepatitis A and hepatitis E virus hepatitis on cirrhosis. Liver Int 2009;29:392–8.

9. Jha AK, Nijhawan S, Rai RR, et al. Etiology, clinical profile, and inhospital mortality of acute-on-chronic liver failure: a prospective study. Indian J Gastroenterol 2013; 32:108–14.

10. Gupta E, Ballani N, Kumar M, et al. Role of non-hepatotropic viruses in acute sporadic viral hepatitis and acute-on-chronic liver failure in adults. Indian J Gastroenterol 2015;34:448–52.

11. Samala N, Abdallah W, Poole A, et al. Insight into an acute hepatitis A outbreak in Indiana. J Viral Hepat 2021;28:964–71.

12. Clària J, Stauber RE, Coenraad MJ, et al. Systemic inflammation in decompensated cirrhosis: Characterization and role in acute-on-chronic liver failure. Hepatology 2016;64:1249–64.

13. Shi Y, Yang Y, Hu Y, et al. Acute-on-chronic liver failure precipitated by hepatic injury is distinct from that precipitated by extrahepatic insults. Hepatology 2015;62:232–42.

14. Cheemerla S, Balakrishnan M. Global epidemiology of chronic liver disease. Clin Liver Dis 2021;17:365–70.

15. Organization W.H., Interim guidance for country validation of viral hepatitis elimination. 2021. Available at: https://www.who.int/publications/i/item/9789240028 395. Accessed November 8, 2022.

16. Robinson A, Wong R, Gish RG. Chronic hepatitis B virus and hepatitis D virus: new developments. Clin Liver Dis 2023;27:17–25.

17. Ward JW, Hinman AR. What is needed to eliminate hepatitis B virus and hepatitis C virus as global health threats. Gastroenterology 2019;156:297–310.

18. Sonderup MW, Spearman CW. Global disparities in hepatitis B elimination—a focus on Africa. Viruses 2022;14:82.

19. Jindal A, Kumar M, Sarin SK. Management of acute hepatitis B and reactivation of hepatitis B. Liver Int 2013;33:164–75.

20. Chen L, Zheng CX, Lin MH, et al. Distinct quasispecies characteristics and positive selection within precore/core gene in hepatitis B virus HBV associated acute-on-chronic liver failure. J Gastroenterol Hepatol 2013;28:1040–6.

21. Li Q., Wang J., Lu M., et al., Acute-on-chronic liver failure from chronic-Hepatitis-B, who is the behind scenes, *Front Microbiol*, 11, 2020, 1-13.

22. Tan W, Xia J, Dan Y, et al. Genome-wide association study identifies HLA-DR variants conferring risk of HBV-related acute-on-chronic liver failure. Gut 2018;67: 757–66.

23. Reddy KR, Beavers KL, Hammond SP, et al. American Gastroenterological Association Institute guideline on the prevention and treatment of hepatitis B virus reactivation during immunosuppressive drug therapy. Gastroenterology 2015;148: 215–9 [quiz: e16-7].

24. Terrault NA, Lok AS, McMahon BJ, et al. Update on prevention, diagnosis, and treatment of chronic hepatitis B: AASLD 2018 hepatitis B guidance. Hepatology 2018;67:1560–99.

25. Huang K-W, Tam K-W, Luo J-C, et al. Efficacy and safety of lamivudine versus entecavir for treating chronic hepatitis B virus–related acute exacerbation and acute-on-chronic liver failure. J Clin Gastroenterol 2017;51:539–47.

26. Lange CM, Bojunga J, Hofmann WP, et al. Severe lactic acidosis during treatment of chronic hepatitis B with entecavir in patients with impaired liver function. Hepatology 2009;50:2001–6.

27. Wan Y-M, Li Y-H, Xu Z-Y, et al. Tenofovir versus entecavir for the treatment of acute-on-chronic liver failure due to reactivation of chronic hepatitis B with genotypes B and C. J Clin Gastroenterol 2019;53:e171–7.

28. Wu T, Li J, Shao L, et al. Development of diagnostic criteria and a prognostic score for hepatitis B virus-related acute-on-chronic liver failure. Gut 2018;67: 2181.
29. Li J, Liang X, You S, et al. Development and validation of a new prognostic score for hepatitis B virus-related acute-on-chronic liver failure. J Hepatol 2021;75: 1104–15.
30. Luo J, Liang X, Xin J, et al. Predicting the onset of hepatitis B virus-related acute-on-chronic liver failure. Clin Gastroenterol Hepatol 2022.
31. Stockdale AJ, Kreuels B, Henrion MYR, et al. The global prevalence of hepatitis D virus infection: systematic review and meta-analysis. J Hepatol 2020;73:523–32.
32. Rizzetto M, Hamid S, Negro F. The changing context of hepatitis D. J Hepatol 2021;74:1200–11.
33. Wedemeyer H, Schöneweis K, Bogomolov P, et al. Safety and efficacy of bulevirtide in combination with tenofovir disoproxil fumarate in patients with hepatitis B virus and hepatitis D virus coinfection (MYR202): a multicentre, randomised, parallel-group, open-label, phase 2 trial. Lancet Infect Dis 2022;23(1):117–29.
34. Horvatits T., Schulze Zur Wiesch J., Lütgehetmann M., et al., The clinical perspective on hepatitis E, *Viruses*, 11, 2019, 1-19.
35. Kumar A, Saraswat VA. Hepatitis E and acute-on-chronic liver failure. J Clin Exp Hepatol 2013;3:225–30.
36. Zhang X, Ke W, Xie J, et al. Comparison of effects of hepatitis E or A viral superinfection in patients with chronic hepatitis B. Hepatol Int 2010;4:615–20.
37. Kamar N, Dalton HR, Abravanel F, et al. Hepatitis E virus infection. Clin Microbiol Rev 2014;27:116–38.
38. Kamar N, Izopet J, Tripon S, et al. Ribavirin for chronic hepatitis E virus infection in transplant recipients. N Engl J Med 2014;370:1111–20.
39. Goyal R, Kumar A, Panda SK, et al. Ribavirin therapy for hepatitis E virus-induced acute on chronic liver failure: a preliminary report. Antivir Ther 2012;17:1091–6.
40. Kamani L, Padhani ZA, Das JK. Hepatitis E: genotypes, strategies to prevent and manage, and the existing knowledge gaps. JGH Open 2021;5:1127–34.
41. Dang H, Yeo YH, Yasuda S, et al. Cure with interferon-free direct-acting antiviral is associated with increased survival in patients with hepatitis C virus-related hepatocellular carcinoma from both east and west. Hepatology 2020;71:1910–22.
42. Tillmann HL, Thompson AJ, Patel K, et al. A polymorphism Near IL28B is associated with spontaneous clearance of acute hepatitis C virus and jaundice. Gastroenterology 2010;139:1586–92.e1.
43. Torres HA, Hosry J, Mahale P, et al. Hepatitis C virus reactivation in patients receiving cancer treatment: a prospective observational study. Hepatology 2018;67:36–47.
44. Hu J, Zhao H, Lou D, et al. Human cytomegalovirus and Epstein-Barr virus infections, risk factors, and their influence on the liver function of patients with acute-on-chronic liver failure. BMC Infect Dis 2018;18:1–8.
45. Ichai P, Roque Afonso AM, Sebagh M, et al. Herpes simplex virus-associated acute liver failure: a difficult diagnosis with a poor prognosis. Liver Transplant 2005;11:1550–5.
46. Ge J, Pletcher MJ, Lai JC, et al. Outcomes of SARS-CoV-2 infection in patients with chronic liver disease and cirrhosis: a national COVID cohort collaborative study. Gastroenterology 2021;161:1487–501. e5.
47. Kim D, Adeniji N, Latt N, et al. Predictors of outcomes of COVID-19 in patients with chronic liver disease: US multi-center study. Clin Gastroenterol Hepatol 2021;19:1469–79.e19.

48. Satapathy SK, Roth NC, Kvasnovsky C, et al. Risk factors and outcomes for acute-on-chronic liver failure in COVID-19: a large multi-center observational cohort study. Hepatology International 2021;15:766–79.

49. Sarin SK, Choudhury A, Lau GK, et al. Pre-existing liver disease is associated with poor outcome in patients with SARS CoV2 infection; the APCOLIS Study (APASL COVID-19 Liver Injury Spectrum Study). Hepatology International 2020; 14:690–700.

50. Lim H, Palaiodimos L, Berto CG, et al. Remdesivir in the treatment of COVID-19: a propensity score-matched analysis from a public hospital in New York city assessing renal and hepatic safety. J Clin Med 2022;11:3132.

51. John BV, Deng Y, Schwartz KB, et al. Postvaccination COVID-19 infection is associated with reduced mortality in patients with cirrhosis. Hepatology 2022.

Drug-Induced Acute-on-Chronic Liver Failure

Challenges and Future Directions

Jiayi Ma, MD[a], Marwan Ghabril, MD[b], Naga Chalasani, MD[b,*]

KEYWORDS

- Acute-on-chronic liver failure • Chronic liver disease • Drug-induced liver injury

KEY POINTS

- Drug-induced liver injury (DILI) can be severe and lead to significant liver injury and acute liver failure.
- Acute-on-chronic liver failure (ACLF) occurs in patients with underling chronic liver disease and carries a high risk of short-term mortality.
- Drug-induced ACLF (DI-ACLF) can be challenging to diagnose due to the lack of a gold-standard diagnostic test for DILI.
- There is geographic variability in the underlying liver conditions and types of implicated agents in DI-ACLF.
- Underlying liver disease may be associated with more severe DILI, and DI-ACLF is associated with high mortality.

INTRODUCTION

The impact of drug-induced liver injury (DILI) is global as it is observed in all age groups and races and across multiple continents. It is associated with a wide range of therapeutic drugs and increasingly with herbal and dietary supplements (HDS), even in Western populations.[1–6] DILI is an unpredictable idiosyncratic reaction with serious morbidity and mortality and is a major reason for drug attrition during drug development. It is estimated to develop in approximately 19 cases per 100,000 persons after exposure to drugs that are otherwise safe for the vast majority of individuals.[7,8] The severity of DILI can range from asymptomatic transaminitis to acute liver failure and death, though a sizable proportion of patients develop jaundice, abdominal pain, and/or nausea.[1]

[a] Gastroenterology and Hepatology, Indiana University School of Medicine, 702 Rotary Circle, Suite 225, Indianapolis, IN 46202, USA; [b] Gastroenterology and Hepatology, Indiana University School of Medicine & Indiana University Health, 702 Rotary Circle, Suite 225, Indianapolis, IN 46202, USA
* Corresponding author. 702 Rotary Circle, Suite 225, Indianapolis, IN 46202.
E-mail address: nchalasa@iu.edu

Clin Liver Dis 27 (2023) 631–648
https://doi.org/10.1016/j.cld.2023.03.007
1089-3261/23/© 2023 Elsevier Inc. All rights reserved.

Acute-on-chronic liver failure (ACLF) was first systematically defined by the CANONIC study of the European Association for the Study of the Liver in 2013.[9] In this seminal study, ACLF was defined as new decompensation of underlying cirrhosis with organ failure, other than liver failure. ACLF was most commonly precipitated by infections or gastrointestinal bleeding; however, other liver insults leading to ACLF including DILI are recognized. Regardless of precipitating factors, patients with ACLF suffer from severe illness, frequently require critical care, and carry very high mortality rates.

DILI leading to ACLF, or drug-induced ACLF (DI-ACLF), is therefore a clinically important entity that draws on our understanding of both DILI and ACLF and the challenges inherent to both clinical entities. Considerations of DI-ACLF also raise questions as to whether DILI carries a different risk for ACLF outcomes compared with other precipitating factors, and whether underlying liver disease including cirrhosis alters the risk for and the natural history of DILI. The key aspects of both DILI and ACLF provide important context to how DI-ACLF may be defined and characterized and are further discussed.

DRUG-INDUCED LIVER INJURY
The Adjudication of Drug-Induced Liver Injury

A critical feature of DILI is that it lacks a diagnostic gold standard and can only be made through a process of excluding competing etiologies of liver injury. As a result, the diagnosis of DILI is expressed as the probability of DILI, as reflected by multiple causality assessment methods described in the field. Although this is also true for intrinsic DILI or dose-dependent liver injury seen with known hepatotoxins such as acetaminophen, it is most challenging for idiosyncratic DILI, where normally safe doses of an implicated agent lead to liver injury. In all cases, the key components of the presentation are considered including (1) latency (time from initial exposure to the onset of liver injury), (2) dechallenge (the course of liver injury after withdrawal of the implicated agent), (3) an understanding of the expected features of liver injury commonly seen with an implicated agent, and importantly (4) laboratory and imaging studies to exclude competing etiologies. Multiple societies from North America, Europe, and Asia have established guidelines for the diagnosis and treatment of DILI.[10–12] Here, we highlight the most common diagnostic approaches and summarize the potential impact of underlying liver disease, a requirement for ACLF, on the risk of DILI.

Important DILI causality assessment methods include the following.

1. Additive or algorithmic scoring systems are used to quantitively assess causality in cases of suspected DILI. The most frequently used of these is the Roussel Uclaf Causality Assessment Method (RUCAM) developed by the Council for International Organizations of Medical Sciences which provides an ordinal scale of probabilities for DILI (definite, probable, possible, unlikely, and excluded).[13] The key domains of RUCAM and other structured methodologies are summarized in **Table 1**. Notable among these is the recently introduced Revised Electronic Causality Assessment Method (RECAM), available online (http://gihep.com/dili-recam/) allowing semiautomated scoring and categorization of the probability of DILI.[14] It must be emphasized that these scores are designed to complement and not replace clinical assessment in diagnosing DILI.
2. Expert opinion, attained through consensus adjudication by three experienced clinicians using a semi-structured qualitative approach. This was developed by the US Drug-Induced Liver Injury Network (DILIN).[15] It also provides an ordinal scale

Table 1
The key domains used by structured algorithmic scoring systems for adjudication of drug-induced liver injury

Components	RUCAM[13]	CDS[45]	DDW-J (Modification of RUCAM)[46,47]	RECAM[14] (Available Online, Semi-automated)
Clinical risk factors such as age, gender, and alcohol use	Yes	Yes	Yes	No
Liver injury pattern, latency, dechallenge, rechallenge	Yes	Yes	Yes	Yes
Laboratory and imaging studies to exclude competing etiologies of liver injury	Yes	Yes	Yes	Yes
Concomitant medications	Yes	No	Yes	No
Extrahepatic manifestations	No	Yes	No	No
Other	NA		Drug lymphocyte stimulation test results, peripheral eosinophilia	LiverTox risk score for the implicated agent Requires hepatitis E IgM and hepatitis C RNA testing

Abbreviations: CDS, Maria-Victorino Clinical Diagnostic Scale; DDW-J, Digestive Disease Week Japan 2004 score; IgG, immunoglobulin M; NA, not applicable; RECAM, revised electronic causality assessment method; RNA, ribonucleic acid; RUCAM, Roussel Uclaf Causality Assessment Method.

of probabilities of DILI (definite, highly likely, probable, possible, and unlikely). Although the need for three experts renders this impractical for all cases of suspected DILI, it is reliable and useful in clinical research. The LiverTox Web site is a critical and immensely practical repository of cumulative expertise in DILI relating to individual agents and classes of drugs and HDS.[6] It is a crucial resource for educating clinicians and aiding them in considering the probability of DILI on a case-by-implicated-agent-case basis.

The Pattern of Liver Injury and Outcomes

The pattern of liver injury in DILI is determined by the R-ratio (the ratio of serum alanine transferase to alkaline phosphatase values, both expressed as multiples of upper limit of normal) at the onset of injury. Hepatocellular injury ($R > 5$) is more common than cholestatic ($R < 2$) and mixed (R between 2–5), it occurs in younger patients who are more likely to be female and is associated with higher mortality and need for liver transplantation (LT).[1] This is epitomized by Hy's law describing mortality rates of 10% in DILI with alanine transferase elevations greater than three times upper limit of normal and jaundice (bilirubin >2 times the upper limit of normal).[16] DILI accounted for 11.1% of acute liver failures in the United States. Acute Liver Failure Study Group cohort with a predominance of female patients (70%) and hepatocellular injury pattern (78%) in further support of these important associations.[17]

The Impact of Underlying Liver Disease on Risk of Drug-Induced Liver Injury

Chronic liver disease (CLD) is a prerequisite for ACLF and may also contribute to the risk of DILI, although the infrequency of DILI per drug exposure makes it difficult to study this association prospectively. Whether underlying CLD predisposes to DILI is controversial and may be compound and liver disease etiology-specific. For example, it has been shown that statin hepatotoxicity is not more common in patients with suspect fatty liver disease.[18] On the other hand, patients with suspected fatty liver disease had an increased risk of suspected DILI in a large population-based study.[19] Other data on nonalcoholic fatty liver disease suggest a fourfold increased odds of developing DILI related to antihypertensives, antimicrobials and other agents, with a close association with central obesity.[20] In addition, obesity is associated with increased prevalence and severity of halothane and methotrexate DILI, whereas diabetes mellitus (another risk factor for nonalcoholic fatty liver disease) seems to be a risk factor for severe DILI.[21]

There is also evidence of an increased risk of DILI with other underlying chronic liver conditions. For example, in a systematic review of prospective studies, patients with viral hepatitis had 3.4 higher odds of developing suspected DILI, whereas in other studies, viral hepatitis was associated with higher rates of antituberculosis and highly active antiretroviral therapy-related DILI.[11,22] Alcohol use, a risk factor for liver disease, is also considered a risk factor for DILI in RUCAM and its use seems to be a risk factor for isoniazid, methotrexate, and halothane hepatotoxicity.[23]

In addition to a potential increased risk of DILI, patients with underlying CLD are at risk for a worse prognosis with DILI. A significant proportion (10%) of patients enrolled in DILIN had underlying CLD and they had a threefold higher rate of mortality.[1] The rate of underlying CLD among patients in the Spanish Registry of DILI was 6.3% with an approximately fourfold increased risk of liver-related death due to DILI.[24] In aggregate, these data suggest that underlying CLD may predispose to increased frequency and severity of DILI, although this statement should be tempered by the limited data.

ACUTE-ON-CHRONIC LIVER FAILURE
Definitions of Acute-on-Chronic Liver Failure

ACLF is a recently recognized syndrome among patients with cirrhosis or CLD characterized by new organ failures (hepatic, brain, circulatory, renal, respiratory, and coagulation) and high short-term mortality. To discuss DI-ACLF, we must first define ACLF, but like DILI, it lacks gold-standard diagnostic biomarkers and is a clinical diagnosis. In addition, the definitions of ACLF differ across the globe, even though all definitions incorporate some common themes including (1) underlying liver disease (although not all guidelines require cirrhosis), (2) an acute hepatic insult from either a hepatic (alcohol, viral hepatitis, or DILI) or extrahepatic (infection, variceal bleeding) precipitating event, (3) organ failure highlighted by new or acute hepatic decompensations (with or without extrahepatic organ failures depending on definitions), and (4) high short-term risk of mortality. An important difference in the definitions of ACLF is that cirrhosis is not a prerequisite in the Asia Pacific Association for the Study of the Liver (APASL),[25] the World Gastroenterology Organization (WGO),[26] and the American College of Gastroenterology (ACG) definitions.[27] In contrast, it is a requirement in the seminal European and North American studies describing ACLF.[9,28] The key features of the definitions and scoring of ACLF used by the aforementioned guidelines and studies are summarized in **Table 2**. An inclusive definition of ACLF as proposed by the WGO Working Group, and recently adopted by the ACG, seems to encompass the greatest range of patients and time frames meeting the key tenants of ACLF as a guide for management and further study.[26,27]

DRUG-INDUCED ACUTE-ON-CHRONIC LIVER FAILURE

DI-ACLF has been explored in a number of studies using the definitions outlined previously. Overall, DI-ACLF comprises a small number of overall ACLF cases, with antituberculosis drugs and HDS making up the majority of implicated agents. These findings are summarized in **Table 3** and are discussed in more detail below.

Asian Pacific Association for Study of the Liver Defined Drug-Induced Acute-on-Chronic Liver Failure

There are limited data describing DI-ACLF with the largest study coming from Asia. To date, three studies using the APASL criteria have described DI-ACLF. The first study is a prospective single-center study from India in which 213 consecutively enrolled patients with all-cause ACLF were included for analysis.[29] Within the cohort, 112 had undiagnosed underlying CLD while 101 presented with known underlying cirrhosis. DI-ACLF caused by antituberculosis drugs was the precipitating agent in 11 (5.2%) patients, including 8 patients with CLD and 3 with cirrhosis. Cryptogenic cirrhosis was the cause of CLD in 8 of the 11 cases. During follow-up, 5 (45.5%) patients with DI-ACLF survived while 6 died.[29]

A more recent study described the etiologies and clinical course of ACLF in 10 tertiary centers in India.[30] A total of 1049 patients with ACLF were included. Among them, 60 (5.7%) patients had DI-ACLF, with the most common agents being antituberculosis drugs. Seventeen of the 60 patients with DI-ACLF also had sufficient data to quantify organ failures according to the Chronic Liver Failure modified Sequential Organ Failure Assessment (CLIF-SOFA) score developed by the CANONIC study.[9] Non-survivors had significantly higher CLIF-SOFA scores than survivors, with a median score of 9 versus 7, respectively. Patients with DI-ACLF experienced 35% short-term mortality.[30]

Finally, in the largest study to date specifically on DI-ACLF, 3132 patients from the multinational APASL Research Consortium database were identified and prospectively

Table 2
Key features of the criteria for and definitions of acute-on-chronic liver failure used by liver disease societies and seminal studies globally

Liver Disease Society or Consortia	ACG Guideline[27]	APASL Consensus[25]	EASL-CLIF Study[9]	NACSELD Study[28]	WGO Proposal[26]
Time interval defining acuity of the event	3 mo	4weeks	4 wk	30 d	3 mo
Underlying liver disease allowed or included					
Chronic liver disease without cirrhosis	Yes	Yes	No	No	Yes (Type A ACLF)
Cirrhosis, compensated	Yes	Yes	Yes	No	Yes (Type B ACLF)
Cirrhosis, decompensated	Yes	No	Yes	Yes with infection	Yes (Type C ACLF)
Organ failure criteria	Hepatic and extrahepatic organ failure	Liver failure includes coagulopathy and HE	Extrahepatic organ failures include coagulopathy and HE Grades ACLF 0–3 based on number of organ failure	Extrahepatic organ failures include coagulopathy and HE 2 or more organ failures needed	Hepatic failure (jaundice and prolonged INR) and at least 1 extrahepatic organ failure
Liver (Bilirubin)	Threshold not specified	Bilirubin ≥ 5 mg/dL	Bilirubin ≥ 12 mg/dL	Not included	Threshold not specified
Coagulation (INR)	Threshold not specified	INR ≥ 1.5	INR ≥ 1.5	Not included	Threshold not specified
Brain (HE)	Threshold not specified	New HE, West Haven grade 3–4	HE, West Haven grade 3–4	HE, West Haven grade 3–4	Threshold not specified
Kidney	Threshold not specified	AKIN criteria	RRT or Creatinine≥ 2 mg/dL	RRT	Threshold not specified

Circulation	Threshold not specified	Not included	Pressors used	Mean arterial pressure< 60 mm Hg or 40 mm Hg reduction in systolic blood pressure despite adequate fluid resuscitation and cardiac output	Threshold not specified
Respiratory	Threshold not specified	Not included	$PaO_2/FiO_2 \leq 200$ or $SpO_2/FiO_2 \leq 214$ or mechanical ventilation	Mechanical ventilation	Threshold not specified
Other	-	New ascites	-	-	-
Exclusion criteria	Not specified	Prior hepatic decompensation or infection	HIV infection, HCC beyond Milan criteria	HIV infection, active malignancies, and previous transplant recipients	Not specified

Abbreviations: ACG, American College of Gastroenterology; AKIN, acute kidney injury network criteria; APASL, Asia Pacific Association for Study of the Liver; EASL-CLIF, European Association for Study of the Liver Chronic Liver Failure; HCC, hepatocellular carcinoma; HE, hepatic encephalopathy; HIV, human immunodeficiency virus; INR, international normalized ratio; NACSELD, North American Consortium for Study of End-Stage Liver Disease; RRT, renal replacement therapy; WGO, World Gastroenterology Organization working party.

Table 3
Selected characteristics and features of studying evaluating drug-induced acute on chronic liver failure

Study	Location	Number of Patients Studied	Definition of ACLF Used	Proportion DI-ACLF	Implicated Agents	Underlying Liver Disease	Mortality Rates	Comment
Shalimar et al,[29] 2016	India, single center	213	APASL	11/132, 5.2%	Antituberculosis drugs	40% alcohol, 24% HBV, 20% cryptogenic	In hospital: Overall: 43% AT drugs: 55%	Acute hepatic insult due to antituberculosis drugs did not independently predict mortality.
Shalimar et al,[30] 2016	India, multicenter	1049 consecutive patients, 381 with complete data	APASL	17/381, 4.5%	Antituberculosis drugs, antiepileptics	52% alcohol, 21% cryptogenic, 16% viral	In hospital: Overall: 148/381, 39% Drugs: 6/17, 34%	Acute hepatic insult due to DI-ACLF did not independently predict mortality compared with other precipitants.
Devarbhavi et al,[10] 2021	Asia, multinational	3132	APASL	329/3132, 11%	Antituberculosis drugs, CAMs, methotrexate (n = 2), antiepileptic drug (n = 1)	29% alcohol, 26% cryptogenic, 17% HBV, 17% NASH	90-d: Non-DI-ACLF: 39% DI-ACLF: 47%	DI-ACLF frequently presented with jaundice (100%), ascites (88%), and encephalopathy (47%) Arterial lactate and total bilirubin were independent predictors of mortality in DI-ACLF.

Study	Location	N	Criteria			Etiology	Outcomes	Conclusions
Shi et al,[33] 2015	China, single center	322	EASL-CLIF	10/322 (2.5%)	Not specified	64% HBV, 11% alcohol, 14% both	90-d: Hepatic ACLF (including DI): 59%[a] Extrahepatic ACLF: 68%[a]	Extrahepatic ACLF had significantly higher 90 d and 1 y mortality vs hepatic ACLF.
Li et al,[34] 2016	China, single center	300	EASL-CLIF	7/300 (2.3%)	Not specified	100% HBV	90-d: ACLF: 50%[a] No ACLF: 4.6%[a]	Overall rates of hepatotoxic drug or herb intake prior to admission did not differ significantly between patients presenting with ACLF vs no ACLF. The use of hepatotoxic drugs and herbs was not found to be an independent predictor of developing ACLF during hospitalization.

(continued on next page)

Table 3
(continued)

Study	Location	Number of Patients Studied	Definition of ACLF Used	Proportion DI-ACLF	Implicated Agents	Underlying Liver Disease	Mortality Rates	Comment
Maipang et al,[35] 2019	Thailand, single center	343	EASL-CLIF	3/343 (0.9%)	Not specified	38% HBV, 21% HCV, 20% cryptogenic	90-d: Hepatic ACLF (including DI-ACLF): 73% Extrahepatic ACLF: 59%	Hepatic ACLF had significantly higher 28-d mortality versus extrahepatic ACLF. Mortality at 90-d, 6 mo, and 1-y were similar between the two groups.

Abbreviations: APASL, Asia Pacific Association for Study of the Liver; CAM, complementary and alternative medicine; DI-ACLF, drug-induced acute-on-chronic liver failure; EASL-CLIF, European Association for Study of the Liver Chronic Liver Failure; HBV, hepatitis B virus; HCV, hepatitis C virus; NASH, nonalcoholic steatohepatitis.
[a] Statistically significant.

followed.[31] Among them, 329 (10.5%) patients identified as having DI-ACLF underwent a thorough workup to exclude competing etiologies including viral and autoimmune causes and biliary pathology. A significant portion (27%) of the DI-ACLF subgroup underwent biopsy, with 85% of those biopsies showing cirrhosis. There was a strong temporal relationship between drug exposure and development of ACLF as defined by jaundice and coagulopathy with either ascites or encephalopathy. Of note, patients with previous hepatic decompensation were excluded per the APASL definition of ACLF. Among the 329 patients with DI-ACLF, the most common implicated class of agents were complementary and alternative medicines (CAM, akin to HDS) and antituberculosis drugs making up 236 (72%) and 90 (27%) of the cases, respectively. The remaining cases were from methotrexate ($n = 2$) and anti-epileptic drug ($n = 1$). The median duration of drug exposure was 84 days, and the overall 90-day mortality was 47%, with drug class-specific mortalities being 47%, 46%, and 33% for antituberculosis, CAM, and non-CAM DI-ACLF, respectively.[31]

Comparing DI-ACLF with other causes of ACLF, the investigators noted patients with DI-ACLF were significantly older (47 vs 44 years) and had a higher proportion of female patients (35% vs 12%) and of cryptogenic underlying CLD (72% vs 43%). Clinical presentation at baseline did not differ, with similar rates of jaundice, ascites, and encephalopathy. However, the DI-ACLF group had significantly higher Model for End-Stage Liver Disease (MELD) (30.2 vs 28.9) and 90-day mortality (46.5% vs 38.8%), respectively.[31] When comparing survivors to non-survivors within the DI-ACLF group, the investigators did not find a difference in age, sex, or etiology of underlying liver disease. As one might expect, non-survivors had significantly higher MELD and CLIF-SOFA scores than survivors of DI-ACLF.

Similarly, the investigators also compared the different classes of drugs between antituberculosis drugs and CAM. Aside from a significantly higher proportion of men with CAM DI-ACLF, there were no clinical differences in rates of jaundice, ascites, encephalopathy, MELD, or CLIF-SOFA scores. Regarding prognosis, arterial lactate and total bilirubin were independent predictors of 7-day mortality, and arterial lactate, total bilirubin, international normalized ratio (INR), urea, and the presence of hepatic encephalopathy were independent predictors of 90-day mortality.[31]

European Association for Study of the Liver-Chronic Liver Failure Defined Drug-Induced Acute-on-Chronic Liver Failure

The systematic review and meta-analysis by Mezzano and colleagues included 30 cohort studies from around the world composing of 43,000 patients with ACLF as defined by the European Association for Study of the Liver-Chronic Liver Failure (EASL-CLIF) criteria and 140,000 patients without ACLF.[32] Precipitants for ACLF were divided into alcohol, viral, infection, gastrointestinal bleeding and other, with the other category including DI-ACLF. There was little specified on outcomes among patients with DI-ACLF. Overall, other causes of ACLF made up of 5% of the total global cases. Although there was insufficient detail on the subgroup of patients with DI-ACLF in this meta-analysis, it provided contrasting pictures of ACLF globally. For example, the severity of disease or grade of ACLF differed by region, with ACLF-grade 1 being the most common in South America and ACLF-grade 3 being the most common in Asia. Nevertheless, 90-day mortality rates between South America and South Asia were comparable at 73% and 68%, respectively.

Three other studies have examined DI-ACLF using the EASL-CLIF definition. An earlier prospective cohort study from China included 322 ACLF patients with well-characterized precipitating events.[33] The investigators ascertained the use of hepatotoxic drugs within 3 months of admission. A small proportion of patients had DILI identified as the precipitant of ACLF (2.5%). On admission, the grade of ACLF per CLIF-SOFA for DI-ACLF did not differ significantly from ACLF due to other precipitants, with most patients (67.5%) having ACLF-grade 2. DI-ACLF was categorized as hepatic-ACLF, that is, ACLF precipitated by a hepatic insult and compared with extrahepatic-ACLF. There was little additional detail on patients with DI-ACLF, but this study shed light on potential differences in ACLF outcomes based on hepatic and extrahepatic precipitants. Interestingly, CLIF-SOFA scores were significantly higher in the extrahepatic-ACLF group, leading to significantly higher 90-day and 1-year mortality rates. However, 28-day mortality was comparable between hepatic and extrahepatic ACLF.[33]

In another study, 890 patients with hepatitis B-related cirrhosis and acute decompensation were followed and the investigators compared the clinical course of those with ACLF ($n = 300$) on admission to those without ACLF ($n = 590$).[34] The overall rates of hepatotoxic drug or herbal agent intake within the last 3 months before admission did not differ significantly between the ACLF group (2.3%) and the non-ACLF group (1.4%). Within the ACLF subgroup, the rates of hepatotoxic drug or herbal agent intake were also similar and the rates of grade 1, 2, and 3 DI-ACLF were 1.8%, 0.7%, and 5.1%, respectively. Among the patients without ACLF on admission, the use of hepatotoxic drugs and herbals was not found to be an independent predictor of developing subsequent ACLF during hospitalization.[34]

Lastly, a recent retrospective study from Thailand identified 343 patients with ACLF per the EASL-CLIF definition.[35] Hepatotoxic drugs were the acute precipitant in 3 (0.9%) cases. Similar to the study by Shi and colleagues, the investigators classified ACLF into hepatic ($n = 44$), including drug-induced and extrahepatic-ACLF ($n = 244$). Of note, patients with hepatic-ACLF had significantly higher bilirubin and CLIF-SOFA scores than the non-hepatic ACLF group, with a higher percentage of ACLF-grade 3 and 28-day mortality. In an exploratory analysis, the investigators found that 95% of patients with hepatic-ACLF had extrahepatic organ failure and experienced significantly higher 28-day mortality (69%) than patients with extrahepatic-ACLF (49%).[35]

In an interesting single-center retrospective study from Singapore, the investigators examined ACLF using both APASL and EASL-CLIF criteria.[36] Among 78 patients with ACLF meeting either definition, 49 met both, 14 met APASL only and 15 EASL-CLIF only. Underlying liver disease was more likely viral in the APASL (79%) group versus EASL-CLIF (51%) defined ACLF groups. In total, six (7.7%) patients had traditional Chinese medicine as the precipitating event for ACLF. Clinically, the overall rate of exposure to traditional Chinese medicine was not significantly different between those who died of or survived their ACLF episode, at 11% and 3%, respectively.[36]

North American Consortium for the Study of End-Stage Liver Disease Defined Acute-on-Chronic Liver Failure

The North American Consortium for the Study of End-Stage Liver Disease NACSELD definition was derived prospectively from a hospitalized cohort of patients with cirrhosis and infection. Data are not available on DI-ACLF as DILI was not examined as an acute precipitant of ACLF in this study.[28]

Chinese Society for Hepatology Defined Drug-Induced Acute-on-Chronic Liver Failure

The Chinese Society for Hepatology defines ACLF as an acute decompensation in liver function in patients with diagnosed or undiagnosed CLD with jaundice and coagulopathy.[37] During a 10-year period, a total of 1934 patients with ACLF were prospectively identified in this cross-sectional study, with hepatitis B as the leading precipitant of ACLF (73%). Only 35 (1.8%) cases were drug-induced, and among those herbal or traditional Chinese medications were the most common implicated agents.[37] In a retrospective study using the same definition, 857 Chinese patients with ACLF were identified, 9 (1.1%) of which were related to DILI, though the implicated agents were not specified.[38] Like other studies, little data are shed on patients with DI-ACLF, including mortality, likely due to the limited number of patients with suspected DILI within these cohorts.

In summary, DILI contributes to a limited extent to the burden of ACLF globally. Common themes are evident, including differences among patients with ACLF globally with respect to underlying liver disease (more common viral disease in the east), precipitating factors (viral hepatitis in the east), and class of implicated agents (antituberculosis, HDS, or CAM in the east). However, mortality rates seem to be high regardless of ACLF precipitants.

TREATMENT OF DRUG-INDUCED ACUTE-ON-CHRONIC LIVER FAILURE

The treatment of DI-ACLF is focused on treating the precipitating factor, DILI, and on the management of organ failure and the underlying liver disease. LT may need to be considered as well.

Treatment of Drug-Induced Liver Injury

The mainstay of the treatment of DILI is withdrawal of the offending agent which can result in full recovery in the majority (80%) of patients without long-term complications.[12] The American Association for Study of Liver Disease (AASLD) summarizes general therapies for DILI, beyond drug withdrawal and supportive measures.

A. *N-acetylcysteine*: In adults with non-acetaminophen DILI and acute liver failure, N-acetylcysteine infusion which has been shown to significantly improve transplant-free survival in patients with mild encephalopathy.[39] Of note, NAC was associated with increased mortality in children age less than 2 years with non-acetaminophen DILI and acute liver failure.[40]
B. *Corticosteroids*: Corticosteroids are specifically recommended in patients with checkpoint inhibitor-related DILI and in patients with severe hypersensitivity reactions such as drug reaction with eosinophilia and systemic symptoms. They are also commonly used in cases of DILI with autoimmune hepatitis like features, although there is no prospective randomized data supporting this practice.[12]

The AASLD also summarizes drug-specific interventions for DILI.

A. L-carnitine for valproate hepatotoxicity with hyperammonemia. Short-term use of L-carnitine in acute valproate overdose may be useful in patients with altered mentation and hyperammonemia.[41]
B. Cholestyramine for leflunomide/teriflunomide DILI. Leflunomide is associated with prolonged half-life due to intrahepatic recirculation. To facilitate drug withdrawal cholestyramine is beneficial by augmenting improving drug washout.[42]
C. Penicillin intravenously, silymarin or dialysis for amanita mushroom poisoning. Although there is no definitive antidote for amanita mushroom poisoning, in addition to supportive care, detoxification therapies, and treatments are commonly used. Extracorporeal purification procedures such as dialysis or molecular adsorbent recirculating systems have been used. Pharmacologic therapies to displace amanita from transmembrane transport into hepatic sites have shown efficacy, with agents like penicillin G and silymarin.[43] There may also be a role for NAC as an antioxidant and free radical scavenger.

Treatment of Acute-and-Chronic Liver Failure

Patients with ACLF are critically ill and draw on multidisciplinary expertise in critical care. Although treatment is largely supportive, it remains highly complex and multifaceted. The recent ACG guidelines outline general approaches to management of ACLF, and though not specific to DI-ACLF provide a detailed approach to the principles of management.[27]

Treatment of the Underlying Liver Disease

The acuity of insult in patients with ACLF may be expected to limit the benefits of the treatment of the underlying liver disease. Such treatment options are also likely quite limited outside of previously untreated viral hepatitis such as hepatitis B or previously unrecognized autoimmune hepatitis. Nevertheless, this is an important consideration in a systematic approach to management of DI-ACLF and data are currently lacking.

Liver Transplantation for Drug-Induced-Acute-on-Chronic Liver Failure

There are a number of important considerations in LT for ACLF. Although all patients with ACLF should be considered for LT, one must consider the prognosis of ACLF without LT, where patients with low-grade ACLF may recover, and conversely the potential futility of LT in high-grade ACLF carrying high risk for poor outcomes even with LT. Here, definitions of ACLF that provide grading and prognostic scores such as EASL-CLIF and NAC-SELD are helpful in these considerations. At present, there are no well-defined criteria for LT futility, and the appropriateness of LT should be considered on a case-by-case basis. Another important observation is that MELD does not predict short-term mortality in ACLF as well as it does in other patients with cirrhosis (particularly at relatively low MELD).[44] ACLF does not afford special consideration for organ allocation on the transplant list. Finally, underlying cirrhosis precludes the ability to list patients as status 1a, even if they otherwise meet criteria for acute liver failure as a result of DILI, further limiting organ allocation priority in these patients with high mortality.

SUMMARY

Although DI-ACLF is not common, it is increasingly recognized within the relatively new field of ACLF. Heterogeneity in the field abounds due to challenges in reliably diagnosing DILI and differing diagnostic criteria for ACLF. In global terms, there are differences in underlying chronic liver conditions and precipitating classes of agents in patients with DI-ACLF. The contrasts in DI-ACLF between East and West are driven by different prevalence of viral hepatitis and culturally driven patterns of medication, HDS, or CAM use.

Refinement in adjudication of DILI with more widespread availability of high-quality information on hepatotoxicity, for example, LiverTox, and anticipated assistance from semi-automated scoring systems, for example, RECAM, will aid with timely diagnosis of DILI in patients with ACLF. Conversely wider adoption of more inclusive definitions of ACLF will homogenize reporting in this field and allow for comparative and systemic analysis. In combination, these factors may enhance the volume and quality of data on DI-ACLF and pave the road for a better understanding of potentially unique characteristics, specific needs, and prognosis in this important condition.

CLINICS CARE POINTS

- The treatment of DI-ACLF focuses on treating the precipitating factor, DILI, and on the management of organ failures.

- Withdrawing the offending agent is the mainstay of DILI treatment..
- N-acetylcysteine can be used in adults with non-acetaminophen DILI and acute liver failure to increase transplant-free survival, but it should be avoided in children under the age of 2 with non-acetaminphen DILI and acute liver failure as it has been shown to increase mortality.
- Corticosteroids are recommended in patients with checkpoint inhibitor-related DILI and in patients with drug reaction with eosinophillia and systemic symptoms.-L-carnitine can be used for valproate hepatotoxicity with hyperammonemia.
- Cholestyramine can be used for leflunomide/teriflunomide DILI to facilitate drug washout.
- The treatment of DI-ACLF does not differ from ACLF of other causes and relies on a multidisciplinary approach in critical care.

FINANCIAL SUPPORT

None.

DISCLOSURE

None of the authors have relevant disclosures with the following exceptions. Nonrelevant for Dr N. Chalasani. For disclosure, he reports paid consulting agreements with Abbvie, Zydus, Galectin, Lilly, Boehringer-Ingelheim, Altimmune, Foresite, and Madrigal. He has research support from DSM, the Netherlands, Exact Sciences, and Galectin. He has equity in RestUp, LLC and Avant Sante, LLC.

AUTHOR CONTRIBUTIONS

Study design: All authors. Data analysis: All authors. Article drafting: All authors. Data interpretation and review and revision of the manuscript: All authors.

REFERENCES

1. Chalasani N, Bonkovsky HL, Fontana R, et al. Features and outcomes of 899 patients with drug-induced liver injury: the DILIN prospective study. Gastroenterology 2015;148:1340–13452 e7.
2. Navarro VJ, Khan I, Bjornsson E, et al. Liver injury from herbal and dietary supplements. Hepatology 2017;65:363–73.
3. Medina-Caliz I, Garcia-Cortes M, Gonzalez-Jimenez A, et al. Herbal and dietary supplement-induced liver injuries in the Spanish DILI Registry. Clin Gastroenterol Hepatol 2018;16:1495–502.
4. Andrade RJ, Ortega-Alonso A, Lucena MI. Drug-Induced Liver Injury Clinical Consortia: a global research response for a worldwide health challenge. Expert Opin Drug Metab Toxicol 2016;12:589–93.
5. Shen T, Liu Y, Shang J, et al. Incidence and etiology of drug-induced liver injury in mainland China. Gastroenterology 2019;156:2230–2241 e11.
6. LiverTox: clinical and research information on drug-induced liver injury. Bethesda, MD: National Institutes of Health.
7. Hoofnagle JH, Bjornsson ES. Drug-induced liver injury - types and phenotypes. N Engl J Med 2019;381:264–73.
8. Bjornsson ES, Bergmann OM, Bjornsson HK, et al. Incidence, presentation, and outcomes in patients with drug-induced liver injury in the general population of Iceland. Gastroenterology 2013;144:1419–25, 1425 e1-1425;quiz e19-20.

9. Moreau R, Jalan R, Gines P, et al. Acute-on-chronic liver failure is a distinct syndrome that develops in patients with acute decompensation of cirrhosis. Gastroenterology 2013;144:1426–37, 1437 e1-9.

10. Devarbhavi H, Aithal G, Treeprasertsuk S, et al. Drug-induced liver injury: Asia pacific association of study of liver consensus guidelines. Hepatol Int 2021;15: 258–82.

11. European Association for the Study of the Liver. Electronic address eee, Clinical Practice Guideline Panel: Chair, Panel Members, et al. EASL Clinical Practice Guidelines: drug-induced liver injury. J Hepatol 2019;70:1222–61.

12. Fontana RJ, Liou I, Reuben A, et al. AASLD practice guidance on drug, herbal, and dietary supplement-induced liver injury. Hepatology 2022;77(3):1036–65.

13. Danan G, Benichou C. Causality assessment of adverse reactions to drugs–I. A novel method based on the conclusions of international consensus meetings: application to drug-induced liver injuries. J Clin Epidemiol 1993;46:1323–30.

14. Hayashi PH, Lucena MI, Fontana RJ, et al. A revised electronic version of RUCAM for the diagnosis of DILI. Hepatology 2022;76:18–31.

15. Hayashi PH, Barnhart HX, Fontana RJ, et al. Reliability of causality assessment for drug, herbal and dietary supplement hepatotoxicity in the Drug-Induced Liver Injury Network (DILIN). Liver Int 2015;35:1623–32.

16. Zimmerman HJ. The spectrum of hepatotoxicity. Perspect Biol Med 1968;12: 135–61.

17. Reuben A, Koch DG, Lee WM, et al. Drug-induced acute liver failure: results of a U.S. multicenter, prospective study. Hepatology 2010;52:2065–76.

18. Chalasani N, Aljadhey H, Kesterson J, et al. Patients with elevated liver enzymes are not at higher risk for statin hepatotoxicity. Gastroenterology 2004;126: 1287–92.

19. Lammert C, Imler T, Teal E, et al. Patients with chronic liver disease suggestive of nonalcoholic fatty liver disease may Be at higher risk for drug-induced liver injury. Clin Gastroenterol Hepatol 2019;17:2814–5.

20. Tarantino G, Conca P, Basile V, et al. A prospective study of acute drug-induced liver injury in patients suffering from non-alcoholic fatty liver disease. Hepatol Res 2007;37:410–5.

21. Bessone F, Dirchwolf M, Rodil MA, et al. Review article: drug-induced liver injury in the context of nonalcoholic fatty liver disease - a physiopathological and clinical integrated view. Aliment Pharmacol Ther 2018;48:892–913.

22. Wang NT, Huang YS, Lin MH, et al. Chronic hepatitis B infection and risk of antituberculosis drug-induced liver injury: systematic review and meta-analysis. J Chin Med Assoc 2016;79:368–74.

23. Zimmerman HJ. Effects of alcohol on other hepatotoxins. Alcohol Clin Exp Res 1986;10:3–15.

24. Stephens C, Robles-Diaz M, Medina-Caliz I, et al. Comprehensive analysis and insights gained from long-term experience of the Spanish DILI Registry. J Hepatol 2021;75:86–97.

25. Sarin SK, Choudhury A, Sharma MK, et al. Acute-on-chronic liver failure: consensus recommendations of the Asian Pacific association for the study of the liver (APASL): an update. Hepatol Int 2019;13:353–90.

26. Jalan R, Yurdaydin C, Bajaj JS, et al. Toward an improved definition of acute-on-chronic liver failure. Gastroenterology 2014;147:4–10.

27. Bajaj JS, O'Leary JG, Lai JC, et al. Acute-on-chronic liver failure clinical guidelines. Am J Gastroenterol 2022;117:225–52.

28. Bajaj JS, O'Leary JG, Reddy KR, et al. Survival in infection-related acute-on-chronic liver failure is defined by extrahepatic organ failures. Hepatology 2014; 60:250–6.
29. Shalimar, Kumar D, Vadiraja PK, et al. Acute on chronic liver failure because of acute hepatic insults: etiologies, course, extrahepatic organ failure and predictors of mortality. J Gastroenterol Hepatol 2016;31:856–64.
30. Shalimar, Saraswat V, Singh SP, et al. Acute-on-chronic liver failure in India: the indian national association for study of the liver consortium experience. J Gastroenterol Hepatol 2016;31:1742–9.
31. Devarbhavi H, Choudhury AK, Sharma MK, et al. Drug-induced acute-on-chronic liver failure in Asian patients. Am J Gastroenterol 2019;114:929–37.
32. Mezzano G, Juanola A, Cardenas A, et al. Global burden of disease: acute-on-chronic liver failure, a systematic review and meta-analysis. Gut 2022;71:148–55.
33. Shi Y, Yang Y, Hu Y, et al. Acute-on-chronic liver failure precipitated by hepatic injury is distinct from that precipitated by extrahepatic insults. Hepatology 2015;62:232–42.
34. Li H, Chen LY, Zhang NN, et al. Characteristics, diagnosis and prognosis of acute-on-chronic liver failure in cirrhosis associated to hepatitis B. Sci Rep 2016;6:25487.
35. Maipang K, Potranun P, Chainuvati S, et al. Validation of the prognostic models in acute-on-chronic liver failure precipitated by hepatic and extrahepatic insults. PLoS One 2019;14:e0219516.
36. Selva Rajoo A, Lim SG, Phyo WW, et al. Acute-on-chronic liver failure in a multi-ethnic Asian city: a comparison of patients identified by Asia-pacific association for the study of the liver and European association for the study of the liver definitions. World J Hepatol 2017;9:1133–40.
37. Qin G, Shao JG, Zhu YC, et al. Population-representative incidence of acute-on-chronic liver failure: a prospective cross-sectional study. J Clin Gastroenterol 2016;50:670–5.
38. Xia Q, Dai X, Zhang Y, et al. A modified MELD model for Chinese pre-ACLF and ACLF patients and it reveals poor prognosis in pre-ACLF patients. PLoS One 2013;8:e64379.
39. Lee WM, Hynan LS, Rossaro L, et al. Intravenous N-acetylcysteine improves transplant-free survival in early stage non-acetaminophen acute liver failure. Gastroenterology 2009;137:856–64, 864 e1.
40. Squires RH, Dhawan A, Alonso E, et al. Intravenous N-acetylcysteine in pediatric patients with nonacetaminophen acute liver failure: a placebo-controlled clinical trial. Hepatology 2013;57:1542–9.
41. Lheureux PER, Penaloza A, Zahir S, et al. Science review: carnitine in the treatment of valproic acid-induced toxicity – what is the evidence? Crit Care 2005; 9:431.
42. Laub M, Fraser R, Kurche J, et al. Use of a cholestyramine washout in a patient with septic shock on leflunomide therapy:A case report and review of the literature. J Intensive Care Med 2016;31:412–4.
43. Santi L, Maggioli C, Mastroroberto M, et al. Acute liver failure caused by amanita phalloides poisoning. Int J Hepatol 2012;2012:487480.
44. Abdallah MA, Kuo YF, Asrani S, et al. Validating a novel score based on interaction between ACLF grade and MELD score to predict waitlist mortality. J Hepatol 2021;74:1355–61.
45. Maria VA, Victorino RM. Development and validation of a clinical scale for the diagnosis of drug-induced hepatitis. Hepatology 1997;26:664–9.

46. Hanatani T, Sai K, Tohkin M, et al. A detection algorithm for drug-induced liver injury in medical information databases using the Japanese diagnostic scale and its comparison with the Council for International Organizations of Medical Sciences/the Roussel Uclaf Causality Assessment Method scale. Pharmacoepidemiol Drug Saf 2014;23:984–8.

47. Takikawa H, Takamori Y, Kumagi T, et al. Assessment of 287 Japanese cases of drug induced liver injury by the diagnostic scale of the International Consensus Meeting. Hepatol Res 2003;27:192–5.

Nonviral or Drug-Induced Etiologies of Acute-on-Chronic Liver Failure (Autoimmune, Vascular, and Malignant)

Suzanne A. Elshafey, MD, MPH, Robert S. Brown Jr, MD, MPH*

KEYWORDS

- Acute on chronic • Liver failure • Budd–Chiari syndrome • Portal vein thrombosis
- Autoimmune hepatitis • Malignancy

KEY POINTS

- After common reasons are excluded, patients should be evaluated for additional causes of acute-on-chronic liver failure including vascular etiologies, autoimmune hepatitis, and malignancy-related causes.
- The mainstay of therapy for Budd–Chiari syndrome and portal vein thrombosis is anticoagulation; advanced interventional therapies should be considered in patients with significant decompensation.
- Malignancy-related acute-on-chronic liver failure has a poor prognosis with limited treatment options.

INTRODUCTION

Most cases of acute-on-chronic liver failure (ACLF) are due to infection, alcohol, and viral etiologies. However, the additional causes of ACLF include vascular, autoimmune hepatitis (AIH), and malignancy. These causes are rare but important to consider in patients who present with acute liver decompensation as they have both therapeutic and prognostic significance.

VASCULAR

Vascular causes of ACLF are relatively uncommon. The liver's dual blood supply is a protective factor, but in patients with chronic liver disease and underlying cirrhosis,

Division of Gastroenterology and Hepatology, Weill Cornell Medicine, 1305 York Avenue, 4th Floor, New York, NY 10021, USA
* Corresponding author.
E-mail address: Rsb2005@med.cornell.edu
Twitter: @drbobbybrown (R.S.B.)

Clin Liver Dis 27 (2023) 649–657
https://doi.org/10.1016/j.cld.2023.03.008
1089-3261/23/© 2023 Elsevier Inc. All rights reserved.

vascular insults can contribute to significant decompensation and rapid deterioration. Vascular etiologies include Budd–Chiari syndrome (BCS) and portal vein thrombosis (PVT).

BCS is defined by hepatic venous outflow obstruction, classically resulting from thromboses of one or more of the hepatic veins as they drain into the inferior vena cava. The prevalence of BCS is estimated to be 1 per million per year.[1] In a retrospective, population-based study, cirrhosis was present in 18.7% ($n = 1577$) of patients presenting with BCS from 1998 to 2017.[2] In a small, single-center retrospective cohort study, 26 patients (55.3%) had underlying cirrhosis. The presence of cirrhosis at diagnosis was a significant predictor of poor prognosis (need for liver transplantation or death) with an odds ratio of 6.25 (95% CI 1.19–32.72, $P = 0.030$).[3] The etiology is most commonly thrombotic in nature secondary to hypercoagulable states and myeloproliferative disorders including polycythemia vera, Janus tyrosine kinase 2 mutations, antiphospholipid syndrome, antithrombin deficiency, factor V Leiden mutation, lupus anticoagulant, protein C/S deficiency, among others. Although uncommon in Western countries, membranous obstruction of the inferior vena cava accounts for a significant number of BCS cases in Africa and Asia. Other causes include infections and malignancy.

Clinical features represent sequelae of impaired hepatic venous drainage, increased sinusoidal pressure, and portal hypertension. Patients can present with new or worsening ascites, hepatomegaly, pain, and/or gastrointestinal bleeding. Clinical presentation can vary depending on the disease duration and severity. Chronic untreated BCS can itself cause chronic liver disease. Patients with subacute or chronic progression may present insidiously due to the development of portal and hepatic venous collaterals. The triad of acute liver failure (ALF), tender hepatomegaly, and ascites should raise suspicion for BCS, which may be confounded or absent in patients with underlying liver disease. Laboratories may show minimal or no transaminase elevation. Paracentesis protein studies may offer a diagnostic clue. As with other causes of portal hypertensive (sinusoidal or post-sinusoidal) source of ascites, the serum-ascites albumin gradient is greater than or equal to 1.1. In early BCS, the ascitic total protein is typically greater than 2.5 g/dL but often is lower in late BCS.

Doppler ultrasound is the preferred initial diagnostic modality. Contrast-enhanced computed tomography (CT) or MRI can also be performed to confirm the diagnosis. Hepatic venography can be performed in cases where the diagnosis remains unclear. Liver biopsy is generally not indicated. If BCS is diagnosed, workup for an underlying cause should be pursued. An underlying disorder can be identified in the majority of cases. Evaluation includes serologic and imaging workup for acquired and inherited thrombotic conditions as well as space occupying or compressive lesions.

If BCS diagnosis is confirmed or clinical suspicion is high, anticoagulation should be initiated immediately to treat existing thrombus and prevent clot extension/propagation. Additional treatments depend on clinical, patient, and anatomic factors. A step-wise approach is recommended.[4] Additional treatments include thrombolysis, angioplasty/stenting, and transjugular intrahepatic portosystemic shunt (TIPS) or surgical shunting. In severe cases of fulminant liver failure, evaluation for liver transplantation may be considered. Treatment of underlying and predisposing conditions should also be pursued. TIPS has emerged as a treatment of choice when medical therapy alone is not sufficient. In a cohort of 157 patients with BCS, 62 patients underwent TIPS (39.5%) for refractory ascites, liver failure, and portal hypertension (eg, variceal) bleeding. Four of the patients subsequently underwent rescue liver transplantation but of the remaining 58 patients, 48 (83%) were alive after a median follow-up of 51 months (range, 0.3–69 months). Ten patients died within 5.8 months (range, 0.2–39 months). One, 3-, and 5-year survival and orthotopic liver transplantation (OLT)-free survival of patients treated with TIPS was 88%, 83%, and 72% and 85%, 78%, and 72%, respectively. When comparing overall survival or transplant-free survival, no differences were observed in patients with TIPS performed before or after the first month after diagnosis.[5] Although histologic data were only available for 39 study patients, evidence of cirrhosis was present in seven patients (18%).[6]

PVT can be complete or partial and most commonly occurs in the presence of cirrhosis or underlying advanced liver disease. Cirrhosis is an independent risk factor for thrombosis due to perturbations in flow and alterations in hemostatic cascades. In patients with cirrhosis (and without hepatocellular carcinoma), PVT has a prevalence of 10% to 25%.[7] The thrombus may be isolated to the portal vein or it may extend to involve the splenic or mesenteric veins. Factor V Leiden G1691A mutation and prothrombin G20210A mutation have been identified in patients with cirrhosis and PVT.[8,9]

Clinical presentation most commonly includes exacerbation of underlying cirrhosis and portal hypertension including acute variceal hemorrhage (most common), hepatic encephalopathy, renal failure including hepatorenal syndrome, and/or ascites. Pain is less likely unless concomitant mesenteric ischemia is present due to involvement of the superior mesenteric vein and its tributaries. Diagnosis can be made on Doppler ultrasound or contrast-enhanced cross-sectional imaging. Cavernous transformation (formation of multiple small collateral vessels) is characteristic of chronic PVT and not typically seen in acute presentations. In clinically stable patients, upper endoscopy should be performed to assess for high-risk varices, followed by endoscopic variceal ligation if indicated or nonselective beta-blocker prophylaxis.

In patients with no other indication for TIPS, anticoagulation is the mainstay of therapy. Anticoagulation should be initiated in patients with cirrhosis and acute or subacute occlusive PVT who do not have contraindications (**Fig. 1**). The decision to treat with anticoagulation should consider patient factors, comorbidities, bleeding risk (prior history of bleeding and severe thrombocytopenia <50,000/mm^3) and transplantation potential, among other considerations. Anticoagulation agents include low molecular weight heparin (LMWH), direct-acting oral anticoagulants (DOACs), and vitamin K antagonists (VKA). In critically ill patients with acute decompensation, LMWH or unfractionated heparin (UFH) may be prudent in the event of bleeding complications due to the drug half-life and availability of reversal agents. In patients with concomitant severe renal impairment or evolving renal failure, UFH may be the preferred agent although baseline prolonged activated partial thromboplastin time can make dosing and adjustment challenging.

The primary challenge in VKA use is that in patients with cirrhosis or advanced liver disease, the baseline prothrombin time is typically prolonged, leading to possible drug underdosing. The target treatment international normalized ratio is typically narrow (2.0–3.0, target 2.5). Further, dose response can be variable and require multiple adjustments and frequent monitoring.

Clinical interest in the use of DOACs in patients with cirrhosis is growing, but randomized controlled studies examining their use and comparing them to other agents in patients with cirrhosis are lacking. Martinez and colleagues[10] described a case of a 55-year-old man with Child-Pugh class A cirrhosis and acute PVT extending to the superior mesenteric vein treated with 6 weeks of rivaroxaban with complete resolution of the clot on follow-up CT scan and no bleeding complications during the treatment period. Similar outcomes have been described in additional case studies in patients with Child-Pugh class A cirrhosis and acute PVT.[11,12] However, these cases described DOAC use in patients with relatively low MELD and preserved renal function. DOAC-related bleeding maybe particularly challenging in patients with underlying advanced

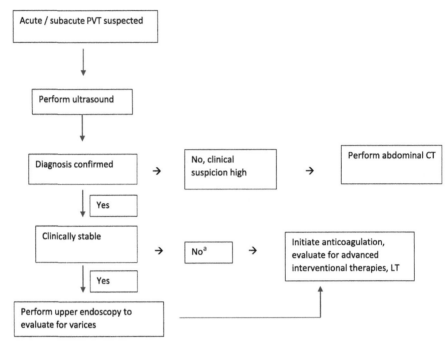

Fig. 1. Algorithm for diagnosis and treatment of PVT. [a]Significant decompensation with rapid decline, organ failure, suspected secondary to thrombosis.

liver disease. Select antidotes are available (andexanet alfa), but the cost is high and they may not be accessible at all centers. Prothrombin complex concentrate, which contains concentrated clotting factors, can be used but has the potential risk of thromboses at higher doses. In a small cohort study comparing rates of bleeding in patients with cirrhosis treated with DOACs versus traditional anticoagulation (warfarin and LMWH), no statistically significant difference in bleeding events between the two groups was observed.[13] DOAC use is an evolving area of research in the literature and warrants further investigation. Apixaban may be the preferred agent due to lower rates of bleeding complications in other indications.

Duration of therapy for PVT is a minimum of 6 months. Owing to the risk of rethrombosis, continued anticoagulation beyond this time frame should be considered in patients undergoing evaluation for liver transplantation if no adverse events (eg, bleeding) have occurred during the treatment period.

In a multicenter retrospective case series of treatment of nonmalignant PVT with either warfarin or LMWH in 55 patients with cirrhosis, partial or complete recanalization was achieved in 33 patients (60%). The risk of recurrent thrombosis after complete recanalization is high when anticoagulation therapy is discontinued (38.5%, median time 1 month after anticoagulation cessation). The single factor significantly associated with successful recanalization was early anticoagulation initiation (within 14 days, $P = 0.04$).[14]

Interventional treatments such as TIPS, transjugular/transhepatic thrombolysis, and surgical or interventional thrombectomy can be considered in patients with significant decompensation and severe complications of portal hypertension including refractory ascites, variceal bleeding, and organ decompensation. In a study assessing 70 consecutive patients with cirrhosis and non-tumor PVT treated with TIPS for portal hypertension complications, complete recanalization occurred in 57% of patients. Thirty-eight (95%) patients with complete recanalization after TIPS placement maintained a patent portal vein (mean follow-up of 20.7 months).[15] Ongoing anticoagulation post-TIPS is usually required to maintain TIPS patency but may be lower risk due to resolution/reduction of portal hypertension with successful TIPS.

Transhepatic and transjugular directed thrombolysis for the treatment of acute PVT has been described in case reports. In a retrospective study of 20 patients with acute or subacute PVT and/or mesenteric vein thrombosis, 15 of 20 patients (75%) experienced some degree of lysis. Three patients experienced complete lysis and 12 patients experienced partial lysis. The complication rate was high and 12 patients (60%) developed major complications including need for transfusion and one patient death[16] (see **Fig. 1**).

AUTOIMMUNE

AIH is characterized by an inflammatory injury of the liver. Incidence ranges from 0.7 per 100,000 (Israel) to 2 per 100,000 (New Zealand).[17,18] Although the exact etiology is not known, genetic predisposition and susceptibility alleles in varying populations have been identified. The mechanism is postulated to involve interplay of genetic predisposition, environmental trigger, and immune system dysregulation. The disease primarily affects middle-aged women in the fourth to sixth decade of life, but it can present at any age in either gender. In its chronic form, AIH can lead to advanced liver disease and cirrhosis. Approximately one-third of people with AIH have cirrhosis at the time of presentation.[19] African American patients are more likely to have cirrhosis (57% compared with 38%) and more advanced fibrosis at initial presentation compared with non-African Americans.[20] Patients (and their family members) may have other coexisting autoimmune disorders including autoimmune thyroiditis, Grave's disease, rheumatoid arthritis, and celiac disease.

AIH can present on a clinical spectrum with significant heterogeneity. In patients who remain undiagnosed for years and present with a chronic, insidious form, systemic symptoms such as fatigue, arthralgias, and malaise may be reported. An acute flare of the condition can present with features of ALF superimposed on a cirrhotic or fibrotic liver. Mortality is increased in patients with underlying cirrhosis. In a population-based study in Sweden, AIH individuals with cirrhosis on biopsy had a higher risk of death when compared with matched general population reference individuals (hazard ratio [HR] 4.55, 95% confidence interval [CI] 3.95–5.25).[21] Patients with cirrhosis at baseline have been found to have poorer 10-year survival (61.9% [CI 44.9%–78.9%]) than those without cirrhosis at presentation (94.0% [CI 87.4%–100%]) ($P = .003$) regardless of whether symptomatic at the time of presentation or whether they received immunosuppressive therapy.[22]

Diagnosis is made using a combination of serologic markers, laboratory tests, and liver biopsy. In patients with cirrhosis or advanced disease, elevations in hepatocellular markers (alanine aminotransferase [ALT] and aspartate aminotransferase) are less marked. Bilirubin is often elevated, typically less than three times the upper limit of normal. Alkaline phosphatase elevation may be present, less than twice the upper limit of normal. Hypergammaglobulinemia, particularly immunoglobulin G (IgG), is characteristic. IgM and IgA levels are typically normal. Serologic markers include antinuclear antibody (ANA), smooth muscle antibodies (ASMA), soluble liver antigen, and antibodies to liver-kidney microsomal type 1 (anti-LKM 1). Type 1 AIH is the more frequent type (accounts for 90% of cases) and is associated with positive ANA and ASMA. Type 2 AIH is associated with anti-LKM 1 and anti-liver cytosol type 1 antibody.

Liver biopsy is typically required for diagnosis and has the added benefit of guiding treatment. The hallmark histologic finding on liver biopsy is interface hepatitis (hepatitis at the portal–parenchymal interface). However, this finding is not specific and can be seen in other processes including drug-induced or viral-mediated liver injury. Additional classic findings include a plasma cell-rich lymphoplasmocytic infiltration of the portal tract and hepatocellular rosette formation. Centrilobular zone 3 necrosis may be seen more commonly in patients with acute onset of disease and less in those with cirrhosis (38% vs 10%).[23] Drug-induced hepatitis with immune-mediated mechanisms can mimic AIH on histology. An elevated IgG level and elevated serologic markers (autoantibodies), which are unlikely in drug-induced hepatitis, can be helpful in distinguishing the two entities.

A simplified scoring system was developed in 2008 using a previously validated scoring criteria developed by the International Autoimmune Hepatitis Group (IAHG), which was initially developed for research trials. The scoring system (**Table 1**) evaluates serologic parameters in conjunction with liver histology and exclusion of other etiologies (eg, viral hepatitis). The scoring system has both a high sensitivity (95%) and specificity (90%) and is best used in conjunction with clinical judgement.[24,25] A score- ≥ 6 indicates probable AIH and a score ≥ 7 indicates definite AIH.

Treatment of AIH consists primarily of immunosuppression with systemic steroids and azathioprine. Patients with early inflammatory disease respond best to therapy and can have long-term control of disease. Advanced fibrosis or cirrhosis secondary to AIH is also an indication for treatment. However, steroid treatment is likely to be of little clinical benefit in patients with decompensated cirrhosis or "burned out" inactive disease on histology as assessed by the hepatic activity index. In patients presenting with ACLF, clinical evaluation should be undertaken to rule out infectious etiologies before initiation of immunosuppression.

Prednisolone or prednisone therapy is administered for induction using weight-based dosing (0.5–1 mg/kg/day) followed by the addition of azathioprine 1 to 2 mg/kg. In cases of severe liver decompensation, higher initial steroid doses can be used and delayed azathioprine initiation until clinical response is seen. Improvement in ALT and IgG levels indicate treatment response. In patients with AIH and liver failure, a 1 to 2 week trial of steroids is reasonable, followed by liver transplant (LT) evaluation if no improvement is seen. In a retrospective study of patients with AIH-related ALF, use of glucocorticoids did not improve overall survival (60% with steroids vs 73% without steroids; $P = 0.27$). Steroid use was significantly associated with lower overall survival in high-MELD patients.[26]

Table 1
Simplified autoimmune hepatitis scoring system from the International Autoimmune Hepatitis Group [24]

Parameters	Value	Points
ANA or SMA	$\geq$1:40	1
ANA or SMA *Or* anti-LKM1 Or SLA	$\geq$1:80 $\geq$1:40 Positive	2
IgG	>Upper limit of normal (ULN) >1.10 times ULN	1 2
Absence of viral hepatitis	Yes	2
Liver histology	Compatible with AIH Typical of AIH	1 2

MALIGNANT

The liver is the most common site of metastatic disease in solid tumors, but ACLF secondary to malignancy is relatively rare. Malignant causes of ACLF are primarily related to bulky metastatic disease involvement or diffuse infiltration. Primary malignancies include breast cancer causing pseudocirrhosis, colon cancer, leukemia, and lymphoma.[27] Hematologic malignancies are the most common, primarily non-Hodgkin lymphoma such as diffuse large B cell lymphoma.[28] Patients may also present acutely with liver failure after resection of liver metastases. Malignancy is an added risk factor for thrombosis including BCS and PVT, which can contribute to an acute presentation.

Clinical presentation includes jaundice, hepatic encephalopathy, massive hepatomegaly, and/or splenomegaly. Laboratory values may reveal elevated tumor markers and elevation in alkaline phosphatase and bilirubin in a patient with a history of known cancer, although mixed patterns of injury are possible. In patients with lymphoma, an elevated lactate dehydrogenase may be seen. Diagnosis can be confirmed on imaging with expert radiology review. Infiltrative disease of the liver may be more challenging to detect on imaging. Liver biopsy may be required in certain cases, especially when patients present without known history of malignancy and imaging is nondiagnostic.

Treatment options are limited and typically involve treatment of the underlying malignancy and/or palliative care. The clinical course is often marked by rapid clinical deterioration with multiorgan failure and death. In a case series of 27 patients with malignant infiltration presenting as ALF, 24 patients (89%) died within 3 weeks of onset of liver failure.[29] Liver transplantation for colorectal liver metastases in select cases has been performed, although not typically after the cascade of rapid liver and organ failure has commenced.

SUMMARY

Vascular, AIH and malignancy are relatively uncommon etiologies of ACLF. Among the vascular causes, BCS and PVT are the main causes. Anticoagulation is the mainstay of therapy but patients with liver failure may require interventional therapies and evaluation for transplantation. AIH should be considered in patients with concomitant autoimmune disease and systemic symptoms. Malignant causes can be secondary to infiltration or bulky metastatic disease and have a poor prognosis with high mortality.

CLINICS CARE POINTS

- Noninvasive Doppler ultrasound is the diagnostic test of choice for vascular etiologies of acute-on-chronic liver failure (ACLF).

- Anticoagulation is the mainstay of therapy in Budd–Chiari syndrome and portal vein thrombosis.

- The decision to treat with anticoagulation should consider patient factors, comorbidities, bleeding risk (prior history of bleeding and severe thrombocytopenia <50,000/mm³), and transplantation potential.

- AIH primarily affects middle-aged women in the fourth to sixth decade of life; patients (and their family members) may have other coexisting autoimmune disorders.

- Positive autoantibodies and elevated immunoglobulin G are characteristic of autoimmune hepatitis (AIH). Liver biopsy shows interface hepatitis.

- Treatment of AIH consists primarily of immunosuppression with systemic steroids and azathioprine.

- Malignancy-related infiltration or bulky disease can present with ACLF and is often fatal.

DISCLOSURE

The authors have nothing to disclose.

REFERENCES

1. Li Y, De Stefano V, Li H, et al. Epidemiology of Budd-Chiari syndrome: a systematic review and meta-analysis. Clin Res Hepatol Gastroenterol 2019;43(4): 468–74.
2. Alukal JJ, Zhang T, Thuluvath PJ. A nationwide analysis of Budd-Chiari syndrome in the United States. J Clin Exp Hepatol 2021;11(2):181–7.
3. Pavri TM, Herbst A, Reddy R, et al. Budd-Chiari syndrome: a single-center experience. World J Gastroenterol 2014;20(43):16236–44.
4. Northup PG, Garcia-Pagan JC, Garcia-Tsao G, et al. Vascular liver disorders, portal vein thrombosis, and procedural bleeding in patients with liver disease: 2020 practice guidance by the American Association for the study of liver diseases. Hepatology 2021;73(1):366–413.
5. Seijo S, Plessier A, Hoekstra J, et al. Good long-term outcome of Budd-Chiari syndrome with a step-wise management. Hepatology 2013;57(5):1962–8.
6. Darwish Murad S, Plessier A, Hernandez-Guerra M, et al. Etiology, management, and outcome of the Budd-Chiari syndrome. Ann Intern Med 2009;151(3):167–75.
7. Tsochatzis EA, Senzolo M, Germani G, et al. Systematic review: portal vein thrombosis in cirrhosis. Aliment Pharmacol Ther 2010;31(3):366–74.
8. Amitrano L, Brancaccio V, Guardascione MA, et al. Portal vein thrombosis after variceal endoscopic sclerotherapy in cirrhotic patients: role of genetic thrombophilia. Endoscopy 2002;34(7):535–8.
9. Erkan O, Bozdayi AM, Disibeyaz S, et al. Thrombophilic gene mutations in cirrhotic patients with portal vein thrombosis. Eur J Gastroenterol Hepatol 2005; 17(3):339–43.
10. Martinez M, Tandra A, Vuppalanchi R. Treatment of acute portal vein thrombosis by nontraditional anticoagulation. Hepatology 2014;60(1):425–6.
11. Yang H, Kim SR, Song MJ. Recurrent acute portal vein thrombosis in liver cirrhosis treated by rivaroxaban. Clin Mol Hepatol 2016;22(4):499–502.
12. Intagliata NM, Maitland H, Northup PG, et al. Treating thrombosis in cirrhosis patients with new oral agents: ready or not? Hepatology 2015;61(2):738–9.
13. Intagliata NM, Henry ZH, Maitland H, et al. Direct oral anticoagulants in cirrhosis patients pose similar risks of bleeding when compared to traditional anticoagulation. Dig Dis Sci 2016;61(6):1721–7.
14. Delgado MG, Seijo S, Yepes I, et al. Efficacy and safety of anticoagulation on patients with cirrhosis and portal vein thrombosis. Clin Gastroenterol Hepatol 2012; 10(7):776–83.
15. Luca A, Miraglia R, Caruso S, et al. Short- and long-term effects of the transjugular intrahepatic portosystemic shunt on portal vein thrombosis in patients with cirrhosis. Gut 2011;60(6):846–52.
16. Hollingshead M, Burke CT, Mauro MA, et al. Transcatheter thrombolytic therapy for acute mesenteric and portal vein thrombosis. J Vasc Interv Radiol 2005; 16(5):651–61.

17. Ngu JH, Bechly K, Chapman BA, et al. Population-based epidemiology study of autoimmune hepatitis: a disease of older women? J Gastroenterol Hepatol 2010; 25(10):1681–6.
18. Delgado JS, Vodonos A, Malnick S, et al. Autoimmune hepatitis in southern Israel: a 15-year multicenter study. J Dig Dis 2013;14(11):611–8.
19. European association for the study of the liver. EASL clinical practice guidelines: autoimmune hepatitis. J Hepatol 2015;63(4):971–1004.
20. Verma S, Torbenson M, Thuluvath PJ. The impact of ethnicity on the natural history of autoimmune hepatitis. Hepatology 2007;46(6):1828–35.
21. Sharma R, Verna EC, Söderling J, et al. Increased mortality risk in autoimmune hepatitis: a nationwide population-based cohort study with histopathology. Clin Gastroenterol Hepatol 2021;19(12):2636–47.e13.
22. Feld JJ, Dinh H, Arenovich T, et al. Autoimmune hepatitis: effect of symptoms and cirrhosis on natural history and outcome. Hepatology 2005;42(1):53–62.
23. Hofer H, Oesterreicher C, Wrba F, et al. Centrilobular necrosis in autoimmune hepatitis: a histological feature associated with acute clinical presentation. J Clin Pathol 2006;59(3):246–9.
24. Hennes EM, Zeniya M, Czaja AJ, et al. Simplified criteria for the diagnosis of autoimmune hepatitis. Hepatology 2008;48(1):169–76.
25. Czaja AJ. Performance parameters of the diagnostic scoring systems for autoimmune hepatitis. Hepatology 2008;48(5):1540–8.
26. Karkhanis J, Verna EC, Chang MS, et al. Steroid use in acute liver failure. Hepatology 2014;59(2):612–21.
27. Wendon J, Panel members, Cordoba J, Dhawan A, et al. Clinical Practice Guidelines Panel, EASL Clinical Practical Guidelines on the management of acute (fulminant) liver failure. J Hepatol 2017;66(5):1047–81.
28. Bernardo S, Carvalhana S, Antunes T, et al. A rare cause of acute liver failure- a case report. BMC Gastroenterol 2017;17(1):166.
29. Rich NE, Sanders C, Hughes RS, et al. Malignant infiltration of the liver presenting as acute liver failure. Clin Gastroenterol Hepatol 2015;13(5):1025–8.

Acute on Chronic Liver Failure in Patients with Alcohol-Associated Hepatitis
A Review

Camille A. Kezer, MD, Douglas A. Simonetto, MD,
Vijay H. Shah, MD*

KEYWORDS

- Acute on chronic liver failure • Acute liver failure • Alcohol-associated liver disease
- Alcohol • Cirrhosis • Chronic liver disease • Inflammation • Cytokine
- Immune system

KEY POINTS

- ACLF is a process where patients with chronic liver disease or cirrhosis develop rapid decompensation in liver function with extrahepatic organ failures.
- ACLF can be precipitated by a variety of insults, both hepatic and systemic; these include alcohol-associated hepatitis which results in unique pathophysiology related to the immune response.
- Treatment of alcohol-associated hepatitis ACLF centers on supportive care at this time.

OVERVIEW OF ACUTE ON CHRONIC LIVER FAILURE
Background

Liver failure is an increasingly common cause of morbidity and mortality and can broadly be divided into acute liver failure (ALF), acute on chronic liver failure (ACLF), and acute decompensation in end-stage liver disease.[1] **Fig. 1** summarizes a comparison of the types of liver failure. In contrast to ALF wherein there is no preexisting liver disease, ACLF is a distinct disease process in which patients with either chronic liver disease or cirrhosis undergo a rapid decompensation in hepatic function accompanied by extrahepatic organ failure.[2] Furthermore, ACLF differs from the natural history of cirrhosis, which progresses irreversibly to end-stage disease; in ACLF, there is a component of reversibility with early identification and aggressive support.[3] The accurate diagnosis of ACLF is critical because it is associated with high short-term

Division of Gastroenterology and Hepatology, Mayo Clinic, 200 First Street Southwest, Rochester, MN, USA
* Corresponding author.
E-mail address: shah.vijay@mayo.edu

Clin Liver Dis 27 (2023) 659–670
https://doi.org/10.1016/j.cld.2023.03.009
1089-3261/23/© 2023 Elsevier Inc. All rights reserved.

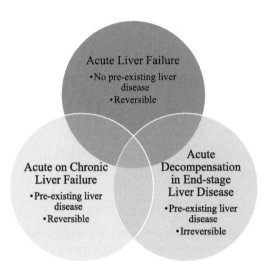

Fig. 1. Comparison of types of liver failure.

mortality. The CANONIC trial, a study of more than 1300 patients hospitalized with cirrhosis and acute decompensation in 8 European countries, found the 28-day mortality rate in patients with ACLF to be 34%.[4]

Variability in Definitions

Despite the acceptance of the concept of ACLF, there is a variety of definitions of ACLF in the literature. Four distinct definitions of ACLF have been proposed by different groups including North American, European, Asian Pacific, and Chinese groups.[5] The North American Consortium for the Study of End-stage Liver Disease defines ACLF as decompensated cirrhosis with 2 or more organ system failures (organ systems include kidney, brain, circulation, and respiration).[5,6] The European Association for the Study of Liver (EASL)—Chronic Liver Failure Consortium defines ACLF as patients with acutely decompensated cirrhosis and failure of 1 of 6 major organ systems (organ systems include liver, kidney, brain, coagulation, circulation, and respiration) with greater than 15% 28-day mortality.[2,4,5] The Asian Pacific Association for the Study of Liver (APASL) ACLF Research Consortium defines ACLF as patients with compensated cirrhosis or noncirrhotic chronic liver disease with a first episode of acute liver deterioration due to an acute hepatic insult, and while they may develop extrahepatic organ failures, these are not included in the definition.[1,5] The Chinese Group on the Study of Severe Hepatitis B defines ACLF in patients with hepatitis B virus (HBV) as acute decompensation of HBV-related chronic liver disease, with or without cirrhosis, with failure of 1 of the 6 major organ systems (organ systems include liver, kidney, brain, coagulation, circulation, and respiration).[5,7] The North American, European, and Chinese consortia all include intrahepatic and extrahepatic causes of ACLF and consider both hepatic and extrahepatic organ failures.[5] The APASL considers patients with cirrhosis and noncirrhotic chronic liver disease but excludes patients with extrahepatic causes of ACLF and those with kidney, circulatory, or respiratory failures are excluded as well.[5]

Due to the variability in classification of ACLF including the definition of chronic liver disease and cirrhosis, timing of precipitating injury, inclusion of organ failures, whether intrahepatic or extrahepatic, the World Gastroenterology Organization proposed a more unified definition of ACLF.[2] They define ACLF as "a syndrome in patients with chronic liver disease with or without previously diagnosed cirrhosis characterized by acute hepatic decompensation resulting in liver failure (jaundice and prolongation of the international normalized ratio), and one or more extrahepatic organ failures, that is associated with increased risk for mortality within a period of 28 days and up to 3 months from onset."[2,8,9]

Pathophysiology of Acute on Chronic Liver Failure

The pathophysiology of ACLF has been described using a 4-part model, the PIRO concept of ACLF (**Fig. 2**), consisting of predisposition, injury, response, and organ failure.[2,10] In this model, there is a predisposing factor to ACLF such as underlying cirrhosis. There is then an injury by a precipitating event. There is a variety of insults, both hepatic and systemic, which can precipitate ACLF. Hepatic insults include alcohol-associated hepatitis (AH), drug-induced liver injury, viral hepatitis, portal vein thrombosis, and ischemic hepatitis.[10] Extrahepatic insults include trauma, surgery, variceal bleeding, and infection.[10] The precipitating event is estimated to be identifiable in approximately 50% of patients.[2] This precipitating event leads to an inflammatory response and ultimately organ failure.[10] The remainder of this review will focus on ACLF in patients with AH.

PRECIPITANTS OF ACUTE ON CHRONIC LIVER FAILURE IN PATIENTS WITH ALCOHOL-ASSOCIATED LIVER DISEASE
Alcohol Consumption

In the CANONIC European observational study, active heavy alcohol consumption, considered as more than 14 drinks per week in women and more than 21 drinks per week in men, within the preceding 3 months was considered the second most frequent event precipitating ACLF, second only to bacterial infection.[4,11] It is unknown

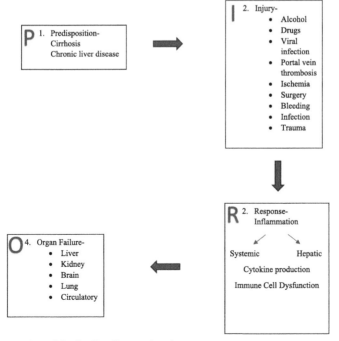

Fig. 2. The 4-part model of ACLF disease development.

whether the alcohol consumption is a precipitant independent of AH because few liver biopsies are done in most studies evaluating patients with ACLF.[11] Therefore, at this time, it remains uncertain whether ACLF is a form of alcohol-associated liver disease (ALD) or a part of the natural history of severe AH.[11] It is clear, however, that AH is a common precipitant of ACLF and pertains a poor prognosis in these patients.

Alcohol-Associated Hepatitis

Severe AH is a common precipitant of ACLF. In the predicting acute-on-chronic liver failure in cirrhosis (PREDICT) study., a multicenter, prospective cohort of 1273 patients with acute decompensation of cirrhosis, 71% of patients with ACLF had identifiable precipitants, 97% of which were bacterial infection or severe AH alone or in combination with other events.[12] The CANONIC European observational study demonstrated heavy active alcohol use as the second most frequent precipitating event for ACLF when one was identified, accounting for approximately 25% of cases, second only to bacterial infection, which accounted for 33% of cases.[4,13] Furthermore, this study showed that patients with alcohol-associated cirrhosis and active heavy alcohol use were younger and had more severe laboratory derangements including higher bilirubin, international normalized ratio (INR), aspartate aminotransferase, γ-glutamyltransferase, and leukocyte count.[4] The CANONIC study also identified alterations in inflammatory cytokine profiles wherein patients with ACLF had severe elevations in both pro and anti-inflammatory cytokines.[14] Furthermore, within ACLF, the changes in cytokines differed based on the presence of severe AH.[14] This suggests that ACLF in AH is a unique process wherein there is concomitant proinflammatory and anti-inflammatory cascades, making the risk of infection high.[15]

ACLF can be diagnosed at the time of AH diagnosis or can develop during the course of treatment of AH.[13,16] A study of 165 patients with biopsy-proven severe AH with Maddrey discriminant function of 32 or greater showed a prevalence of ACLF of 48% and a mortality rate of 47% at 6 months.[16] A retrospective analysis of patients with ACLF precipitated by severe AH in the intensive care unit (ICU) sought to evaluate changes related to ALD prevalence related to the coronavirus disease 2019 (COVID-19) pandemic.[17] In this study, 820 patients were admitted with gastroenterological or hepatological disease, and 237 patients met criteria for ACLF. They noted a moderate increase in ACLF cases in 2020 compared with 2017 to 2019. Notably, AH precipitated 57% of cases of ACLF in 2020 compared with 24% to 27% of cases in 2017 to 2019.[17] This study highlights the increasing prevalence of alcohol-associated ACLF and subsequent relevance of AH as a precipitant of ACLF, particularly in the setting of the COVID-19 pandemic and subsequent changes in patterns of alcohol consumption.

Bacterial Infection

Not only can AH serve as the precipitant for ACLF but patients with ALD are also prone to the development of other precipitants of ACLF. A study comparing patients with ACLF, sepsis, and stable cirrhosis found that patients with ACLF and sepsis had severely reduced production of tumor necrosis factor alpha (TNF-α) and human leukocyte antigen-DR isotype expression compared with those with cirrhosis, suggesting that patients with ACLF and severe sepsis demonstrate similar profiles of immune depression.[18] The EASL guidelines defined precipitating bacterial events as those diagnosed or solved within 48-hour of the development of acute decompensation. Bacterial infections included spontaneous bacterial peritonitis, UTI, bacteremia, pneumonia, bronchitis, skin and soft tissue infection, cholangitis, spontaneous bacterial empyema, secondary peritonitis, and *Clostridium difficile* infection.[12,19] A study of

165 patients with biopsy-proven severe AH found that 48% presented with ACLF and 18% developed ACLF; previous infection was the only independent risk factor for the development of ACLF.[16]

PATHOPHYSIOLOGY

The hallmark of ACLF is presence of organ failure and inflammation; however, the pathophysiology of this disease process is poorly understood.[11] Below, we will explore the current understanding of the development of ACLF.

Systemic and Hepatic Inflammation

Multiple studies demonstrate the role of systemic inflammation in the development of ACLF, particularly in patients with alcohol-associated ACLF.[4,11,20,21] In the CANONIC study, patients with ACLF had significantly higher white blood cell counts and C-reactive protein levels, and these differences persisted even when patients with infection were excluded. Additionally, the degree of organ failure as quantified by the chronic liver failure-sequential organ failure assessment (CLIF-SOFA) score and leukocytosis was associated with mortality in this cohort.[4] This leukocytosis is predominantly secondary to neutrophilia.[11] A study of patients with ACLF compared with patients with chronic hepatitis B and healthy controls found that the neutrophil to lymphocyte ratio was significantly higher in those with ACLF and that elevations in the neutrophil to lymphocyte ratio were associated with severity of liver disease and 3-month mortality.[11,22]

The CANONIC study also demonstrated that patients without earlier acute decompensation who developed ACLF had a more difficult course with higher numbers of organ failures, leukocyte count, and mortality compared with those patients with ACLF who had a history of decompensation.[4] Therefore, it seems that ACLF not only causes a dramatic immune response but also promotes immune tolerance, which is a host defense strategy with the purpose of reducing host susceptibility to damage.[23,24] A study of 60 patients with alcohol-associated cirrhosis comparing those with stable disease, those with acute decompensation in the absence of ACLF, and those with ACLF found that patients with ACLF had significantly higher hepatic vein pressure gradients with reduction in hepatic blood flow and increased intrahepatic resistance, and that this was correlated with mortality. The study also found that the degree of intrahepatic resistance was associated with inflammatory markers, norepinephrine levels, serum creatinine, and degree of encephalopathy.[25]

Although complex, the mechanism of immune response to alcohol is quite similar to that of infection.[24] In AH, tissue necrosis or immune-system mediated damage causes necrotic cells to release damage/danger-associated molecular patterns (DAMPs).[24] These DAMPs interact with toll-like receptors that subsequently trigger the innate immune response priming antigen-specific adaptive immunity. DAMPs also activate inflammasomes, which are groups of protein complexes that lead to cytokine cascade activation.[24]

Cytokine Involvement

There is a paucity of literature on the inflammatory cytokines involved in ACLF. A study comparing patients with decompensated cirrhosis with ACLF, without ACLF, and healthy controls found distinct cytokine profiles between the groups.[26] They found that patients with decompensated cirrhosis in the absence of ACLF had altered cytokine profiles and that these alterations were further deranged in the presence of ACLF.[26] Specifically, patients with ACLF had alterations in cytokines related to chemotaxis and migration of leukocytes, especially monocytes and macrophages.[26]

This study further investigated cytokine profiles to see if the cytokine alterations in ACLF were related to bacterial infection by comparing those patients with ACLF to the subset of patients without ACLF who had bacterial infections. They found that the cytokine profiles were similarly different between those with ACLF and those without ACLF but with infection as in comparing those with and without ACLF, suggesting that the cytokine profile in ACLF is largely unrelated to bacterial infection.[26] They also found that some of the cytokines correlated with 90-day mortality.[26] One of the specific cytokines found to be significantly decreased in patients with ACLF was granulocytes-macrophage colony-stimulating factor (GM-CSF). Reduced GM-CSF was also found to be associated with higher short-term mortality.[26]

A study comparing cytokine profiles among patients with ACLF found that the cytokine alterations were different based on the ACLF precipitant.[14] For example, patients with ACLF with active alcohol use had higher levels of interleukin-8 (IL-8) compared with ACLF precipitated by other causes or an unknown cause.[14] This elevation in IL-8 was attributed largely to the increased levels of IL-8 seen in patients with AH.[14] IL-8 functions as a chemoattractant for neutrophils in acute liver inflammation and is strongly activated in chronic liver disease where it functions in the recruitment and activation of hepatic macrophages.[27] Further studies are needed to delineate the specific cytokine milieu in ACLF precipitated by alcohol.

Immune Cell Dysfunction

Innate immunity

The liver is integral in immune regulation and host defense, serving both to protect against infection and to prevent excessive inflammatory responses.[28] In patients with ACLF, there are alterations in both the innate and adaptive immune system that lead to organ dysfunction and predispose patients to opportunistic infections.[28] There is often disruption of the gut epithelial barrier in patients with liver disease; this can be via direct cellular toxicity in the case of alcohol consumption.[28] Excess alcohol consumption increases intestinal permeability to lipopolysaccharide, resulting in increased toll-like receptor 4 signaling, TNF-α production, and Kupffer cell-mediated hepatocyte injury.[28,29]

The various immune cells of the innate immune system are affected in patients with liver disease. For example, neutrophil function has been shown to be deranged in patients with AH.[30,31] This neutrophil dysfunction, including decreased phagocytosis, in AH has been associated with increased infection, organ failure, and mortality.[31] Granulocyte colony-stimulating factor (G-CSF) administration has been shown to increase neutrophil phagocytosis in patients with ALF and may be useful in the prevention of infection and treatment in these patients.[32] Interestingly, recent studies have shown that the administration of G-CSF decreases bacterial infections and mortality in patients with ACLF.[26,33] Macrophages and dendritic cells are important antigen-presenting cells in the liver, which exhibit dysfunction in liver disease.[28] In the early stages of cirrhosis or ACLF, macrophages exhibit a hyperinflammatory response but as the disease progresses, the immune response becomes diminished and the macrophages become less responsive.[28] Further investigation is needed as to the role of monocytes, macrophages, and neutrophils and whether administration of colony-stimulating factors is a potential treatment option for patients with ACLF.[26]

Adaptive immunity

Cirrhosis and liver disease also lead to dysregulation of the adaptive immune system. Patients with ALD have reduced numbers of B cells.[34] A study of patients with ACLF demonstrated a large increase in mononuclear myeloid-derived suppressor cells resulting in diminished T cell function and increased susceptibility to bacterial infection.[28,35] A recent study exploring the role of the adaptive immune system in the development of ACLF found that there were significantly reduced numbers of innate and adaptive immune cells before ACLF development.[36] In this study, CD4 and CD8 T cell functional ability to produce proinflammatory cytokines was significantly reduced in patients with acute decompensation of cirrhosis and ACLF.[36] Further studies are needed to evaluate the role of the adaptive immune system in the development and natural history of ACLF in patients with AH.

TREATMENT

There is currently no targeted therapy for patients with ACLF, and the principle of treatment is to diagnose and treat any precipitating event and provide supportive care.[37] **Table 1** summarizes treatment options.

Supportive measures

Aggressive supportive care is the cornerstone of treatment of patients with ACLF. This includes admission to ICUs, which should not be withheld or delayed, due to existing liver disease or concern regarding prognosis in the setting of multiorgan failure.[38–40] Organ failures should be treated; these include acute kidney injury (AKI), hemodynamic instability requiring vasopressor support, blood product administration if indicated, respiratory failure necessitating oxygen supplementation and ventilation.[38] Patients who develop AKI may progress to hepatorenal syndrome (HRS). There is a paucity of literature on the role of renal replacement therapy (RRT) in patients with ACLF; however, RRT in patients with type 1 HRS has not been shown to impact short-term and long-term mortality but does lead to longer hospitalizations.[38,41]

Treat underlying infection

As previously outlined, infection is very common as either a precipitant or a complication during the disease course of ACLF; a study of more than 400 patients with ACLF found that 37% presented with a bacterial infection at the time of ACLF diagnosis and 46% of the remaining patients with ACLF developed infection in the subsequent 4 weeks.[42] Therefore, all patients presenting with ACLF, regardless of precipitant, should have a thorough evaluation for possible sources of infection and there should be a low threshold for initiation of empiric antibiotics.[5]

Steroids

Steroids remain the mainstay of treatment of patients with severe AH. The American Association for the Study of Liver Diseases guidelines recommend that patients with

Table 1 Treatment options for patients with alcohol-associated acute on chronic liver failure	
Treatment	
Supportive cares	• Diagnose and treat any precipitating event • Treat organ failures, including ICU interventions
Infection	• Evaluate for sources of infection • Consider initiation of empiric antibiotics if indicated
Steroids	• Consider steroid initiation in patients with AH with MELD >20 or an MDF ≥32
Transplant	• Evaluate patients for transplant candidacy
Experimental treatments	• Evaluate for clinical trial enrollment

AH with a Model for End Stage Liver Disease (MELD) greater than 20 or a Maddrey Discriminant Function (MDF) of 32 or greater be initiated on corticosteroid treatment. The Lille model is a dynamic tool used to determine steroid responsiveness in patients with AH.[43] A study comparing steroid responsiveness in patients with severe AH with and without ACLF found that patients with ACLF were significantly less likely to respond to steroids.[16] The number of organ failures was inversely correlated with steroid responsiveness.[16] In this study, the infection rate was significantly higher in patients with ACLF who were nonresponders to steroids as compared with patients with ACLF who were responders to steroids.[16] Further studies are needed to evaluate the risks and benefits of steroid administration in patients with ACLF.

Transplant

Liver transplant has been shown to improve survival in patients with ACLF.[44,45] However, patients with higher grades of ACLF have been shown to have more complications of liver transplant as well as longer hospitalizations.[45] Although retrospective studies do show liver transplant as a promising treatment of patients with ACLF, prospective studies are needed to further evaluate liver transplant as a treatment of ACLF.

Experimental Treatments

Stem cell technology is currently being studied as a potential treatment modality that can promote liver regeneration for patients with ACLF. There are phase II clinical trials (NCT04229901, NCT02946554) exploring the efficacy of stem cell therapy in the treatment of ACLF.[46] Currently, there is inconsistent evidence for the role of G-CSF in treatment of ACLF. A single-center prospective study of 47 patients with ACLF randomly assigned to receive either placebo plus standard of care versus G-CSF found that G-CSF treatment resulted in higher median leukocyte and neutrophil counts at 1 week, significantly increased survival at 60 days, and was associated with significantly reduced rates of HRS, hepatic encephalopathy, and sepsis.[33] Another study of patients with ACLF, this a prospective multicenter study of 176 patients, showed no significant difference in 90-day, 360-day, or overall survival with the addition of G-CSF.[47] Subgroup analysis evaluating patients with alcohol-associated ACLF also did not show any difference in survival with the administration of G-CSF.[47] Further studies are needed to explore novel therapies for ACLF and to further investigate the clinical significance of stem cell therapy in the treatment of ACLF.

PROGNOSIS

Numerous scoring systems attempting to prognosticate patients with ACLF exist. The Sequential Organ Failure Assessment (SOFA) score was developed to assess organ dysfunction and failure over time in critically ill patients.[48,49] The diagnosis of ACLF in the CANONIC study relied upon the CLIF-SOFA, which is an adaptation of the SOFA score for patients with cirrhosis.[50] The CLIF-SOFA score consists of 6 subscores and is based on expert opinion rather than studies.[50] Therefore, in an effort to simplify the CLIF-SOFA score for patients with ACLF, the CLIF Consortium ACLF score (CLIF-C ACLFs) was developed. Again, the CANONIC database was used for score derivation. The CLIF-C ACLFs includes an organ failure score, age, and white blood cell count to predict mortality.[14] The acute physiology and chronic health evaluation (APACHE) III score has been studied in ACLF.[51] Other scores developed for the assessment of liver disease including the Age, serum Bilirubin, INR, Creatinine (ABIC) score, Glasgow Alcoholic Hepatitis Score, MELD, Model for End Stage Liver Disease-Sodium (MELD-Na), MDF have also been evaluated in the prognostication of ACLF. A study comparing 8 prognostic scores in the prediction of overall survival in patients with ACLF admitted to an ICU found the APACHE III and CLIF-C ACLFs to be significantly more accurate than other models including the MELD.[51] A study of patients with alcohol-related ACLF comparing the APACHE II, MELD, MELD-Na, MDF, ABIC, CLIF-C, and CLIF-C ACLF scores found the CLIF-C ACLF and APACHE II were most accurate in predicting in-hospital, 90-day, and 1-year mortality.[52] Although numerous prognostic models exist, further studies are needed to maximize prognostication, particularly as liver transplant is increasingly being considered as a treatment option for patients with ACLF.

SUMMARY

ACLF is a distinct disease process accountable for significant morbidity and mortality. Alcohol is a major precipitant of ACLF and the current literature supports that the precipitant of ACLF does affect the pathophysiology of the disease course, including in patients with ALD. Therefore, further studies are needed to understand the immune response unique to patients with alcohol-associated ACLF as well as the natural history of the disease, wherein it remains unclear if ACLF is a form of ALD or if it is part of the trajectory of severe AH. Nevertheless, AH is an important and well-recognized precipitant of ACLF and pertains a poor prognosis.

CLINICS CARE POINTS

- Several definitions of ACLF exist, however the World Gastroenterology Organization has proposed a unified definition of ACLF as "a syndrome in patients with chronic liver disease with or without previously diagnosed cirrhosis characterized by acute hepatic decompensation resulting in liver failure (jaundice and prolongation of the international normalized ratio), and one or more extrahepatic organ failures, that is associated with increased risk for mortality within a period of 28 days and up to 3 months from onset."

- The pathophysiology of ACLF can be summarized by using a 4-part model, the PIRO concept of ACLF, which consists of Predisposition, Injury, Response, Organ failure.

- ACLF can be precipitated by a variety of systemic and hepatic insults, often not identifiable, but alcohol-associated hepatitis is a common precipitant alone and in conjunction with the development of other precipitants of ACLF such as bacterial infection.

- There are a variety of scoring systems used to prognosticate patients with ACLF, this is of increasing clinical significance as treatments beyond supportive care such as clinical trials and liver transplant are being considered for patients with ACLF.

DISCLOSURE

None.

CONFLICTS OF INTEREST

The authors have declared no conflicts of interest.

REFERENCES

1. Sarin SK, Kedarisetty CK, Abbas Z, et al. Acute-on-chronic liver failure: consensus recommendations of the asian pacific association for the study of the liver (APASL) 2014. Hepatology International 2014;8(4):453–71.

2. Asrani SK, Simonetto DA, Kamath PS. Acute-on-Chronic liver failure. Clin Gastroenterol Hepatol 2015;13(12):2128–39.
3. Olson JC, Kamath PS. Acute-on-chronic liver failure: concept, natural history, and prognosis. Curr Opin Crit Care 2011;17(2):165–9.
4. Moreau R, Jalan R, Gines P, et al. Acute-on-Chronic liver failure is a distinct syndrome that develops in patients with acute decompensation of cirrhosis. Gastroenterology 2013;144(7):1426–37.e9.
5. Zaccherini G, Weiss E, Moreau R. Acute-on-chronic liver failure: definitions, pathophysiology and principles of treatment. JHEP Rep 2020;3(1):100176.
6. Bajaj JS, O'Leary JG, Reddy KR, et al. Survival in infection-related acute-on-chronic liver failure is defined by extrahepatic organ failures. Hepatology 2014; 60(1):250–6.
7. Wu T., Li J., Shao L., et al., Development of diagnostic criteria and a prognostic score for hepatitis B virus-related acute-on-chronic liver failure, Gut, 67 (12), 2018, 2181.
8. Jalan R., Yurdaydin C., Bajaj J.S., et al., Toward an improved definition of acute-on-chronic liver failure, Gastroenterology, 147 (1), 2014, 4–10.
9. Kamath PS. Acute on chronic liver failure. Clinical liver disease 2017;9(4):86–8.
10. Jalan R, Gines P, Olson JC, et al. Acute-on chronic liver failure. J Hepatol 2012; 57(6):1336–48.
11. Gustot T, Jalan R. Acute-on-chronic liver failure in patients with alcohol-related liver disease. J Hepatol 2019;70(2):319–27.
12. Trebicka J., Fernandez J., Papp M., et al., PREDICT identifies precipitating events associated with the clinical course of acutely decompensated cirrhosis, J Hepatol, 74 (5), 2021, 1097–1108.
13. Gustot T, Fernandez J, Garcia E, et al. Clinical course of acute-on-chronic liver failure syndrome and effects on prognosis. Hepatology 2015;62(1):243–52.
14. Clària J., Stauber R.E. , Coenraad M.J., et al., Systemic inflammation in decompensated cirrhosis: characterization and role in acute-on-chronic liver failure, Hepatology, 64 (4), 2016, 1249–1264.
15. Gustot T, Fernandez J, Szabo G, et al. Sepsis in alcohol-related liver disease. J Hepatol 2017;67(5):1031–50.
16. Sersté T., Cornillie A., Njimi H., et al., The prognostic value of acute-on-chronic liver failure during the course of severe alcoholic hepatitis, J Hepatol, 69 (2), 2018, 318–324.
17. Görgülü E, Gu W, Trebicka J, et al. Acute-on-chronic liver failure (ACLF) precipitated by severe alcoholic hepatitis: another collateral damage of the COVID-19 pandemic? Gut 2021;2021:325278.
18. Wasmuth HE, Kunz D, Yagmur E, et al. Patients with acute on chronic liver failure display 'sepsis-like' immune paralysis. J Hepatol 2005;42(2):195–201.
19. EASL Clinical Practice Guidelines for the management of patients with decompensated cirrhosis. J Hepatol 2018;69(2):406–60.
20. Michelena J, Altamirano J, Abraldes JG, et al. Systemic inflammatory response and serum lipopolysaccharide levels predict multiple organ failure and death in alcoholic hepatitis. Hepatology 2015;62(3):762–72.
21. Jalan R., Stadlbauer V., Sen S., et al., Role of predisposition, injury, response and organ failure in the prognosis of patients with acute-on-chronic liver failure: a prospective cohort study, Crit Care, 16 (6), 2012, R227.
22. Chen L, Lou Y, Chen Y, et al. Prognostic value of the neutrophil-to-lymphocyte ratio in patients with acute-on-chronic liver failure. Int J Clin Pract 2014;68(8): 1034–40.

23. Medzhitov R, Schneider DS, Soares MP. Disease tolerance as a defense strategy. Science 2012;335(6071):936–41.
24. Laleman W, Claria J, Van der Merwe S, et al. Systemic inflammation and acute-on-chronic liver failure: too much, not enough. Can J Gastroenterol Hepatol 2018;2018:1027152.
25. Mehta G, Mookerjee RP, Sharma V, et al. Systemic inflammation is associated with increased intrahepatic resistance and mortality in alcohol-related acute-on-chronic liver failure. Liver Int 2015;35(3):724–34.
26. Solé C, Solà E, Morales-Ruiz M, et al. Characterization of inflammatory response in acute-on-chronic liver failure and relationship with prognosis. Sci Rep 2016; 6(1):32341.
27. Zimmermann HW, Seidler S, Gassler N, et al. Interleukin-8 is activated in patients with chronic liver diseases and associated with hepatic macrophage accumulation in human liver fibrosis. PLoS One 2011;6(6):e21381.
28. Hensley MK, Deng JC. Acute on chronic liver failure and immune dysfunction: a mimic of sepsis. Semin Respir Crit Care Med 2018;39(05):588–97.
29. Seki E, Brenner DA. Toll-like receptors and adaptor molecules in liver disease: update. Hepatology 2008;48(1):322–35.
30. Tritto G, Bechlis Z, Stadlbauer V, et al. Evidence of neutrophil functional defect despite inflammation in stable cirrhosis. J Hepatol 2011;55(3):574–81.
31. Mookerjee R.P., Stadlbauer V., Lidder S., et al., Neutrophil dysfunction in alcoholic hepatitis superimposed on cirrhosis is reversible and predicts the outcome, *Hepatology*, 46 (3), 2007, 831–840.
32. Rolando N, Clapperton M, Wade J, et al. Administering granulocyte colony-stimulating factor to acute liver failure patients corrects neutrophil defects. Eur J Gastroenterol Hepatol 2000;12(12):1323–8.
33. Garg V, Garg H, Khan A, et al. Granulocyte colony–stimulating factor mobilizes CD34+ cells and improves survival of patients with acute-on-chronic liver failure. Gastroenterology 2012;142(3):505–12.e1.
34. Laso FJ, Madruga JI, López A, et al. Distribution of peripheral blood lymphoid subsets in alcoholic liver cirrhosis: influence of ethanol intake. Alcohol Clin Exp Res 1996;20(9):1564–8.
35. Bernsmeier C, Triantafyllou E, Brenig R, et al. CD14(+) CD15(-) HLA-DR(-) myeloid-derived suppressor cells impair antimicrobial responses in patients with acute-on-chronic liver failure. Gut 2018;67(6):1155–67.
36. Rueschenbaum S, Ciesek S, Queck A, et al. Dysregulated adaptive immunity is an early event in liver cirrhosis preceding acute-on-chronic liver failure. Front Immunol 2020;11:534731.
37. Kumar R, Mehta G, Jalan R. Acute-on-chronic liver failure. Clinical medicine (London, England) 2020;20(5):501–4.
38. Gambino C, Piano S, Angeli P. Acute-on-Chronic liver failure in cirrhosis. J Clin Med 2021;10(19):4406.
39. Karvellas C.J., Garcia-Lopez E., Fernandez J., et al., Dynamic prognostication in critically ill cirrhotic patients with multiorgan failure in ICUs in europe and North America: a multicenter analysis, *Crit Care Med*, 46 (11), 2018, 1783–1791.
40. Karvellas CJ, Bagshaw SM. Advances in management and prognostication in critically ill cirrhotic patients. Curr Opin Crit Care 2014;20(2):210–7.
41. Zhang Z., Maddukuri G., Jaipaul N., et al., Role of renal replacement therapy in patients with type 1 hepatorenal syndrome receiving combination treatment of vasoconstrictor plus albumin, *J Crit Care*, 30 (5), 2015, 969–974.

42. Fernández J., Acevedo J., Wiest R., et al., Bacterial and fungal infections in acute-on-chronic liver failure: prevalence, characteristics and impact on prognosis, *Gut*, 67 (10), 2018, 1870.

43. Louvet A, Naveau S, Abdelnour M, et al. The Lille model: a new tool for therapeutic strategy in patients with severe alcoholic hepatitis treated with steroids. Hepatology 2007;45(6):1348–54.

44. Sundaram V., Jalan R., Wu T., et al., Factors associated with survival of patients with severe acute-on-chronic liver failure before and after liver transplantation, *Gastroenterology*, 156 (5), 2019, 1381–1391.e3.

45. Artru F, Louvet A, Ruiz I, et al. Liver transplantation in the most severely ill cirrhotic patients: a multicenter study in acute-on-chronic liver failure grade 3. J Hepatol 2017;67(4):708–15.

46. Khanam A, Kottilil S. Acute-on-Chronic liver failure: pathophysiological mechanisms and management. Front Med 2021;8:752875.

47. Engelmann C., Herber A., Ildh T., et al., O10 Granulocyte-Colony Stimulating Factor (G-CSF) to treat acute-on-chronic liver failure; results of the first multicenter randomized trial (GRAFT study), *Gut*, 70 (Suppl 3), 2021, A6.

48. Vincent J-L, de Mendonça A, Cantraine F, et al. Use of the SOFA score to assess the incidence of organ dysfunction/failure in intensive care units: results of a multicenter, prospective study. Crit Care Med 1998;26(11):1793–800.

49. Ferreira FL, Bota DP, Bross A, et al. Serial evaluation of the SOFA score to predict outcome in critically ill patients. JAMA 2001;286(14):1754–8.

50. Jalan R., Saliba F., Pavesi M., et al., Development and validation of a prognostic score to predict mortality in patients with acute-on-chronic liver failure, *J Hepatol*, 61 (5), 2014, 1038–1047.

51. Chen B.H., Tseng H.J., Chen W.T., et al., Comparing eight prognostic scores in predicting mortality of patients with acute-on-chronic liver failure who were admitted to an ICU: a single-center experience, *J Clin Med*, 9 (5), 2020, 1540.

52. Sonika U., Jadaun S., Ranjan G., et al., Alcohol-related acute-on-chronic liver failure—comparison of various prognostic scores in predicting outcome, *Indian J Gastroenterol*, 37 (1), 2018, 50–57.

The Clinical Spectrum and Manifestations of Acute-on-Chronic Liver Failure

Andrew R. Scheinberg, MD, Paul Martin, MD, FRCP, FRCPI*,
Kalyan Ram Bhamidimarri, MD, MPH

KEYWORDS

- Acute-on-chronic liver failure • Acute decompensation • Cirrhosis
- Liver transplantation • Chronic liver disease

KEY POINTS

- ACLF is a complex syndrome found in the patient with acutely decompensated CLD characterized by at least two severe extra-hepatic organ failures (renal, neurologic, cardiopulmonary, and coagulopathy) associated with high short-term mortality.
- Early recognition and prompt administration of specific and supportive therapies is key to reducing the morbidity and mortality in ACLF.
- CLIF-C ACLFs should be used at time of diagnosis and again calculated at day 3 to 7 to determine a patient's overall prognosis and liver transplant candidacy while the MELD-Na continues to be utilized for liver transplant allocation.
- Palliative care principles in conjunction with a multi-disciplinary approach should be utilized at the time diagnosis and throughout the hospital course.

INTRODUCTION

It is estimated that there are at least 30,000 ACLF hospitalizations in the United States each year costing about 2 billion dollars.[1] The features of ACLF can be identified in approximately 20% to 40% of hospitalized patients with cirrhosis.[2] Overt acute hepatic decompensation (AD) occurs in patients with cirrhosis and is characterized with development of ascites, esophageal variceal bleeding, hepatic encephalopathy (HE), or spontaneous bacterial peritonitis (SBP). On the other hand, acute-on-chronic liver failure (ACLF) is characterized by the presence of AD with extrahepatic organ failures.[2,3] When compared with admissions for acute hepatic decompensation, patients with ACLF have higher costs of admissions and longer length of stay.[4]

Division of Digestive Health and Liver Diseases, University of Miami Miller School of Medicine, Miami, 1120 Northwest 14th Street, Miami, FL 33136, USA
* Corresponding author. Miller School of Medicine, University of Miami, 1120 Northwest 14th Street, Miami, FL 33136.
E-mail address: pmartin2@med.miami.edu

Clin Liver Dis 27 (2023) 671–680
https://doi.org/10.1016/j.cld.2023.03.010
1089-3261/23/© 2023 Elsevier Inc. All rights reserved.

Despite advances in supportive care, ACLF remains associated with high morbidity, mortality, and an overall poor prognosis.[4,5]

CLINICAL MANIFESTATIONS OF ACUTE-ON-CHRONIC LIVER FAILURE

ACLF results from a cascade of dysregulated immune response and inflammation resulting in organ failure(s). Manifestations of ACLF include diminished renal function, cognitive dysfunction, cardiopulmonary instability, and dysregulation of coagulation homeostasis. Grade of ACLF is used to categorize severity and prognosticate the patient with ACLF as outlined in **Table 1**.

Patients hospitalized with an acute decompensation with evidence of acute kidney injury (AKI), sepsis, infection, or other manifestations of organ failures should be considered at risk for the development of ACLF.[6] Although the overall treatment plan for ACLF will be discussed in another chapter, here the authors discuss the clinical manifestations of ACLF and its management emphasizing correction of metabolic derangements, improvement in hemodynamic instability, and introduction of high-protein nutritional support combined with organ-specific supportive care.[7,8]

Renal

Renal impairment is the most common extrahepatic manifestation of ACLF and portends a worse prognosis when present.[9,10] Hepatorenal syndrome (HRS) is the result of a complex dynamic shift in vasoregulation, in which portal hypertension results in a reduced arterial blood volume triggering a reflexive compensatory vasoconstrictive response including renal vasculature resulting in renal hypoperfusion. Renal impairment in a patient with cirrhosis is associated with decreased survival.[11]

Serum creatinine is not a reliable reflection of GFR; therefore, newer criteria for HRS include measuring urine output and changes in serum creatinine from baseline values, as outlined in **Table 2**. Recent nomenclature changes based on recommendations from the International Club of Ascites recommend replacing the term HRS type 1 with HRS-AKI and are based on changes in creatinine or urine output. Patients with ACLF and kidney dysfunction typically fall into the HRS-AKI category. HRS type 2 is now replaced by HRS-non-AKI (HRS-NAKI), which is subdivided into HRS-acute kidney disease (HRS-AKD) and HRS-chronic kidney disease (HRS-CKD) and is based on gomlerular filtration rate (GFR) and chronicity of injury (greater than 7 days but either less than or greater than 3 months).[12,13] HRS-NAKI etiologies include prerenal azotemia, parenchymal kidney disease, and allergic interstitial nephritis.[12] As the prevalence of nonalcoholic fatty liver disease/metabolic-associated fatty liver disease continues to rise, HRS-CKD is becoming more apparent in patients with cirrhosis due to shared risk factors such as diabetes.[12]

Table 1				
Grades of acute-on-chronic liver failure				
No ACLF	**ACLF Grade 1**		**ACLF Grade 2**	**ACLF Grade 3**
No OF	Single kidney failure		2 OFs	3 or more OFs
Single non-kidney OF without kidney disease or without brain dysfunction	Single non-kidney OF with kidney disease or with brain dysfunction			

Abbreviations: ACLF, acute-on-chronic liver failure; OF, organ failure.

Table 2 Classification of hepatorenal syndrome		
Type of HRS		**Definition**
HRS-AKI		Absolute increase in sCr $\geq$0.3 mg/dl within 48 h and/or Urinary output $\leq$ 0.5 ml/kg
HRS-NAKI	HRS-AKD	eGFR <60 ml/min per 1.73 m^{2}for <3 months in the absence of other structural causes
	HRS-CKD	eGFR <60 ml/min per 1.73 m^2 for $\geq$3 months in the absence of other structural causes

Abbreviations: eGFR, estimated glomerular filtration rate; HRS, hepatorenal syndrome; HRS-AKD, HRS-acute kidney disease; HRS-AKI, HRS-acute kidney injury; HRS-CKD, HRS-chronic kidney disease; HRS-NAKI, HRS-non-AKI; sCr, serum creatinine.

The diagnostic workup for the evaluation of AKI includes urinalysis, measurement of urine electrolytes, and renal ultrasonography. HRS-AKI requires aggressive management that begins with the removal of possible offending agents, including diuretics or other nephrotoxic agents, followed by fluid expansion with albumin (1 g/kg up to 100 g per day for at least 2 consecutive days) with monitoring of intravascular volume. Last, withdrawal of beta-blockers should be considered in patients with AKI who are also diagnosed with SBP or those with refractory ascites.[14,15]

HRS-AKI can be confirmed by the persistence of renal dysfunction despite fluid challenge and the absence of other forms of AKI. Vasoconstrictor therapy is well established in the treatment of HRS-AKI and to improve overall patient prognosis.[16,17] If the creatinine fails to improve after a fluid challenge with albumin, treatment should be initiated with terlipressin (recently approved by the US Food and Drug Administration) or alternatively with norepinephrine.[9,17,18] Before the approval of terlipressin, Midodrine and octreotide with albumin were routinely used in clinical practice in the United States which demonstrated improved survival.[19] If kidney function progresses, renal replacement therapy should be initiated. It is also important to note for patients diagnosed with SBP, albumin is recommended to prevent HRS-AKI and/or the development of ACLF. Last, patients with ACLF and on-going renal dysfunction or HRS-CKD should be evaluated for simultaneous liver kidney transplant candidacy based on existing Organ Procurement and Transplantation Network criteria.[20,21]

Brain
HE results from buildup of toxins including ammonia combined with systemic inflammation. Cerebral astrocytes metabolize ammonia via glutamine synthetase into glutamine resulting in astrocyte swelling and cerebral dysfunction.[22] HE presents on a spectrum from covert or minimal HE to overt HE (excessive sleepiness, confusion, obtundation, or coma). There are several precipitating factors that could lead to acute HE such as: dehydration, nonadherence to medications, electrolyte derangements, sepsis, and opioid/sedative use.[7] Although the serum level of ammonia does not correlate with cerebral dysfunction, the lack of hyperammonemia in a confused patient with cirrhosis should prompt a search for an alternative diagnosis.[23] Abrupt changes in mentation with new focal neurologic deficits warrant a search for other causes such as cerebral vascular accident (CVA) or intracranial bleed or central nervous system (CNS) neoplasms. Moreover, the workup of confusion in the patient with cirrhosis should include evaluation of blood count, electrolytes, thyroid-stimulating hormone level,

vitamin B12 and folate levels, as well as an infectious workup. Patients with alcohol use disorder may be malnourished with vitamin deficiencies and present with metabolic encephalopathy.

Patients with cirrhosis and HE have an overall worse prognosis than those without HE, irrespective of the presence of ACLF.[22,24] Most diagnostic criteria for ACLF incorporate the West Haven Criteria for grading of HE, as outlined in **Table 3**. Patients are categorized as having minimal HE to grades I–IV. Minimal HE is subtle and typically requires the use of validated neuropsychiatric diagnostic tests for its recognition.[25] Grade I HE is characterized by diminished attention span or lack of awareness. Grade II HE is characterized by lethargy, disorientation, and personality changes or behavior problems. Grade III HE is present when a patient is somnolent but responsive to stimuli, confused, or demonstrating bizarre behavior. Grade IV HE is coma with patients who are not responsive to verbal or physical stimuli.[25]

Although the data are limited and mainly based on animal studies, the presence of HE in the setting of ACLF is believed to be represent a different phenotype from patients without ACLF. Specifically, Cordoba and colleagues analyzed the EASL-CLIF acute-on-chronic liver failure (CANONIC) study cohort and found HE with ACLF occurred more frequently in younger patients with cirrhosis, with alcohol use disorder, and in the presence of infections or hyponatremia.[24] They also found the presence of HE in the setting of ACLF portended an extremely poor prognosis compared with those without ACLF presumably due to the upregulated immune response and inflammatory environment that ultimately affects brain function and other organs.[24]

Management of HE involves close monitoring for airway compromise, and in cases of severe neurologic impairment, artificial ventilation/endotracheal intubation should be performed. A routine use of sedatives and narcotics should be avoided; however, when indicated propofol or dexmedetomidine may be used.[26,27] Close attention should be paid to patient's glucose and electrolyte disturbances and promptly corrected if abnormal.

Lactulose and rifaximin, a nonabsorbable antibiotic, are the usual therapies effective for HE. Lactulose prevents absorption of ammonia in the colon, and AASLD guidelines recommend lactulose dosing be titrated to a goal of two to three bowel movements per day.[6,23] Patients unable to obtain per oral lactulose may receive enemas. Monitoring for diarrhea volume is important as to not induce hypovolemia or hypernatremia which may further worsen mental status. Although the MELD score does not account for HE or affect a patient's position on the transplant waitlist, liver transplantation should be explored for any patient with grade III/IV HE.[22] Although HE is not a standard established criteria for MELD exception points, if a transplant center feels a patient's MELD does not reflect their acuity, an MELD exception request may be submitted to the National Liver Review Board. The presence of HE portends a worse prognosis and is associated with an increased risk of mortality.[22]

Table 3	
West haven criteria for grade of hepatic encephalopathy	
Grade	**Manifestations**
Minimal	Subtle requires the use of validated neuropsychiatric diagnostic tests
I	Diminished attention span or lack of awareness
II	Lethargy, disorientation, and personal/behavior changes
III	Somnolent but responsive to verbal/painful stimuli
IV	Coma, unresponsive

Coagulopathy

Patients with advanced chronic liver disease have a dynamic coagulation cascade that can fluctuate between a pro-thrombotic state and an increased bleeding risk.[28,29] Vitamin K-dependent clotting factors including V, VII, IX, and X combined with antithrombotic protein C and S may all be affected in the patient with cirrhosis. In addition, prothrombotic von Willebrand factor and factor VIII are increased in cirrhosis as these are derived from the endothelium and not the liver. Patients with ACLF may have coagulopathy in addition to pancytopenia secondary to nutritional deficiencies, sepsis, impaired synthesis of clotting factors, and diminished thrombopoiesis.

Standard assays for coagulation do not always reflect the risk of bleeding.[30] Patients with ACLF may require invasive procedures such as placement of central venous catheters, hemodialysis catheters, or performing a paracentesis or thoracentesis that may be delayed or avoided in the setting of perceived coagulopathy. Thromboelastography more accurately measures the risk of bleeding compared with international normalized ratio (INR) and will help determine the need for blood products.[31–33]

Vitamin K administration is indicated if nutritional deficiency is suspected. The routine administration of platelets or fresh frozen plasma to correct perceived coagulopathy is not recommended due to risks of transfusion-associated circulatory overload, transfusion-associated lung injury, development of antibodies, transfusion reactions, and increasing portal pressure.[7]

Cardiopulmonary Support

The hemodynamic compromise associated with ACLF requires aggressive fluid resuscitation while balancing the avoidance of fluid overload. There should also be a low threshold to initiate vasopressor support to maintain an appropriate mean arterial pressure (MAP). Given the lower arterial pressures generally found in patients with cirrhosis, a goal MAP of greater than 60 mm Hg is reasonable.[6,30]

Crystalloid infusions remain the mainstay of fluid resuscitation.[34] Albumin due to its anti-inflammatory properties and ability to improve oncotic pressure is effective in improving AKI.[35] The use of albumin infusions to maintain a serum albumin level greater than 3.0 g/dL to prevent infection and kidney dysfunction is no longer recommended as a randomized clinical trial published in 2020 showed no benefit.[36,37] Current AASLD and EASL guidelines should be followed regarding the use of albumin for patients with ACLF.[38,39]

Inpatient Care

Given the high morbidity and mortality associated with ACLF, monitoring the patient's hospital course is essential, as outlined in **Fig. 1**. Although ACLF grade 1 may be managed on a regular floor, patients with ACLF grades 2–3 are ideally managed in the intensive care unit. Empiric broad-spectrum antibiotics are appropriate in the setting of worsening ACLF grade, but they must be tailored or withdrawn depending on the clinical scenario. Avoiding hepatotoxic agents as well as proton pump inhibitors (PPIs) may limit further deterioration or development of infection.

Sarcopenia and malnutrition are common in patients with chronic liver disease (CLD). Anorexia, malabsorption, alcohol use, systemic inflammatory response syndrome (SIRS), and infections also contribute to malnutrition in ACLF.[40] Increased rates of metabolism in cirrhosis which when combined with a poor nutritional intake with a catabolic state accentuate sarcopenia.[40] A thorough nutritional evaluation on

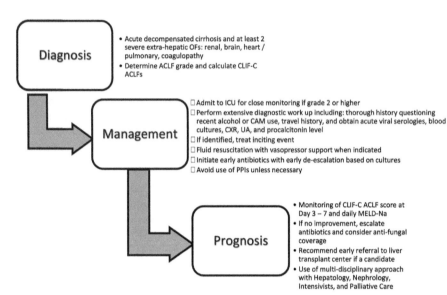

Fig. 1. Flowchart for the management of the patient with ACLF.

admission is warranted along with specific therapy. High-protein diets should be used and efforts should be made to avoid extensive fasting periods. In the ICU, target protein goals are 1.2 to 2.0 g/kg/day for these patients.[40] Patients who are unable to achieve adequate oral intake should start enteral nutrition within 24 to 48 hours of admission to the ICU.

Monitoring the Patient with Acute-on-Chronic Liver Failure

Chronic liver failure consortium (CLIF-C) ACLF score at admission is a good predictor of patient's overall prognosis. However, given the dynamic nature of ACLF, periodic reassessments of ACLF grades during the hospitalization is a better predictor of overall trajectory. Gustot observed that recalculating the ACLF grade at day 3 to 7 of the patient's stay was crucial to predict prognosis. Daily monitoring of ACLF grades in the patient's trajectory are helpful tools to determine escalation of care possibly in favor of transplant or de-escalation of care favoring palliative care measures.[41] In addition, serial CLIF-C ACLFs computed at 48 hours, 3 to 7 days, and 8 to 15 days after diagnosis better predicted prognosis than when calculated at diagnosis and when compared with MELD and model for end stage liver disease - sodium (MELD-Na) scores.[42]

Patients with ACLF grade 2 or above who show improvement in grade to less than 2 can have their care de-escalated from the ICU. However, in those with persistent, ACLF grade 2 or higher should be referred early to a liver transplant center. Transplant-free survival at 28 and 90 days was significantly higher for those with no ACLF or ACLF grade 1 at day 3 to 7, whereas it was extremely low for those with ACLF grade 2 or 3.[42,43]

Owing to the significant mortality associated with ACLF, it is important to involve palliative care "principles" at the time of diagnosis.[44,45] Palliative care may offer a multitude of services for the patient with ACLF including symptom management, assistance with patient family meetings, and facilitating end-of-life discussions with an emphasis on understanding and respecting a patient's cultural, social, and religious attitudes and preferences.[46] Formal palliative care consultations should be used for patients with ACLF grade 2 or higher at or beyond day 3 of admission in the ICU, ACLF patients who are not liver transplant candidates, and patients with a CLIF-C score greater than 70.[45] Further research is ongoing to better elucidate the role for palliative care not only in patients with ACLF but also in those with chronic liver disease.

Prevention of Acute-on-Chronic Liver Failure

The use of nonselective beta-blockers (NSBB) is essential for management of patients with portal hypertension to help minimize risk of a variceal bleed. The CANONIC study demonstrated that patients taking an NSBB had lower grades of ACLF at time of diagnosis, were less likely to progress to a more severe ACLF grade, and showed improvement in 28-day mortality indicating there may be a protective effect of the treatment with NSBBs.[47] Although not statistically significant, the prevalence of renal dysfunction was also lower in the patients treated with NSBBs.[47] Although there are no specific recommendations for the initiation of NSBB for patients with ACLF, physicians should always weigh the benefits and risks of stopping NSBB.[10,34,47]

Lastly, the use of statins in patients with chronic liver disease remains an area of investigation. In one animal study, rats with cirrhosis that developed ACLF had less inflammation and liver damage when given simvastatin.[48] In a retrospective Veteran Affairs cohort study, the use of statins was associated with a reduced risk of developing ACLF in patients with cirrhosis.[49] Despite an overstated concern about drug-induced liver injury, the potential benefit in chronic liver disease outweighs the risk.

SUMMARY

ACLF is a complex syndrome in acutely decompensated chronic liver disease characterized by at least failure of two additional organs and is associated with high short-term mortality. This necessitates measures including monitoring of patients in the ICU and initiating antibiotics early in the hospital course. CLIF-C ACLFs should be used at the time of diagnosis and again calculated at day 3 to 7 to determine a patient's overall prognosis and liver transplant candidacy, whereas the MELD-Na continues to be used for liver transplant allocation.

Although there is agreement on the urgency necessary to recognize, diagnose, and initiate treatment of ACLF to minimize morbidity and mortality, this may also require the development of a unifying definition for ACLF. Although there are specific treatments for several acute insults that result in ACLF, it is essential to manage the cascade of downstream immune dysregulation with supportive care and early referral for liver transplantation. Moreover, despite the abundant evidence for the role of systemic inflammation in the ACLF syndrome, it is clear that further understanding of the immunologic cascade, dysregulation, and response, specifically the roles of pathogen associated molecular patterns (PAMPs) and damage associated molecular patterns (DAMPs), remains incredibly important and may lend insight into possible therapeutic targets in the future. Last, as liver transplantation is the only definitive treatment of ACLF, there continues to be ongoing debate regarding the utility of the MELD score and the role for ACLF exception points as the MELD score may underestimate a patient's acuity and also fails to incorporate all present organ failures.

CLINICS CARE POINTS

- Acute-on-chronic liver failure (ACLF) is a complex syndrome found in the patient with acutely decompensated CLD characterized by at least two severe extrahepatic organ failures (renal, neurologic, cardiopulmonary, and coagulopathy) associated with high short-term mortality.

- Early recognition and prompt administration of specific and supportive therapies is key to reducing the morbidity and mortality in ACLF.
- CLIF-C ACLFs should be used at the time of diagnosis and again calculated at day 3 to 7 to determine a patient's overall prognosis and liver transplant candidacy, whereas the MELD-Na continues to be used for liver transplant allocation.
- Palliative care principles in conjunction with a multidisciplinary approach should be used at the time of diagnosis and throughout the hospital course.

CONFLICT OF INTEREST

All authors declare no conflict of interest.

REFERENCES

1. Allen AM, Kim WR, Moriarty JP, et al. Time trends in the health care burden and mortality of acute on chronic liver failure in the United States. Hepatology 2016; 64(6):2165–72.
2. Moreau R, Gao B, Papp M, et al. Acute-on-chronic liver failure: a distinct clinical syndrome. J Hepatol 2021;75(Suppl 1):S27–35.
3. Ferstl P, Trebicka J. Acute decompensation and acute-on-chronic liver failure. Clin Liver Dis 2021;25(2):419–30.
4. Jalan R, Perricone G, Moreau R, et al. Acute-on-Chronic liver failure: a new disease or an old one hiding in plain sight? Clin Liver Dis 2020;15(S1):S45–51.
5. Arroyo V, Moreau R, Jalan R. Acute-on-Chronic liver failure. N Engl J Med 2020; 382(22):2137–45.
6. Arroyo V, Moreau R, Kamath PS, et al. Acute-on-chronic liver failure in cirrhosis. Nat Rev Dis Prim 2016;2(1):16041.
7. Bernal W, Jalan R, Quaglia A, et al. Acute-on-chronic liver failure. Lancet 2015; 386(10003):1576–87.
8. Sarin SK, Choudhury A. Acute-on-chronic liver failure: terminology, mechanisms and management. Nat Rev Gastroenterol Hepatol 2016;13(3):131–49.
9. Jindal A, Bhadoria AS, Maiwall R, et al. Evaluation of acute kidney injury and its response to terlipressin in patients with acute-on-chronic liver failure. Liver Int 2016;36(1):59–67.
10. Moreau R, Jalan R, Gines P, et al. Acute-on-chronic liver failure is a distinct syndrome that develops in patients with acute decompensation of cirrhosis. Gastroenterology 2013;144(7):1426–37, 1437.e1–9.
11. Davenport A, Sheikh MF, Lamb E, et al. Acute kidney injury in acute-on-chronic liver failure: where does hepatorenal syndrome fit? Kidney Int 2017;92(5): 1058–70.
12. Gupta K, Bhurwal A, Law C, et al. Acute kidney injury and hepatorenal syndrome in cirrhosis. World J Gastroenterol 2021;27(26):3984–4003.
13. Angeli P, Garcia-Tsao G, Nadim MK, et al. News in pathophysiology, definition and classification of hepatorenal syndrome: a step beyond the International Club of Ascites (ICA) consensus document. J Hepatol 2019;71(4):811–22.
14. Mandorfer M, Bota S, Schwabl P, et al. Nonselective β blockers increase risk for hepatorenal syndrome and death in patients with cirrhosis and spontaneous bacterial peritonitis. Gastroenterology 2014;146(7):1680–90.e1.
15. Mandorfer M, Reiberger T. Beta blockers and cirrhosis, 2016. Dig Liver Dis 2017; 49(1):3–10.

16. Sanyal AJ, Boyer TD, Frederick RT, et al. Reversal of hepatorenal syndrome type 1 with terlipressin plus albumin vs. placebo plus albumin in a pooled analysis of the OT-0401 and REVERSE randomised clinical studies. Aliment Pharmacol Ther 2017;45(11):1390–402.
17. Cavallin M, Kamath PS, Merli M, et al. Terlipressin plus albumin versus midodrine and octreotide plus albumin in the treatment of hepatorenal syndrome: a randomized trial. Hepatology 2015;62(2):567–74.
18. de Mattos ÂZ, de Mattos AA, Ribeiro RA. Terlipressin versus noradrenaline in the treatment of hepatorenal syndrome: systematic review with meta-analysis and full economic evaluation. Eur J Gastroenterol Hepatol 2016;28(3):345–51.
19. Esrailian E, Pantangco ER, Kyulo NL, et al. Octreotide/midodrine therapy significantly improves renal function and 30-day survival in patients with type 1 hepatorenal syndrome. Dig Dis Sci 2007;52(3):742–8.
20. Singal AK, Kuo Y-F, Kwo P, et al. Impact of medical eligibility criteria and OPTN policy on simultaneous liver kidney allocation and utilization. Clin Transplant 2022;36(7):e14700.
21. Hussain SM, Sureshkumar KK. Refining the role of simultaneous liver kidney transplantation. J Clin Transl Hepatol 2018;6(3):289–95.
22. Romero-Gómez M, Montagnese S, Jalan R. Hepatic encephalopathy in patients with acute decompensation of cirrhosis and acute-on-chronic liver failure. J Hepatol 2015;62(2):437–47.
23. Vilstrup H, Amodio P, Bajaj J, et al. Hepatic encephalopathy in chronic liver disease: 2014 practice guideline by the American association for the study of liver diseases and the European association for the study of the liver. Hepatology 2014;60(2):715–35.
24. Cordoba J, Ventura-Cots M, Simón-Talero M, et al. Characteristics, risk factors, and mortality of cirrhotic patients hospitalized for hepatic encephalopathy with and without acute-on-chronic liver failure (ACLF). J Hepatol 2014;60(2):275–81.
25. Weissenborn K. Hepatic encephalopathy: definition, clinical grading and diagnostic principles. Drugs 2019;79(Suppl 1):5–9.
26. Bajaj JS, O'Leary JG, Lai JC, et al. Acute-on-Chronic liver failure clinical guidelines. Am J Gastroenterol 2022;117(2):225–52.
27. Karvellas CJ, Francoz C, Weiss E. Liver transplantation in acute-on-chronic liver failure. Transplantation 2021;105(7):1471–81.
28. Campello E, Zanetto A, Bulato C, et al. Coagulopathy is not predictive of bleeding in patients with acute decompensation of cirrhosis and acute-on-chronic liver failure. Liver Int 2021;41(10):2455–66.
29. Blasi A, Patel VC, Adelmeijer J, et al. Mixed fibrinolytic phenotypes in decompensated cirrhosis and acute-on-chronic liver failure with hypofibrinolysis in those with complications and poor survival. Hepatology 2020;71(4):1381–90.
30. Bernal W, Karvellas C, Saliba F, et al. Intensive care management of acute-on-chronic liver failure. J Hepatol 2021;75(Suppl 1):S163–77.
31. De Pietri L, Bianchini M, Montalti R, et al. Thrombelastography-guided blood product use before invasive procedures in cirrhosis with severe coagulopathy: a randomized, controlled trial. Hepatology 2016;63(2):566–73.
32. Kumar M, Ahmad J, Maiwall R, et al. Thromboelastography-Guided blood component use in patients with cirrhosis with nonvariceal bleeding: a randomized controlled trial. Hepatology 2020;71(1):235–46.
33. Blasi A, Calvo A, Prado V, et al. Coagulation failure in patients with acute-on-chronic liver failure and decompensated cirrhosis: beyond the international normalized ratio. Hepatology 2018;68(6):2325–37.

34. Nadim MK, Durand F, Kellum JA, et al. Management of the critically ill patient with cirrhosis: a multidisciplinary perspective. J Hepatol 2016;64(3):717–35.

35. Fernández J, Clària J, Amorós A, et al. Effects of albumin treatment on systemic and portal hemodynamics and systemic inflammation in patients with decompensated cirrhosis. Gastroenterology 2019;157(1):149–62.

36. China L, Freemantle N, Forrest E, et al. A randomized trial of albumin infusions in hospitalized patients with cirrhosis. N Engl J Med 2021;384(9):808–17.

37. Chalasani NP, Hayashi PH, Bonkovsky HL, et al. ACG Clinical Guideline: the diagnosis and management of idiosyncratic drug-induced liver injury. Am J Gastroenterol 2014;109(7):950–66 [quiz: 967].

38. EASL clinical practice guidelines on the management of ascites, spontaneous bacterial peritonitis, and hepatorenal syndrome in cirrhosis. J Hepatol 2010; 53(3):397–417.

39. Biggins SW, Angeli P, Garcia-Tsao G, et al. Diagnosis, evaluation, and management of ascites, spontaneous bacterial peritonitis and hepatorenal syndrome: 2021 practice guidance by the American association for the study of liver diseases. Hepatology 2021;74(2):1014–48.

40. Lai JC, Tandon P, Bernal W, et al. Malnutrition, frailty, and sarcopenia in patients with cirrhosis: 2021 practice guidance by the American association for the study of liver diseases. Hepatology 2021;74(3):1611–44.

41. Gustot T, Fernandez J, Garcia E, et al. Clinical Course of acute-on-chronic liver failure syndrome and effects on prognosis. Hepatology 2015;62(1):243–52.

42. Jalan R, Saliba F, Pavesi M, et al. Development and validation of a prognostic score to predict mortality in patients with acute-on-chronic liver failure. J Hepatol 2014;61(5):1038–47.

43. Engelmann C, Thomsen KL, Zakeri N, et al. Validation of CLIF-C ACLF score to define a threshold for futility of intensive care support for patients with acute-on-chronic liver failure. Crit Care 2018;22(1):254.

44. Bajaj JS, Moreau R, Kamath PS, et al. Acute-on-Chronic liver failure: getting ready for prime time? Hepatology 2018;68(4):1621–32.

45. Patel K, Tandon P, Hernaez R. Palliative care in the patient with acute-on-chronic liver failure. Clin Liver Dis 2022;19(5):198–202.

46. Hernaez R, Patel A, Jackson LK, et al. Considerations for prognosis, goals of care, and specialty palliative care for hospitalized patients with acute-on-chronic liver failure. Hepatology 2020;72(3):1109–16.

47. Mookerjee RP, Pavesi M, Thomsen KL, et al. Treatment with non-selective beta blockers is associated with reduced severity of systemic inflammation and improved survival of patients with acute-on-chronic liver failure. J Hepatol 2016;64(3):574–82.

48. Tripathi DM, Vilaseca M, Lafoz E, et al. Simvastatin prevents progression of acute on chronic liver failure in Rats with cirrhosis and portal hypertension. Gastroenterology 2018;155(5):1564–77.

49. Mahmud N, Chapin S, Goldberg DS, et al. Statin exposure is associated with reduced development of acute-on-chronic liver failure in a Veterans Affairs cohort. J Hepatol 2022;76(5):1100–8.

Prognostic Models in Acute-on-Chronic Liver Failure

Daniela Goyes, MD[a], Hirsh D. Trivedi, MD[b], Michael P. Curry, MD[c],*

KEYWORDS

- Acute-on-chronic liver disease • End-stage liver disease • Scoring system
- Liver transplant

INTRODUCTION

Acute-on-chronic liver failure (ACLF) is a clinical syndrome characterized by severe hepatic dysfunction leading to multiorgan failure in patients with end-stage liver disease (ESLD). There are multiple definitions of ACLF across different international societies. The three most widely accepted consensus-based definitions are from Asian Pacific Association for the Study of the Liver (APASL), the European Association for the Study of the Liver-Chronic Liver Failure (EASL-CLIF), and the North-American Consortium for the Study of End-Stage Liver Disease (NACSELD) and are shown in **Table 1**. The inconsistent definitions and grading of ACLF, however, does introduce heterogeneity into studies that evaluate outcomes of ACLF, making comparison among studies difficult.

Overall, ACLF is associated with an exceedingly high mortality rate. In fact, mortality from ACLF grade 3 is higher than patients with Model for End-Stage Liver Disease (MELD) score of 40 or above and parallels the mortality rate of patients listed for liver transplant as a Status 1A designation.[1] The heightened mortality risk associated with ACLF grade 3 has significant implications in liver transplant (LT) allocation. Clinician awareness of this potentially futile clinical syndrome is paramount when treating patients with ESLD.

Unfortunately, the definition and grading of ACLF varies making diagnosis and management challenging. An accurate more consistent prognostic scoring system would allow for better characterization of ACLF severity and identify who is a suitable candidate for LT. Until a more consistent definition is developed, understanding the implications of currently existing prognostic models is essential. This review aims to provide insights into the common prognostic models that define and grade ACLF and in turn help inform timely implementation of important therapeutic strategies to improve clinical outcomes.

[a] Department of Medicine, Loyola Medicine - MacNeal Hospital, Berwyn, IL, USA; [b] Karsh Division of Gastroenterology and Hepatology, Cedars-Sinai Medical Center, Los Angeles, CA, USA; [c] Department of Medicine and Division of Gastroenterology, Beth Israel Deaconess Medical Center, Boston, MA, USA
* Corresponding author. 110 Francis Street, Suite 8E, Boston, MA 02215.
E-mail address: mcurry@bidmc.harvard.edu

Clin Liver Dis 27 (2023) 681–690
https://doi.org/10.1016/j.cld.2023.03.011
1089-3261/23/© 2023 Elsevier Inc. All rights reserved.
liver.theclinics.com

Table 1
Consensus-based definitions

		APASL[7]	EASL-CLIF[15]	NACSELD[10]
Data source		5200 cases by major hepatology centers across Asia	1343 patients admitted to 21 hospitals across Europe (CANONIC study)	2675 patients from 14 tertiary care hepatology centers
Inclusion criteria		Non-cirrhotic chronic liver disease and compensated cirrhosis	Compensated and decompensated cirrhosis	Decompensated cirrhosis
Exclusion criteria		Prior hepatic decompensation	HCC outside Milan criteria	HIV infection, prior organ transplant, and disseminated malignancies
Definition of ACLF		Acute hepatic insult manifesting as jaundice and coagulopathy complicated within 4 wk by ascites and/ or encephalopathy in a patient with previously diagnosed or undiagnosed chronic liver disease	Acute decompensation, including the development of ascites, encephalopathy, gastrointestinal hemorrhage, and/ or bacterial infections followed by one or more organ failures	Presence of at least two severe extrahepatic organ failures including shock, grade 3–4 hepatic encephalopathy, renal replacement therapy, or mechanical ventilation
Organ failure definition	*Liver*	Total bilirubin $\geq$5 mg/dL and INR $\geq$1.5	Bilirubin >12 mg/dL	
	Kidney	Serum creatinine $\geq$ 0.3 mg/dL or greater ($\geq$26.4 μmol/L) Increase in serum creatinine of $\geq$ 50% Urine output <0.5 mL/kg/h for more than 6 h	Creatinine $\geq$2.0 mg/ dL or dialysis	Dialysis
	Brain	West Haven hepatic encephalopathy grade 3–4	West Haven hepatic encephalopathy grade 3–4	West Haven hepatic encephalopathy grade 3–4
	Coagulation	INR $\geq$1.5	INR $\geq$2.5	
	Circulation		Use of vasopressors, MAP <60 mm Hg	Use of vasopressors, MAP <60 mm Hg
	Respiration		Pao_2/Fio_2 $\leq$200 or $SpO2/Fio_2$ $\leq$214	Need for mechanical ventilation

Abbreviations: APASL, Asian Pacific Association for the Study of the Liver; EASL, European Association for the Study of the Liver; HCC, hepatocellular carcinoma; HIV, human immunodeficiency virus; INR, international normalized ratio; MAP, mean arterial pressure; NACSELD, North American Consortium for the Study of End-Stage Liver Disease.

BURDEN OF DISEASE

ACLF is associated with increased mortality in patients with ESLD. It is difficult to predict the prevalence of ACLF given the lack of a widely accepted definition. However, in the United States alone, reports estimate the prevalence of ACLF ranges from 10% to 28%,[2] whereas worldwide, ACLF affects approximately 35% of patients admitted with cirrhosis.[3] ACLF grade 1 is the most frequent form of ACLF (44%) worldwide, followed by ACLF grade 2 and ACLF grade 3 (32% and 21%, respectively).[3] Patients with ACLF grade 3, in particular, have a 14-day waitlist mortality of 28% compared with 19% in those listed as Status 1A.[1]

ACLF also places significant financial strain on the health care system through increased resource utilization. Between 2001 and 2011, the proportion of patients with cirrhosis admitted with ACLF increased from 1.5% to 4.9% in the United States according to a study in the National Inpatient Sample database.[4] The mean length of hospital stay was higher for ACLF (16 days) compared with cirrhosis without ACLF (7 days). Furthermore, the mean cost per ACLF hospitalization in 2010 was $55,047, seven times more than the mean cost for pneumonia, one of the most common medical reasons for admissions in the United States. Likewise, the total hospitalization cost for ACLF increased from $320 million in 2001 to $1.6 billion in 2011.[4] The burden of ACLF is rising over time, necessitating a better understanding of how best to manage patients with ACLF.

PREDICTING MORTALITY IN ACUTE-ON-CHRONIC LIVER FAILURE

Although there is a lack of a universal definition for ACLF, the current systems are helpful, prognosticating patients' risk of mortality with ACLF.[5] Understanding the strengths and limitations of each prognostic model is imperative in diagnosing and managing hospitalized patients with ACLF (**Table 2**).

Asian Pacific Association for the Study of the Liver-Acute-on-Chronic Liver Failure Research Consortium

The approach of predicting outcomes in ACLF varies considerably among geographic regions. For instance, the APASL-ACLF Research Consortium (AARC) model is commonly used across Asia and Pacific regions. It is a dynamic bedside tool that uses routine laboratory testing such as serum bilirubin, creatinine, international normalized ratio (INR), lactate, and the presence or absence of hepatic encephalopathy (**Table 3**).[6] Grading of liver failure as per AARC score includes grade I (5–7), II (8–10), and III (11–15).[7] Patients with ACLF and an AARC score of ≥ 10 at presentation should be considered for LT, as their 7-day mortality increases dramatically compared with ACLF patients with a baseline AARC score of less than 10 (20% vs 4%).[7]

Furthermore, AARC score is demonstrably superior to Sequential Organ Failure Assessment (SOFA) (area under the receiving operator curve [AUROC] 0.78 vs 0.72), Chronic Liver Failure Consortium-SOFA (CLIF-C-SOFA) (AUROC 0.75), MELD score (AUROC 0.76), and Acute Physiology and Chronic Health Evaluation (APACHE-II) (AUROC 0.69) for assessing the severity of ACLF.[7] The use of the AARC model in Europe and North America lacks generalizability because of differences in the cohort such as etiology of disease. The most common identifiable triggers of ACLF in Europe and North America are alcohol and bacterial infections, whereas in other countries, hepatitis B virus reactivation accounts for the most common acute insult. Alcohol and bacterial infectious were not predominant causes of ACLF among the APASL cohort.[6,8,9]

Table 2
Comparison of prognostic value among scoring systems in predicting mortality of acute-on-chronic liver failure

	AARC	NACSELD	EASL-CLIF
30-d mortality[a,36]			
Accuracy (AUROC)	78	80	77.3
Sensitivity	89.3	89	87.5
Specificity	57	62	58.3
Positive predictive value	79.4	80.9	79.6
Negative predictive value	74	72.5	71.4
90-d mortality[13]			
Accuracy (AUROC)	-	86.2	88.7
Sensitivity	-	36	85
Specificity	-	100	89.8
Positive predictive value	-	100	71.4
Negative predictive value	-	85	95.2

Abbreviations: AARC, Asian Pacific Association for the Study of the Liver-ACLF Research Consortium; ACLF, acute-on-chronic liver failure; EASL-CLIF, European Association for the Study of the Liver-Chronic Liver Failure; NACSELD, North American Consortium for the Study of End-Stage Liver Disease.
[a] Discrimination was given as a c-index and calibration was represented as accuracy, sensitivity, specificity, positive predictive value, and negative predictive value.

The North-American Consortium for the Study of End-Stage Liver Disease Systems and the European Association for the Study of the Liver-Chronic Liver Failure

The NACSELD and the EASL-CLIF systems are commonly used in the Western countries. The NACSELDs definition of ACLF includes two or more extrahepatic organ failures.[10] Standard organ failure definitions have been used by the NACSELD criteria including hepatic encephalopathy grade 3 or 4 by West Haven Criteria,[11] need for renal replacement therapy,[12] need for bilevel positive airway pressure or mechanical ventilation, a mean arterial pressure less than 60 mm Hg, or a reduction of greater than 40 mm Hg in systolic blood pressure from baseline despite adequate fluid resuscitation.[11]

The NACSELD criteria have demonstrated significantly higher accuracy (92% vs 85.3%), specificity (99.7% vs 84%), and positive predictive value (97.1% vs 50.4%)

Table 3
Asian Pacific Association for the Study of the Liver acute-on-chronic liver failure Research Consortium score[7]

Score	Total Bilirubin (mg/dL)	HE Grade	INR	Lactate (mmol/L)	Creatinine (mg/dL)
1	<15	0	<1.8	<15	<0.7
2	15–25	1–2	1.8–2.5	1.5–2.5	0.7–1.5
3	>25	3–4	>2.5	>2.5	>1.5

Grade I (5–7); grade II (8–10); grade III (11–15).
Abbreviations: HE, hepatic encephalopathy; INR, international normalized ratio.

Table 4
Chronic Liver Failure Consortium-Sequential Organ Failure Assessment[17]

Organ/System	Variable	Score 1	Score 2	Score 3
Liver	Bilirubin (mg/dL)	<6	≥6 and < 12	≥12
Kidney	Creatinine (mg/dL)	<2 mg/dL	≥2 and < 3.5	≥3.5 or renal replacement therapy
Brain	Encephalopathy grade (West Haven)	0	1–2	3–4
Coagulation	INR	<2.0	≥2.0 and < 2.5	≥2.5
Circulatory	MAP (mm Hg)	≥70	<70	Use of vasopressors
Respiratory	Pao_2/Fio_2 or SpO_2/Fio_2	>300 or >357	≤300 and > 200 or >214 and ≤ 357	≤200 or ≤214

Abbreviations: Fio_2, fraction of inspired oxygen; Pao_2, partial pressure of arterial oxygen; SpO_2, pulse oximetric saturation.

in predicting transplant-free survival at 28-day when compared with EASL-CLIF criteria.[13] Nonetheless, the overall accuracy in survival (86.3% vs 88.7%) is comparable between NACSELD and EASL-CLIF criteria when predicting 90-day mortality. Thus, the NACSELD system favors identifying sicker patients with ACLF and excluding them from LT early on, whereas the EASL-CLIF score may be more helpful in prioritizing ACLF patients who may ultimately require LT.[13]

In the EASL-CLIF Acute-on-Chronic Liver Failure in Cirrhosis (CANONIC) study, CLIF-SOFA score was evaluated as a variation of SOFA for patients with cirrhosis.[14] In CLIF-SOFA score, platelet count was replaced by INR, and Glasgow Coma Score was replaced by hepatic encephalopathy grade.[15] Further studies have assessed CLIF-SOFA score's discriminative ability for predicting mortality in ACLF patients. Its predictive accuracy for 28-day mortality (AUROC 0.84) is superior compared with Child-Turcotte-Pugh (CTP) score (AUROC 0.70), MELD-Na (AUROC 0.63), and APACHE-II (AUROC 0.69). However, it is similar to the CLIF-C Organ Failure (CLIF-C OF) (AUROC 0.83), a simplified version of CLIF-SOFA (**Table 4**).[16,17] Moreover, different cutoff values of CLIF-SOFA have been studied to discriminate between patients at the lowest and highest risk of dying within 28 days. A CLIF-SOFA score ≤ 8 has a 97.8% sensitivity, whereas a score ≥ 18 represents a 96.3% specificity in predicting 28-day mortality.[16]

Other Scoring Systems

Other existing prognostic scoring systems for ACLF patients are less than robust. CTP, SOFA, and APACHE-II lack specificity for predicting mortality in ACLF patients.[18] The MELD score is currently used as an organ allocation system to prioritize LT for patients with the most severe disease. However, it fails to incorporate measures of systemic inflammation (ie, C-reactive protein, lactate dehydrogenase, white blood cells count), an important prognostic determinant in ACLF.[19] Studies from the United Network for Organ Sharing (UNOS) database in LT candidates under the MELD score allocation system have shown that ACLF grade 3 patients with MELD-Na score ≥35 have a significantly higher risk for 90-day mortality compared with patients with lower ACLF grades.[20] Furthermore, the CLIF-C OF score has shown to be significantly superior to the MELD score in predicting 28-day (AUROC 0.79) and 90-day mortality (AUROC 0.82).[21]

Transplantation for Acute-on-Chronic Liver Failure-3 Model Score

LT for ACLF grade 3 patients is a controversial procedure. One-year survival rates below 50% have been reported in ACLF grade 3 patients[22,23] prompting their consideration for LT early in the course of their disease. On the other hand, given the organ shortage, such poor outcomes weigh against giving access to organs to ACLF grade 3 patients. The transplantation for ACLF-3 model (TAM) score was developed to discriminate patients who would benefit most from LT from those who are "too sick" for transplant.[24] TAM was based on four factors independently associated with posttransplant mortality that were derived and validated in two independent cohorts. The factors include recipient age $\geq$53 years, arterial lactate level $\geq$4 mmol/L, mechanical ventilation with $Pao_2/Fio_2 \leq 200$ mm Hg, and leukocyte count $\leq$10 g/L.[24] Artzner and colleagues[24] demonstrated a 9.1% 1-year survival rate in those ACLF grade 3 patients who have 3 or 4 risk factors. These patients should be excluded from LT. However, the cohort included only patients who received LT, and therefore, these factors should not be used to include patients for LT but rather can be used to determine which patients to exclude from LT.[24] In addition, a study conducted by Michard and colleagues[25] showed the post-LT survival rate in ACLF grade 3 patients decreased as the TAM score at the time of LT increased; from 100% and 90% survival for patients with TAM scores of 0 and 1, respectively, to 10% and 0% for patients with TAM scores of 3 and 4, respectively.[25] The TAM score applied 2 days before LT and at the time of organ offer was more predictive with significantly higher survival rates for patients with TAM scores 0 to 2 of 85% versus TAM scores greater than 2 which had a survival rate of 8%.[25]

MACHINE LEARNING IN PREDICTING MORTALITY FOR ACUTE-ON-CHRONIC LIVER FAILURE

Machine learning (ML) models, a branch of artificial intelligence (AI), use computer-aided systems and algorithms to make predictions from exploratory data analysis.[26] ML models are rapidly evolving in health care and have been expanded to contribute to organ allocation systems and even in prognosticating ACLF patients.

The AARC prospectively collected data from 2481 patients with ACLF according to APASL definition. They developed an AI model using 10 significant factors for the prediction of 30-day mortality in patients with ACLF.[27] Significant covariates included creatinine levels, sodium, INR, leukocytes, and platelet counts; circulatory failure, or hepatic encephalopathy at day 7, and platelet count and the presence of sepsis, both at day 4.[27] The AARC-AI model (AUROC 0.878) was significantly better than day 7 MELD score (AUROC 0.759) in the validation set, showing a 12.8% increase in discrimination, 10.6% increase in accuracy, and a 7% increase in precision.[28] Furthermore, its reliability (AUC 0.965) was confirmed in an external cohort of patients with ACLF in India. However, the AARC-AI model lacks generalizability in Europe and North America because ACLF was defined according to the APASL criteria.[28]

A retrospective study was designed to develop ML models to predict short-term prognosis in patients with ACLF after LT. Four ML models were built to predict 90-day post-LT survival based on the patient's preoperative characteristics. The models used support vector machine (SVM), logistic regression (LR), multilayer perceptron (MLP), and random forest (RF).[29] A total of 132 patients achieving the APASL criteria were eligible for this study. All the patients included in the study also met the EASL-

CLIF consortium ACLF criteria.[29] Among the ML models, the RF model had the highest AUROC (0.94). Followed by MLP (AUROC 0.89), LR (AUROC 0.83), and SVM (AUROC 0.81). Furthermore, ML models had a better performance than conventional models such as MELD score (AUROC 0.704).[29] The future use of ML may enhance the efficiency of allocation and organ utilization among ACLF patients.

MANAGEMENT

The management of ACLF depends on timely diagnosis, prognostication and implementation of therapeutic strategies including treating precipitating causes (ie, infections), providing organ support, and preventing associated complications. Patients with ACLF should be treated in an ICU environment and it is best accomplished by a multidisciplinary team.[5] Liver transplantation should be a strong consideration.

Liver Transplantation for Acute-on-Chronic Liver Failure and Its Implications

One of the characteristic features of ACLF is rapid disease progression associated with high mortality. Some patients require expedited LT assessments, whereas others may be too sick for transplant and require palliative measures.[3] Differentiating who is "too sick" for transplant versus who is a suitable candidate through appropriate use of the available prognostic scores is imperative. In addition, the American College of Gastroenterology recommends early advance care planning in all patients admitted with ACLF, given their high risk of mortality.[5] The UNOS database analyses demonstrated that MELD-Na underestimates the 90-day mortality risk in patients hospitalized with ACLF, particularly in those with MELD-Na less than 30.[30] Therefore, patients with ACLF are at a significant disadvantage to receive timely LT.[1] Experts agree that patients with ACLF should be offered LT if there is more than 50% 5-year survival expectancy and an acceptable quality of life after LT.[31]

Considering the number of organs and which organs are involved in ACLF is also important. For example, the presence of respiratory failure seems to influence post-transplant survival.[32] The need for mechanical ventilation has been associated with lower 1-year survival compared with ACLF patients not on mechanical ventilation at time of LT (75.3% vs 85.4%).[32] Posttransplant survival in ACLF patients with more than three organs involved is associated with the increased risk of infections, hepatic artery thrombosis, biliary, and neurologic complications after LT.[33] The potential advantages of early transplantation are increasingly recognized. A UNOS registry study found LT increases odds of survival for ACLF grade 3 patients, when performed within 30 days of placement on the waitlist compared with greater than 30 days (82.2% vs 78.7%).[32] Further analysis using the same database showed a statistically significant improvement in patient survival among those ACLF grade 3 patients transplanted within 14 days (82.9% vs 78.5%).[34] Other studies support LT after clinical improvement rather than early transplantation. For instance, improvement from ACLF grade 3 to ACLF grade 0 to 2 resulted in greater posttransplant survival (87.6 vs 82.7%) when compared with transplantation of ACLF grade 3 patients within 7 days of listing.[35] Using reliable predictive models is therefore important for determining appropriate patient selection for timely transplantation.

SUMMARY

ACLF is a challenging clinical syndrome with a rapid clinical course and high short-term mortality. There is no single uniform definition of ACLF or consensus in predicting ACLF-related outcomes, which makes comparing studies difficult and standardizing management protocols challenging. A more uniform definition of ACLF is required to consolidate its prediction and help inform therapeutic measures (ie, LT vs palliation) in a timely fashion. Finally, the use of ML models for predictions of outcomes in patients with ACLF could improve the stratification of patients for timely interventions.

CLINICS CARE POINTS

- ACLF is a severe hepatic dysfunction leading to multiorgan failure in patients with ESLD.
- The three most widely accepted consensus-based definitions for ACLF are APASL, EASL-CLIF, and NACSELD.
- Grading of liver failure as per AARC score includes grade I, II, and III. Patients with ACLF and an AARC score of ≥ 10 should be considered for LT.
- Standard organ failure definitions have been used by the NACSELD criteria including hepatic encephalopathy grade 3 or 4 by West Haven Criteria, need for renal replacement therapy, need for bilevel positive airway pressure or mechanical ventilation, a mean arterial pressure less than 60 mm Hg, or a reduction of greater than 40 mm Hg in systolic blood pressure from baseline despite adequate fluid resuscitation.
- The TAM was based on four factors independently associated with posttransplant mortality. The factors include recipient age ≥53 years, arterial lactate level ≥4 mmol/L, mechanical ventilation with Pao2/Fio2 ≤ 200 mm Hg, and leukocyte count ≤10 g/L.
- The potential advantages of early transplantation are increasingly recognized.

FINANCIAL SUPPORT

H.D. Trivedi receives support from 2021 Advanced Transplant Hepatology Award. M.P. Curry receives research funding from Sonic Incytes, Gilead, and Mallinckrodt, as well as consulting fees from Gilead, Sonic Incytes, Mallinckrodt, and Alexion. This work was completed independent of the above funding sources.

CONFLICT OF INTEREST

The authors declare no conflicts of interest that pertain to this work.

REFERENCES

1. Sundaram V., Shah P., Wong R., et al., Patients with acute on chronic liver failure grade 3 have greater 14-day waitlist mortality than status-1a patients, *Hepatology*, 70 (1), 2019, 334–345.
2. Hernaez R., Kramer J., Yan L., et al., Prevalence and short-term mortality of acute-on-chronic liver failure: a national cohort study from the USA, *J Hepatol*, 70 (4), 2019, 639–647.
3. Mezzano G., Juanola. A., Cardenas A., et al., Global burden of disease: acute-on-chronic liver failure, a systematic review and meta-analysis, *Gut*, 71 (1), 2022, 148–155.
4. Allen AM, Kim WR. Epidemiology and healthcare burden of acute-on-chronic liver failure. Semin Liver Dis 2016;36(2):123–6.
5. Bajaj J.S., O'Leary J.G., Lai J.C., et al., Acute-on-Chronic liver failure clinical guidelines, *Am J Gastroenterol*, 117 (2), 2022, 225–252.
6. Choudhury A, Jindal A, Maiwall R, et al. Liver failure determines the outcome in patients of acute-on-chronic liver failure (ACLF): comparison of APASL ACLF

research consortium (AARC) and CLIF-SOFA models. Hepatol. Int 2017;11(5): 461–71.

7. Sarin S.K., Choudhury A., Sharma M.K., et al., Acute-on-chronic liver failure: consensus recommendations of the Asian Pacific association for the study of the liver (APASL): an update, *Hepatol Int*, 13 (4), 2019, 353–390.

8. Shalimar, Kumar D, Vadiraja PK, et al. Acute on chronic liver failure because of acute hepatic insults: etiologies, course, extrahepatic organ failure and predictors of mortality. J Gastroenterol Hepatol 2016;31(4):856–64.

9. Bajaj J.S., O'Leary J.G., Reddy K.R., et al., Survival in infection-related acute-on-chronic liver failure is defined by extrahepatic organ failures, *Hepatology*, 60 (1), 2014, 250–256.

10. O Leary J.G., Reddy K.R., Garcia-Tsao G., et al., NACSELD acute-on-chronic liver failure (NACSELD-ACLF) score predicts 30-day survival in hospitalized patients with cirrhosis, *Hepatology*, 67 (6), 2018, 2367–2374.

11. Bajaj J.S., Leary J.G.O., Reddy K.R., et al., Failure is defined by extra-hepatic organ failures, *Hepatology*, 60 (1), 2014, 250–256.

12. Angeli P., Gines P., Wong F., et al., Diagnosis and management of acute kidney injury in patients with cirrhosis: revised consensus recommendations of the International Club of Ascites, *Gut*, 64 (4), 2015, 531–537.

13. Cao Z., Liu Y., Cai M., et al., The use of NACSELD and EASL-CLIF classification systems of ACLF in the prediction of prognosis in hospitalized patients with cirrhosis, *Am J Gastroenterol*, 115 (12), 2020, 2026–2035.

14. Ferreira FL. Serial evaluation of the SOFA score. October 2001;286(14):1754–8.

15. Arroyo V, Moreau R, Jalan R, et al. Acute-on-chronic liver failure: a new syndrome that will re-classify cirrhosis. J Hepatol 2015;62(S1):S131–43.

16. Maipang K., Potranun P., Chainuvati S., et al., Validation of the prognostic models in acuteon-chronic liver failure precipitated by hepatic and extrahepatic insults, *PLoS One*, 14 (7), 2019, 1–16.

17. Jalan R., Saliba F., Pavesi M., et al., Development and validation of a prognostic score to predict mortality in patients with acute-on-chronic liver failure, *J Hepatol*, 61 (5), 2014, 1038–1047.

18. Wlodzimirow KA, Eslami S, Abu-Hanna A, et al. A systematic review on prognostic indicators of acute on chronic liver failure and their predictive value for mortality. Liver Int 2013;33(1):40–52.

19. Cai YJ, Dong JJ, Dong JZ, et al. A nomogram for predicting prognostic value of inflammatory response biomarkers in decompensated cirrhotic patients without acute-on-chronic liver failure. Aliment Pharmacol Ther 2017;45(11):1413–26.

20. Sundaram V., Shah P., Mahmud N., et al., Patients with severe acute-on-chronic liver failure are disadvantaged by model for end-stage liver disease-based organ allocation policy, *Aliment Pharmacol Ther*, 52 (7), 2020, 1204–1213.

21. Barosa R, Roque-Ramos L, Patita M, et al. CLIF-C ACLF score is a better mortality predictor than MELD, MELD-Na and CTP in patients with acute on chronic liver failure admitted to the ward. Rev. Esp. Enfermedades Dig 2017;109(6):399–405.

22. Umgelter A, Lange K, Kornberg A, et al. Orthotopic liver transplantation in critically ill cirrhotic patients with multi-organ failure: a single-center experience. Transplant Proc 2011;43(10):3762–8.

23. Levesque E, Winter A, Noorah Z, et al. Impact of acute-on-chronic liver failure on 90-day mortality following a first liver transplantation. Liver Int 2017;37(5):684–93.

24. Artzner T., Michard B., Weiss E., et al., Liver transplantation for critically ill cirrhotic patients: stratifying utility based on pretransplant factors, *Am J Transplant*, 20 (9), 2020, 2437–2448.

25. Michard B., Artzner T., Deridder M., et al., Pretransplant intensive care unit management and selection of grade 3 acute-on-chronic liver failure transplant candidates, *Liver Transplant*, 28 (1), 2022, 17–26.

26. Nam D, Chapiro J, Paradis V, et al. Artificial intelligence in liver diseases: improving diagnostics, prognostics and response prediction. JHEP Reports 2022;4(4):100443.

27. Tonon M, Moreau R. Using machine learning for predicting outcomes in ACLF. Liver Int 2022;42(11):2354–5.

28. Verma N., Choudhury A., Singh V., et al., APASL-ACLF Research Consortium-Artificial Intelligence (AARC-AI) model precisely predicts outcomes in acute-on-chronic liver failure patients, *Liver Int*, 43 (2), 2022, 442–451.

29. Yang M., Peng B., Zhuang Q., et al., Models to predict the short-term survival of acute-on-chronic liver failure patients following liver transplantation, *BMC Gastroenterol*, 22 (1), 2022, 1–11.

30. Hernaez R, Liu Y, Kramer JR, et al. Model for end-stage liver disease-sodium underestimates 90-day mortality risk in patients with acute-on-chronic liver failure. J Hepatol 2020;73(6):1425–33.

31. Putignano A, Gustot T. New concepts in acute-on-chronic liver failure: implications for liver transplantation. Liver Transplant 2017;23(2):234–43.

32. Sundaram V., Jalan R., Wu T., et al., Factors associated with survival of patients with severe acute-on-chronic liver failure before and after liver transplantation, *Gastroenterology*, 156 (5), 2019, 1381–1391.e3.

33. Artru F, Louvet A, Ruiz I, et al. Liver transplantation in the most severely ill cirrhotic patients: a multicenter study in acute-on-chronic liver failure grade 3. J Hepatol 2017;67(4):708–15.

34. Choudhary NS, Saraf N, Saigal S, et al. Factors associated with survival of patients with severe acute-on-chronic liver failure before and after liver transplantation: unanswered questions. Gastroenterology 2019;157(4):1162–3.

35. Sundaram V., Kogachi S., Wong R.J., et al., Effect of the clinical course of acute-on-chronic liver failure prior to liver transplantation on post-transplant survival Vinay, *J Hepatol*, 72 (3), 2020, 481–488.

36. Verma N., Dhiman R.K., Singh V., et al., Comparative accuracy of prognostic models for short-term mortality in acute-on-chronic liver failure patients: CAP-ACLF, *Hepatol. Int*, 15 (3), 2021, 753–765.

Hepatic Encephalopathy in Acute-on-Chronic Liver Failure

Bryan D. Badal, MD, Jasmohan S. Bajaj, MD*

KEYWORDS

• Acute-on-chronic liver failure • Encephalopathy • Infections

INTRODUCTION

Acute-on-chronic liver failure (ACLF) is a syndrome with high rate of short-term mortality characterized by the presence of chronic liver disease and extrahepatic organ dysfunction (**Figs. 1** and **2**, **Tables 1** and **2**).[1] In January 2022, the American College of Gastroenterology (ACG) released a guideline for the diagnosis and management of ACLF, defining ACLF as a potentially reversible condition in patients with or without cirrhosis that is associated with the potential for multiorgan failure and high mortality within three months in the absence of treatment of the underlying liver disease, liver support, or liver transplantation.[2] While what constitutes extrahepatic organ dysfunction in ACLF is variable and evolving, the presence of grade III/IV encephalopathy is one commonality among major society definitions of ACLF. Hepatic encephalopathy (HE) is characterized by brain dysfunction due to liver insufficiency or portosystemic shunting.[3] The definition of brain failure or acute HE in the context of ACLF is grade III/IV HE using the West Haven Criteria, according to the European Association for the Study of Liver–Chronic Liver Failure Consortium (EASL-CLIF), North American Consortium for the Study of End-Stage Liver Disease (NACSELD), The Asian Pacific Association for the Study of the Liver, and ACG.[3–6]

PATHOPHYSIOLOGY OF ACUTE-ON-CHRONIC LIVER FAILURE

While the mechanism behind ACLF has not been fully elucidated, systemic inflammation is recognized as a main driver of ACLF.[7] Systemic inflammation is commonly triggered by infection or liver insult. However, oftentimes, a patient will have no identifiable trigger.

In chronic liver disease or cirrhosis, patients have increased bloodstream exposure to circulating pathogen-associated molecular patterns (PAMPs) as a result of gut

Division of Gastroenterology, Hepatology and Nutrition, Virginia Commonwealth University and Central Virginia Veterans Healthcare System, 1201 Broad Rock Boulevard, Richmond, VA, USA
* Corresponding author.
E-mail address: jasmohan.bajaj@vcuhealth.org

Clin Liver Dis 27 (2023) 691–702
https://doi.org/10.1016/j.cld.2023.03.012
1089-3261/23/© 2023 Elsevier Inc. All rights reserved.

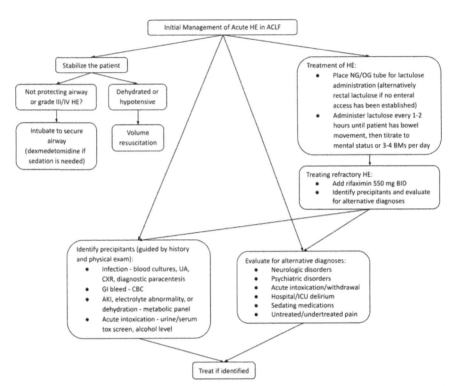

Fig. 1. Management of acute encephalopathy in ACLF. It consists of a four-part approach that should occur in parallel: initial management, evaluate for alternative diagnoses, identify precipitants, and HE therapy. ACLF, acute on chronic liver failure; AKI, acute kidney injury; BID, twice daily; BM, bowel movement; CBC, complete blood count; CXR, chest x ray; GI, gastrointestinal; HE, hepatic encephalopathy; ICU, intensive care unit; NG, nasogastric; OG, orogastric; UA, urinalysis.

microbial dysbiosis and/or increased gut permeability.[8] PAMPs are highly conserved molecular structures expressed by a variety of pathogens that trigger the innate immune system via pattern-recognition receptors (PRRs), leading to a signaling cascade that results in the production and release of inflammatory proteins and cytokines such as tumor necrosis factor-alpha and interleukin 6.[9] The massive inflammatory response that ensues can result in end-organ damage that is witnessed during ACLF. One of the most well-known PAMPs is lipopolysaccharide, which is present on the surface of gram-negative bacteria and activates toll-like receptor 4, initiating the inflammatory cascade. Other PAMPs include similarly well-conserved structures such as peptidoglycan in bacterial cell walls, double-stranded RNA in viruses, and beta-glucan in fungal cell walls. Thus, bacterial, viral, or fungal infections are common triggers of ACLF.

In addition to PAMPs, products of cell death that are produced and accumulate during ACLF itself can trigger inflammation by the release of damage-associated molecular patterns, which are also recognized by PRRs of the innate immune system.[10] The initial insult that damages the liver commonly occurs from alcohol, viral hepatitis exposure or reactivation, or hepatotoxic drugs. The resultant inflammatory cascade results in additional end-organ damage and ultimately end-organ failure.

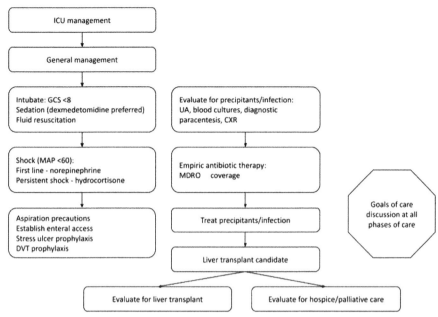

Fig. 2. ICU management of a patient with acute-on-chronic liver failure. The goal of management is to stabilize the patient. Identify and treat precipitants with special attention given to infections. Eligible patients should be considered for transplant evaluation, and if not eligible, they should be considered for hospice or palliative care services. CXR, chest x-ray; DVT, deep venous thrombosis; GCS, Glasgow coma scale; ICU, intensive care unit; MAP, mean arterial pressure; MDRO, multidrug-resistant organism; UA, urinalysis. (*Adapted from* Bajaj et al NEJM 2021.)

Pathophysiology of Hepatic Encephalopathy

Similar to ACLF, HE is a multiorgan phenomenon. It is well established that ammonia plays an important role in the pathogenesis of HE although the mechanism is incompletely understood. Ammonia is the byproduct of amino acid metabolism by gut

Table 1
West Haven Criteria grades of hepatic encephalopathy

	Grade		Description
0 (Minimal)		Covert	Psychomotor or executive function decline on psychometric or neuropsychological testing without clinical manifestations
I			Shortened attention span; lack of awareness
			Cognitive impairment; inability to add or subtract
			Anxiety, irritability, or euphoria
			Altered sleep rhythm
II		Overt	Lethargic or apathetic
			Disoriented to time
			Personality changes; inappropriate behavior
			Dyspraxia or asterixis
III	Brain failure		Somnolent or semi-stuporous, but responsive to stimuli
			Confusion
			Disoriented to time and place; grossly disoriented
			Bizarre behavior
IV			Coma; unresponsive to noxious or painful stimuli

Grades III/IV constitutes brain failure.

Table 2
Glasgow coma scale/score

Behavior	Response	Points
Eye opening	Spontaneously	4
	To voice	3
	To painful stimuli	2
	No eye opening	1
Verbal	Oriented	5
	Confused but conversant	4
	Inappropriate words but intelligible	3
	Unintelligible speech	2
	No verbal response	1
Motor	Obeys commands	6
	Localizes to pain	5
	Withdraws from pain	4
	Abnormal Flexion (decorticate)	3
	Abnormal Extension (decerebrate)	2
	No response	1

bacteria, which enters systemic circulation via the portal vein. Small intestinal bacterial overgrowth, common in cirrhosis, creates an environment of increased ammonia absorption. In cirrhosis, there is decreased metabolism of ammonia via the urea cycle, leading to ammonia entering systemic circulation. Additionally, ammonia is shunted past the liver in patients who form portosystemic collaterals due to portal hypertension, entering systemic circulation and crossing the blood-brain barrier, resulting in neurologic dysfunction. Once ammonia crosses the blood-brain barrier, there are various mechanisms by which ammonia alters brain function. With a rapid influx of ammonia, astrocytes take up the ammonia and is metabolized into glutamine, an osmolyte, resulting in astrocyte edema and swelling.[11] Cerebral edema is a critical component of encephalopathy in acute liver failure and has also been noted in some patients with ACLF although is less clinically relevant in ACLF.[12] Another effect of ammonia entering the blood-brain barrier is an increased concentration of gamma-amino butyric acid, the primary neuro-inhibitory peptide, resulting in depressed neurologic activity.[13] Neurotoxicity from excess ammonia is also exacerbated by the inflammatory cytokines present in ACLF.[14] Inflammation of the blood-brain barrier may also allow ammonia to cross more easily into the brain. The kidneys, which are commonly affected in ACLF, also have an important role in ammonia metabolism. The kidneys facilitate excreting ammonia as urea but can quickly become overburdened by the excess ammonia, excreting it back into systemic circulation. Decreased renal function in the context of ACLF further exacerbates this process.

OUTCOMES OF PATIENTS WITH HEPATIC ENCEPHALOPATHY AND ACUTE-ON-CHRONIC LIVER FAILURE

Multiple studies have described an association between admission for HE and adverse outcomes such as increased mortality. Patients with severe HE (West Haven grade III/IV) as part of the ACLF syndrome have higher mortality than those with HE but who did not meet criteria for ACLF.[15] Additionally, patients with ACLF had higher mortality if they had HE compared to those without HE. A study analyzing 1569 patients enrolled in the NACSELD studied HE in the presence of other extrahepatic organ failures and found HE to be an independent risk factor for mortality. Patients with HE grade III/IV had a mortality rate of 38%.[16] Not only is the presence of HE associated with increased mortality, but the severity is an important risk factor as well. Intensive care unit (ICU) patients with grade IV encephalopathy had a higher mortality rate than those with grade III encephalopathy.[17]

Microbiome

Studies regarding the human microbiome may give insight into complications of cirrhosis, liver disease progression, and the occurrence of ACLF and encephalopathy. Patients with cirrhosis are more prone to dysbiosis than patients without cirrhosis resulting in an increased ratio of potential pathobionts versus commensal bacterial species.[18] Commensal bacteria help maintain the integrity of the intestinal mucosal barrier and reduce the amount of inflammation in the colon. While an increase in potential pathobionts results in increased endotoxemia which ultimately lead to more systemic inflammation, progression of liver disease, and decompensation. There have been several studies documenting differences in the microbiome of patients who develop HE compared to patients with cirrhosis without HE.[19–22]

There have also been studies documenting differences in the microbiome in patients who are admitted with ACLF. In a study, patients who developed ACLF were found to have more dysbiosis and higher rates of endotoxemia than those without ACLF.[18] Two studies found that patients with ACLF had higher proportions of different gram-positive species such as Streptococcaceae and Enterococcaceae and decrease in native bacteria such as Lachnospiraceae.[18,23] There was also a significantly lower amount of Lachnospiraceae in ACLF patients with HE than in those without HE.[23] The role Lachnospiraceae may play in the development of HE during ACLF may be in part as a butyrate producer, and decreased colonic short-chain fatty acids (SCFAs) with decreased Lachnospiraceae as SCFA are associated with decreased colonic pH, maintaining healthy colonocyte, and reducing the absorption of ammonia.[24,25]

PRECIPITANTS
Infections

Infections are one of the most common precipitants of ACLF and can also precipitate HE.[26] Due to the high prevalence of infection, investigation into infection is warranted in patients with ACLF with or without HE and is often a part of the investigation of patients admitted with HE.[27] The inflammatory reaction from infection is a driver of not only ACLF as described previously but also for Grade III/IV encephalopathy. Studies have found bacterial infection and degree of inflammatory reaction to be better predictors of severe HE than serum ammonia levels.[17] A study by Fernandez and colleagues discovered bacterial infections in 37% of patients at initial diagnosis of ACLF.[28] Not only is infection a common precipitant, but it is also an important complication to consider while caring for the patient with ACLF. Of the patients who did not present with bacterial infection, 46% went on to develop a bacterial infection in the 4-week follow-up period.[28]

Serious infections are more common in patients with ACLF than in those admitted with decompensated cirrhosis without ACLF.[28] Patients with bacterial infections and ACLF were more likely to have HE than noninfected patients with ACLF (31% vs 17%) and had higher rates of mortality (51% vs 38%).[28] A large study from the NAC-SELD showed that while the number of organ failures is the strongest predictor of mortality, infection remains an important factor in driving mortality.[29] In this study, patients with HE had a survival rate of 61% with infection, compared to 85% without infection.

In patients meeting NACSELD-ACLF criteria for two or more organ failures, mortality was 59%. Among ACLF patients with infection, there was 52% mortality.[29] In a study by Cordoba and colleagues using the EASL-CLIF Canonic study database when comparing HE among those with and without ACLF, patients with ACLF and HE were found to have higher rates of bacterial infections than those with HE alone.[15]

Special considerations should be made when caring for patients presenting with complications of chronic liver disease such as HE or ACLF. Of particular concern is the rising percentage of multidrug-resistant organism (MDRO) infections in patients with cirrhosis, which varies by region but has been reported to range from 18% in North American centers to as high as 73% in Indian centers.[30] Fungal infections have been reported to occur in 10%-13% of patients and, thus, are important to consider in patients who have presumed infection but fail to respond to empiric antibiotics, as well as those who are culture-negative.[31,32] Patients with fungal infection are more likely to develop ACLF, and those with fungal peritonitis have the highest mortality rate.[32] Rates of both MDRO and fungal infections are increased in secondary infections.

ALCOHOL

Active alcohol use can be a precipitant of both ACLF and HE. Alcohol-associated ACLF with acute encephalopathy occurs in the setting of increased inflammation compared to those without encephalopathy.[33] Alcohol use was identified as either a precipitant or contributing factor in the development of ACLF in most patients in the EASL-CLIF study by Moreau and colleagues.[1] Comparing patients with HE and ACLF to patients with HE alone, Cordoba and colleagues found that patients with both ACLF and HE tend to be younger and more likely to have active alcohol use than patients with HE alone.[15] Additionally, patients with ACLF secondary to alcohol-associated hepatitis are more likely to have received steroids as part of their treatment, with a potential for increased rates and severity of infections.[1]

MANAGEMENT
Diagnosis

Overt HE is a clinical diagnosis, and the West Haven Criteria are considered the gold standard for staging encephalopathy. Glasgow Coma Scale can also be used in assessing the patient with decreased consciousness.[34] Physical examination findings consistent with overt HE include disorientation and asterixis. Decreased levels of arousal ranging from somnolence to stupor or coma are signs of acute encephalopathy or brain failure.[3] While HE is often associated with hyperammonemia, measuring serum ammonia levels is not clinically useful in diagnosing the severity of encephalopathy with chronic liver disease and is not recommended. Many patients with chronic liver disease will have elevated ammonia levels without the evidence of HE, and using serum ammonia as a method to evaluate for HE will too often lead to a misdiagnosis.[35,36] However, a patient with normal serum ammonia is unlikely to have HE.[37] Excluding alternative diagnoses for acute mental status change is critical in making the diagnosis of HE. Brain imaging with magnetic resonance imaging or computed tomography should be considered if presentation is not typical of HE or if there are focal neurologic examination findings.[38]

IDENTIFYING AT-RISK PATIENTS

Patients with ACLF and grade III/IV encephalopathy will more often require an ICU level of care and have higher rates of mortality. The challenges of caring for these patients is that their encephalopathy limits their participation in major decisions such as transplant evaluation or deciding on end-of-life care. Reliable markers to prognosticate which patients are at risk of developing brain failure during admission are crucial. As previously mentioned, differences in microbiome and metabolomics are one potential area for prognostication. Microbiome analysis has shown that patients with higher levels of Proteobacteria and lower Firmicutes have been found to be more prone to encephalopathy.[39] Currently, the ability to analyze patient's microbiome in routine clinical care is limited. However, the difference in microbiome among patients may allow for measurement with serum microbial metabolites as an alternative. One large multicenter study in North America found low levels of levothyroxine in addition to altered profiles of microbial metabolites such as high methyl-4-hydroxybenzoate sulfate, 3-4 dihydroxy butyrate, and lower maltose to be predictive of developing grade III/IV HE.[40] Levothyroxine levels were validated in a local hospital laboratory in this study, and this could be a potential marker to be investigated for predicting grade III/IV HE development during admission.

Management

Initial management of the patient with ACLF and acute HE first requires stabilizing and appropriately triaging the patient. A careful assessment of the patient with a physical examination is paramount, with special focus on the patient's mental status and ability to protect their airway. Patients with grade III/IV encephalopathy and Glasgow coma scale <8 should be intubated to secure the airway, and medications should be administered either intravenously (IV) or via a nasogastric (NG) tube to reduce the risk of aspiration pneumonia.[41] Patients with hypotension or shock should be treated appropriately with IV fluids and may require vasopressors in the event of refractory hypotension despite fluid resuscitation. If there is concern for infection, empiric antibiotics should be initiated immediately after the appropriate cultures are obtained, including a diagnostic paracentesis in patients with ascites. Ultimately, a decision needs to be made as to where to admit the patient and whether they require a more monitored setting than the floors. Patients that meet the criteria for brain failure with grades III/IV encephalopathy are best cared for in an intensive care setting.

The next phase of management should include an assessment for precipitants of HE and possible alternative diagnoses. Common precipitants include infections, gastrointestinal bleeding, electrolyte imbalances, and dehydration secondary to diuretic overuse. Potential sources of infection should be identified with blood cultures, urinalysis and urine culture, chest x-rays, and diagnostic paracentesis to rule out spontaneous bacterial peritonitis in all patients with appreciable ascites. Diagnostic paracentesis should not be delayed, and SBP diagnoses are critical, as mortality rate increases with delay in initiation of antimicrobial therapy. In addition, ascites and blood culture data can be used to tailor antimicrobial therapy. Focal neurologic deficits should prompt the clinician to search for causes of altered mental status other than HE and consider brain imaging. Alcohol levels and drug screens can identify intoxication. Laboratory data including chemistry and complete blood count should be reviewed for abnormalities. As previously mentioned, some patients may have no identifiable precipitant for their ACLF.

Lactulose and rifaximin are cornerstone therapies in the treatment of acute HE due to decompensated cirrhosis or ACLF. In the initial phases of administration, lactulose should be administered rectally or via an NG tube to avoid aspiration until the patient is alert enough for safe oral administration. Lactulose should be titrated to 3-4 loose bowel movements a day. Higher numbers of daily bowel movements put the patient at risk of dehydration and hypernatremia. Rifaximin is a nonabsorbable antibiotic that is used to reduce ammonia-producing gut bacteria. Surprisingly, although lactulose and rifaximin are foundational to HE treatment, in a study using the Canonic database, Cordoba and colleagues found that only 34.3% of patients with HE were receiving lactulose therapy, and only 6.8% of patients were treated with rifaximin or neomycin.[15]

As many patients with acute encephalopathy in the setting of ACLF require intensive care management, providers should be vigilant to avoid and alleviate other contributors to encephalopathy common in the ICU. Pain and irritation from endotracheal tubes are common precipitants of ICU delirium.[42] Studies have shown that using dexmedetomidine may lessen delirium with shorter time to extubation than other commonly used sedatives.[43]

Artificial Liver Support

Extracorporeal liver support systems have been studied for the treatment of ACLF. These liver support systems use dialysis techniques to remove water-soluble or albumin-bound toxins from the serum of patients with ACLF. One of these devices is molecular adsorbent recirculating system (MARS) which has the ability to remove albumin-bound toxins from the serum, as well as reduce serum bilirubin and creatinine. Clinical trials comparing MARS in conjunction with standard HE therapy versus standard therapy alone have shown higher rates of improvement in HE. Banares and colleagues saw a 62.5% rate of improvement in HE in the MARS group compared to 38.2% receiving standard therapy alone.[44] Similarly, Hassanein and colleagues found 62% of patients undergoing treatment with MARS had improvement in their HE by at least 2 grades, compared to 40% in the standard-therapy-alone group.[45] The widespread use of this device has been limited given that in clinical trials, there was no evidence of improved survival in patients with ACLF that receive MARS as part of treatment.[45]

Prometheus (Fresenius, germany) is commercially available fractionated plasma separation device, which fractionates albumin-bound and water-soluble toxins based on size.[46] Albumin- and protein-bound toxins are removed via two adsorbents which are subsequently dialyzed. While Prometheus has been shown to reduce serum bilirubin, creatinine, ammonia, and urea, there was no improvement in survival in patients with ACLF.[47,48] There have not been any studies showing an improvement in HE with Prometheus.[46]

LIVER TRANSPLANT

Given the high mortality rate among patients with ACLF, liver transplantation should be considered in appropriate patients. Despite generally being sicker at time of transplant, patients with ACLF appear to have acceptable outcomes when compared with patients without ACLF undergoing liver transplant. A large multicenter study using NACSELD criteria for ACLF found no difference in mortality outcomes at 3 and 6 months when comparing patients transplanted with and without an episode of ACLF before transplantation.[49] Increasing number of extrahepatic organ failures is associated with worse outcomes after transplant, with the presence of three organ failures being associated with more complications and longer ICU stays after transplantation when compared to patients with two or less organ failures.[50] A meta-analysis of outcomes in patients with ACLF who undergo liver transplant pooled data from 12 studies and identified advanced age, greater than 30 days on waitlist, and mechanical ventilation as risk factors for worse outcomes after transplant.[51] The ACG guideline recommends against transplantation for patients requiring mechanical ventilation for either respiratory or brain failure,[2] further emphasizing maximizing HE therapy in patients that would be considered for liver transplant.

Palliative Care

Given the high rate of short-term mortality with ACLF goals of care, discussions should occur at all stages of the patient's care. The presence of overt encephalopathy only further complicates these discussions as the patient will be unable to participate in these discussions. Approaching end-of-life decisions can be challenging and first required identification of a surrogate decision maker.[52] Special attention should be made to the setting where these discussions occur, allowing for ample time to discuss prognosis and goals and answer questions.[52] Providers should be prepared to discuss treatment options, transplant candidacy, prognosis, and futility when applicable. When available, palliative care consults can be immensely valuable and can result in shorter hospital stays and decreased hospital resource utilization.[53] While some centers will have liver-focused palliative care services, this is unfortunately either unavailable or underutilized at many centers.[54,55]

SUMMARY

Inclusion of HE across all society definitions of ACLF is a sign of the importance of acute encephalopathy in the syndrome. Acute encephalopathy in ACLF occurs in the setting of massive inflammation, and reversible causes should be investigated. HE not only is associated with increased mortality in ACLF but often also interferes or delays evaluation for liver transplant, as the patient will be either too unstable or unable to participate in the evaluation. Given its impact on survival and increased hospital resource utilization, more work is needed to appropriately identify those who are at risk of developing brain failure during admission with better prognostication tools. Additionally, research efforts should include novel treatments for acute encephalopathy in the setting of ACLF. Research into medical therapy managing the encephalopathic patient with ACLF should also identify optimal ICU care such as ventilator management, sedation, and vasopressor support. When transplant is not feasible or futility has been reached, better implementation of palliative care services, including liver-centric palliative care providers, may result in shorter hospital stays, resource utilization, and patient satisfaction.

FUNDING

VA merit review 2I0CX001076 and I01tCX002472.

DISCLOSURE

Grant support to institution: Bausch, Grifols.

REFERENCES

1. Moreau R, et al. Acute-on-chronic liver failure is a distinct syndrome that develops in patients with acute decompensation of cirrhosis. Gastroenterology 2013; 144(7):1426–37, 1437.e1-9.
2. Bajaj JS, et al. Acute-on-Chronic liver failure clinical guidelines. Am J Gastroenterol 2022;117(2):225–52.
3. Vilstrup H, et al. Hepatic encephalopathy in chronic liver disease: 2014 practice guideline by the American Association for the study of liver diseases and the European Association for the study of the liver. Hepatology 2014;60(2):715–35.

4. Sarin SK, et al. Acute-on-chronic liver failure: consensus recommendations of the Asian Pacific association for the study of the liver (APASL): an update. Hepatol Int 2019;13(4):353–90.
5. Jalan R, et al. Development and validation of a prognostic score to predict mortality in patients with acute-on-chronic liver failure. J Hepatol 2014;61(5):1038–47.
6. Bajaj JS, et al. Survival in infection-related acute-on-chronic liver failure is defined by extrahepatic organ failures. Hepatology 2014;60(1):250–6.
7. Trebicka J, et al. The PREDICT study uncovers three clinical courses of acutely decompensated cirrhosis that have distinct pathophysiology. J Hepatol 2020; 73(4):842–54.
8. Bauer TM, et al. Small intestinal bacterial overgrowth in patients with cirrhosis: prevalence and relation with spontaneous bacterial peritonitis. Am J Gastroenterol 2001;96(10):2962–7.
9. Arroyo V, et al. Acute-on-chronic liver failure in cirrhosis. Nat Rev Dis Primers 2016;2:16041.
10. Albillos A, et al. Cirrhosis-associated immune dysfunction. Nat Rev Gastroenterol Hepatol 2022;19(2):112–34.
11. Dabrowska K, et al. Roles of glutamate and glutamine transport in Ammonia neurotoxicity: state of the art and question marks. Endocr Metab Immune Disord: Drug Targets 2018;18(4):306–15.
12. Joshi D, et al. Cerebral oedema is rare in acute-on-chronic liver failure patients presenting with high-grade hepatic encephalopathy. Liver Int 2014;34(3):362–6.
13. Llansola M, et al. Interplay between glutamatergic and GABAergic neurotransmission alterations in cognitive and motor impairment in minimal hepatic encephalopathy. Neurochem Int 2015;88:15–9.
14. Shawcross DL, et al. Systemic inflammatory response exacerbates the neuropsychological effects of induced hyperammonemia in cirrhosis. J Hepatol 2004; 40(2):247–54.
15. Cordoba J, et al. Characteristics, risk factors, and mortality of cirrhotic patients hospitalized for hepatic encephalopathy with and without acute-on-chronic liver failure (ACLF). J Hepatol 2014;60(2):275–81.
16. Bajaj JS, et al. Hepatic encephalopathy is Associated with mortality in patients with cirrhosis independent of other extrahepatic organ failures. Clin Gastroenterol Hepatol 2017;15(4):565–574 e4.
17. Shawcross DL, et al. Infection and systemic inflammation, not ammonia, are associated with Grade 3/4 hepatic encephalopathy, but not mortality in cirrhosis. J Hepatol 2011;54(4):640–9.
18. Bajaj JS, et al. Altered profile of human gut microbiome is associated with cirrhosis and its complications. J Hepatol 2014;60(5):940–7.
19. Bajaj JS, et al. Linkage of gut microbiome with cognition in hepatic encephalopathy. Am J Physiol Gastrointest Liver Physiol 2012;302(1):G168–75.
20. Bajaj JS, et al. Colonic mucosal microbiome differs from stool microbiome in cirrhosis and hepatic encephalopathy and is linked to cognition and inflammation. Am J Physiol Gastrointest Liver Physiol 2012;303(6):G675–85.
21. Bajaj JS, et al. Salivary microbiota reflects changes in gut microbiota in cirrhosis with hepatic encephalopathy. Hepatology 2015;62(4):1260–71.
22. Zhang Z, et al. Large-scale survey of gut microbiota associated with MHE via 16S rRNA-based pyrosequencing. Am J Gastroenterol 2013;108(10):1601–11.
23. Chen Y, et al. Gut dysbiosis in acute-on-chronic liver failure and its predictive value for mortality. J Gastroenterol Hepatol 2015;30(9):1429–37.

24. Wong JM, et al. Colonic health: fermentation and short chain fatty acids. J Clin Gastroenterol 2006;40(3):235–43.
25. Peng L, et al. Butyrate enhances the intestinal barrier by facilitating tight junction assembly via activation of AMP-activated protein kinase in Caco-2 cell monolayers. J Nutr 2009;139(9):1619–25.
26. Merli M, et al. Increased risk of cognitive impairment in cirrhotic patients with bacterial infections. J Hepatol 2013;59(2):243–50.
27. Hung TH, et al. The effect of infections on the mortality of cirrhotic patients with hepatic encephalopathy. Epidemiol Infect 2013;141(12):2671–8.
28. Fernandez J, et al. Bacterial and fungal infections in acute-on-chronic liver failure: prevalence, characteristics and impact on prognosis. Gut 2018;67(10):1870–80.
29. O'Leary JG, et al. NACSELD acute-on-chronic liver failure (NACSELD-ACLF) score predicts 30-day survival in hospitalized patients with cirrhosis. Hepatology 2018;67(6):2367–74.
30. Piano S, et al. Epidemiology and effects of bacterial infections in patients with cirrhosis worldwide. Gastroenterology 2019;156(5):1368–80.e10.
31. Bajaj JS, Kamath PS, Reddy KR. The evolving challenge of infections in cirrhosis. N Engl J Med 2021;384(24):2317–30.
32. Bajaj JS, et al. Prediction of fungal infection development and their impact on survival using the NACSELD cohort. Am J Gastroenterol 2018;113(4):556–63.
33. Mehta G, et al. Systemic inflammation is associated with increased intrahepatic resistance and mortality in alcohol-related acute-on-chronic liver failure. Liver Int 2015;35(3):724–34.
34. Bajaj JS, et al. Review article: the design of clinical trials in hepatic encephalopathy–an International Society for Hepatic Encephalopathy and Nitrogen Metabolism (ISHEN) consensus statement. Aliment Pharmacol Ther 2011;33(7):739–47.
35. Ong JP, et al. Correlation between ammonia levels and the severity of hepatic encephalopathy. Am J Med 2003;114(3):188–93.
36. Gundling F, et al. How to diagnose hepatic encephalopathy in the emergency department. Ann Hepatol 2013;12(1):108–14.
37. Drolz A, et al. Clinical impact of arterial ammonia levels in ICU patients with different liver diseases. Intensive Care Med 2013;39(7):1227–37.
38. Romero-Gomez M, Montagnese S, Jalan R. Hepatic encephalopathy in patients with acute decompensation of cirrhosis and acute-on-chronic liver failure. J Hepatol 2015;62(2):437–47.
39. Bajaj JS, et al. Association between intestinal microbiota collected at hospital Admission and outcomes of patients with cirrhosis. Clin Gastroenterol Hepatol 2019;17(4):756–65.e3.
40. Bajaj JS, et al. Admission serum metabolites and thyroxine predict Advanced hepatic encephalopathy in a multicenter inpatient cirrhosis cohort. Clin Gastroenterol Hepatol 2023;21(4):1031–40.e3.
41. Teasdale G, Jennett B. Assessment of coma and impaired consciousness. A practical scale. Lancet 1974;2(7872):81–4.
42. Burki TK. Post-traumatic stress in the intensive care unit. Lancet Respir Med 2019;7(10):843–4.
43. Nadim MK, et al. Management of the critically ill patient with cirrhosis: A multidisciplinary perspective. J Hepatol 2016;64(3):717–35.
44. Hassanein TI, et al. Randomized controlled study of extracorporeal albumin dialysis for hepatic encephalopathy in advanced cirrhosis. Hepatology 2007;46(6):1853–62.

45. Banares R, et al. Extracorporeal albumin dialysis with the molecular adsorbent re-circulating system in acute-on-chronic liver failure: the RELIEF trial. Hepatology 2013;57(3):1153–62.
46. Larsen FS. Artificial liver support in acute and acute-on-chronic liver failure. Curr Opin Crit Care 2019;25(2):187–91.
47. Krisper P, et al. In vivo quantification of liver dialysis: comparison of albumin dialysis and fractionated plasma separation. J Hepatol 2005;43(3):451–7.
48. Kribben A, et al. Effects of fractionated plasma separation and adsorption on survival in patients with acute-on-chronic liver failure. Gastroenterology 2012;142(4): 782–789 e3.
49. O'Leary JG, et al. Outcomes After listing for liver transplant in patients with Acute-on-chronic liver failure: the multicenter North American Consortium for the study of end-stage liver disease experience. Liver Transpl 2019;25(4):571–9.
50. Sundaram V, et al. Factors Associated with survival of patients with severe Acute-on-chronic liver failure before and After liver transplantation. Gastroenterology 2019;156(5):1381–91.e3.
51. Abdallah MA, et al. Systematic review with meta-analysis: liver transplant provides survival benefit in patients with acute on chronic liver failure. Aliment Pharmacol Ther 2020;52(2):222–32.
52. Hernaez R, et al. Considerations for prognosis, goals of care, and specialty palliative care for hospitalized patients with Acute-on-chronic liver failure. Hepatology 2020;72(3):1109–16.
53. Adejumo AC, et al. Suboptimal use of inpatient palliative care consultation may lead to higher readmissions and costs in end-stage liver disease. J Palliat Med 2020;23(1):97–106.
54. O'Leary JG, et al. Underutilization of hospice in inpatients with cirrhosis: the NAC-SELD experience. Dig Dis Sci 2020;65(9):2571–9.
55. Rush B, et al. Palliative care access for hospitalized patients with end-stage liver disease across the United States. Hepatology 2017;66(5):1585–91.

Bacterial Infections in Acute on Chronic Liver Failure

Simone Incicco, MD, Paolo Angeli, MD, PhD, Salvatore Piano, MD, PhD*

KEYWORDS

- Sepsis • Acute on chronic liver failure • Liver transplantation • Liver cirrhosis
- Septic shock

KEY POINTS

- Bacterial Infections are the most common precipitating event of ACLF. Moreover, in patients with ACLF a state of immune paralysis facilitates the occurrence of bacterial/fungal infections.
- The combination of bacterial infections and ACLF is associated with high mortality rate.
- Bacterial infections should be ruled out in all patients with ACLF.
- Timely administration of an appropriate empirical antibiotic therapy improves survival in patients with ACLF.
- The treatment of infections in patients with ACLF should be aggressive, ensuring coverage also for multidrug-resistant bacteria according to the local epidemiology.

INTRODUCTION

In the last years, the interaction between bacterial infections (BIs) and acute chronic liver failure (ACLF) has emerged as a hot topic in liver disease: BIs have been shown to be the most frequent precipitating events of ACLF[1–4] and to have a huge negative impact on the clinical course of ACLF and patients' outcome.[2,5,6] Furthermore patients with ACLF display features of immune system paralysis[7,8] which increase the occurrence of new bacterial and fungal infections, further aggravating the course of the syndrome.[5] Finally, the increasing spread of multidrug-resistant (MDR) bacteria, especially in nosocomial settings, poses a great challenge in the management of patients with ACLF and BIs.[9–11]

Herein we reviewed the literature on pathophysiology, epidemiology, clinical impact, and treatment strategies of BIs both precipitating and complicating ACLF.

Department of Medicine (DIMED), Unit of Internal Medicine and Hepatology (UIMH), University Hospital of Padova, Via Giustiniani 2, Padova 35128, Italy
* Corresponding author. Department of Medicine (DIMED), Unit of Internal Medicine and Hepatology (UIMH), University Hospital of Padova, Via Giustiniani 2, Padova 35128, Italy.
E-mail address: salvatorepiano@gmail.com

Clin Liver Dis 27 (2023) 703–716
https://doi.org/10.1016/j.cld.2023.03.013
1089-3261/23/© 2023 Elsevier Inc. All rights reserved.

PATHOPHYSIOLOGY OF BACTERIAL INFECTIONS-RELATED ACUTE-ON-CHRONIC LIVER FAILURE

ACLF is characterized by full-blown systemic inflammation whose intensity correlates with the number of organ failures and patients' prognosis.[1,12] Systemic inflammation is thought to cause organ failure through different mechanisms. The first is the nitric oxide (NO)-mediated accentuation of preexisting splanchnic vasodilation and reduction in arterial effective blood volume resulting in the overactivation of endogenous vasoconstrictor systems and tissue hypoperfusion.[13] Furthermore, inflammatory cells and mediators cause immune-mediated tissue damage, a process called immunopathology.[14] Finally, inflammatory cytokines, reactive oxygen species (ROS) and NO can induce mitochondrial dysfunction, compromising cellular energy production through oxidative phosphorylation.[15]

In BI-related ACLF systemic inflammation is induced by pathogen-associated molecular patterns (PAMPs), unique conserved molecular structures that are recognized by pattern recognition receptors (PRRs) expressed in myeloid immune cells, such as Toll- (TLRs) and NOD-like receptors (NLRs).[16] PRRs engagement activates intracellular signaling pathways leading to cytokine production, recruitment and activation of cells of the innate immune system[16] (**Fig. 1**).

Several findings suggest the existence of an excessive inflammatory response to BIs in patients with cirrhosis. Patients with BIs and cirrhosis have higher plasma levels of proinflammatory cytokines than non-cirrhotic patients.[17,18] Ex-vivo studies found that lipopolysaccharide (LPS, a PAMP recognized by TLR4) stimulated production of proinflammatory cytokines (in particular tumor necrosis factor [TNF]-alpha and interleukin [IL]-6) is more pronounced in cells from patients with cirrhosis than in control cells and that monocytes from patients with cirrhosis show defects in negative-feedback mechanisms of TLR4 signaling.[19]

Bacterial Infections as Precipitating Event of Acute-On-Chronic Liver Failure

In the last decade, several studies have shown that BIs are by far the most common precipitating event of ACLF. In the CANONIC study, a European multicenter observational study that defined the diagnostic criteria of the syndrome, ACLF was triggered by BIs in one-third of the patients.[1] In the PREDICT study cohort, ACLF was precipitated by proven BIs in more than 40% of cases.[3] On the other hand, data coming from the GLOBAL study show that, worldwide, almost half (48%) of hospitalized patients with BIs develops ACLF during hospitalization, with the highest rates observed in the Indian subcontinent (75%) and the lowest in Southern Europe (38%).[5]

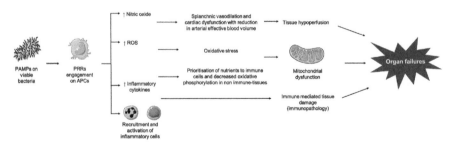

Fig. 1. Pathogenesis of bacterial infections-related ACLF. APCs, antigen-presenting cells; PAMPs, pathogen-associated molecular patterns; PRRs, pattern recognition receptors; RAAS, renin-angiotensin-aldosterone System; ROS, reactive oxygen species; SNS, sympathetic nervous system.

Among BIs, spontaneous bacterial peritonitis (SBP), pneumonia, nosocomial infections, and infections caused by multidrug-resistant (MDR) and extensively drug-resistant (XDR) bacteria are associated with a higher risk of ACLF.[1–3,5,10] Other clinical characteristics associated with the risk of developing ACLF in patients with BIs are ascites, hepatic encephalopathy (HE) and a higher MELD score,[5] while the administration of an appropriate empirical antibiotic therapy has been shown to reduce the risk of ACLF development.[3,5]

Data evaluating the clinical course of ACLF confirmed that when ACLF is precipitated by BIs, the clinical course is far more complex. Indeed, patients with ACLF precipitated by BIs have higher degree of systemic inflammation, a more severe ACLF grade and are more likely to have a worsening of ACLF grade than patients with ACLF not triggered by BIs.[2,3,20] Moreover, the 28-day and 90-day mortality is significantly higher in patients with BIs associated with ACLF than in ACLF not precipitated by BIs.[2,3,6]

BACTERIAL INFECTIONS AS A COMPLICATION OF ACUTE-ON-CHRONIC LIVER FAILURE

BIs are not only the most common precipitating event of ACLF but also an extremely frequent complication of the syndrome. Data from the CANONIC study show that approximately one every two (46%) noninfected patients with ACLF develops BIs within 4 weeks after diagnosis.[2] Furthermore, patients with ACLF are at increased risk of developing invasive fungal infections.[2,21] Bacterial and fungal infections complicating ACLF significantly increase 28-day and 90-day transplant-free mortality rates.[2,21] Risk factors for developing bacterial and fungal infections are higher grade of systemic inflammation (as shown by higher levels of leukocytes and C-reactive protein [CRP]), oxidative stress and higher severity of ACLF at the diagnosis of the syndrome.[2]

The mechanism of the increased risk of BIs in patients with ACLF is likely multifactorial, involving an increase in intestinal permeability, changes in the gut microbiome, immune dysfunction, and invasive procedures.

Systemic inflammation may enhance pathological bacterial translocation in several ways.[22] TNF-alpha, IL-6 and ROS increase intestinal permeability by disrupting epithelial tight-junctions,[23,24] while interferon (IFN)-gamma induces transcytosis of commensal *Escherichia coli* across epithelial cells.[25] The release of norepinephrine at the intestinal mucosa, due to systemic inflammation-related worsening of circulatory dysfunction and homeostatic stimulation of sympathetic nervous system, impairs the local immune system function and induces qualitative and quantitative changes of the intestinal microbiota toward a phenotype associated with bacterial translocation.[26,27]

Recently published metagenomic studies show the existence of marked alterations in gut microbiota in patients with cirrhosis that parallel disease severity and reach their maximum in patients with ACLF.[28] These alterations, characterized by a progressive reduction in gut microbial diversity and enrichment by unusual gut bacteria (particularly *Enterococcus* species), are associated with worse prognosis and development of complications, in particular hepatic encephalopathy and BIs[28,29]. As suggested by experimental models of liver cirrhosis, altered gut microbiota may impair intestinal immune responses and disrupt intestinal barrier function, promoting bacterial translocation.[30]

ACLF is frequently associated with a state of immune paralysis characterized by impaired pathogen-killing activity and ROS release by macrophages and neutrophils.[31,32] Indeed, patients with ACLF have expanded populations of immunoregulatory monocytes and myeloid-derived suppressor cells, which are characterized by a distinct transcriptional profile, altered metabolism and weak antimicrobial immune responses.[33–35]

Finally, patients with ACLF frequently undergo invasive procedures, such as urinary, intra-arterial and central venous catheters and/or requires organ support devices, which are other major factors increasing the risk of BIs in these patients.[36]

PREVENTION OF BACTERIAL INFECTIONS

The prevention of BIs is of utmost importance in improving the prognosis of patients with decompensated cirrhosis. The main current strategy is the use of prophylactic antibiotics targeted at specific subpopulations at high risk of BIs (**Table 1**).[37] However, due to the spread of antibiotic resistance worldwide, nonantibiotic prophylactic strategies are gaining increasing interest.

Antibiotic Prophylaxis

Antibiotic prophylaxis should consider the balance between preventing infections and the risk of selecting MDR bacteria.[38] The universal prophylaxis has not been shown to be useful in patients hospitalized for acute decompensation (AD) of cirrhosis and should be discouraged pending new data.[39] There are only three clinical scenarios in which antibiotic prophylaxis has been shown to be beneficial in patients with cirrhosis, namely, upper gastrointestinal bleeding, secondary prophylaxis of SBP and primary prophylaxis in patients at high risk of developing SBP.

In patients with upper gastrointestinal bleeding, infections are frequent and increase the probability of unsuccessful bleeding control, rebleeding and in-hospital mortality.[40] Antibiotic prophylaxis has been shown to reduce the incidence of BIs, rebleeding, and mortality and should be instituted from admission.[40,41] The administration of intravenous ceftriaxone is now reccomended since it is more effective than norfloxacin

Table 1 Current indications for antibiotic prophylaxis in cirrhosis	
Indication	**Antibiotic and Dose**
Upper gastrointestinal bleeding	Norfloxacin 400 mg/12 h for 5–7 d in patients with preserved liver function; IV Ceftriaxone 1 g/d for 5–7 d in case of: • Advanced liver disease (at least 2 of the following: ascites, malnutrition, Hepatic Encephalopathy, bilirubin > 3 mg/dL); • Ongoing quinolone prophylaxis; • High prevalence of quinolone-resistant bacteria.
Secondary prophylaxis of SBP	Norfloxacin 400 mg/d.
Primary prophylaxis of SBP in patients with low protein ascites (<1.5 g/dL)	Norfloxacin 400 mg/d until liver transplantation, clinical improvement and resolution of ascites in patients with at least one of: • Child-Turcotte-Pugh score ≥9 with serum bilirubin ≥3 mg/dL; • serum creatinine ≥1.2 mg/dL or urea ≥25 mg/dL; serum sodium <130 mmol/L.

Legend: SBP, spontaneous bacterial peritonitis.

in patients with advanced cirrhosis (≥2 of the following: ascites, severe malnutrition, HE, bilirubin >3 mg/dL).[42] Anyway, antibiotic prophylaxis regimen should be adapted to local epidemiology and patterns of antibiotic resistance.[41]

In patients surviving an episode of SBP, norfloxacin reduced the recurrence of SBP.[43] Furthermore, in patients with ascites and the highest risk of developing a first episode of SBP (ascitic fluid protein <1.5 g/dL and at least one of: Child-Turcotte-Pugh score ≥9 with serum bilirubin ≥3 mg/dL; serum creatinine ≥1.2 mg/dL or urea ≥25 mg/dL; serum sodium <130 mmol/L), norfloxacin prophylaxis reduced the incidence of SBP and slightly improved survival.[44] More recently, a post hoc analysis of a randomized placebo-controlled trial confirmed the survival benefit of norfloxacin prophylaxis in patients with Child-Turcotte-Pugh class C and low ascitic fluid protein (<1.5 g/dL).[45] For these reason, current guidelines recommend primary and secondary norfloxacin prophylaxis (400 mg/d) in these patients.[37]

Rifaximin is a nonabsorbable broad-spectrum antibiotic and does not appear to promote the emergence of antibiotic resistance.[46] Nonrandomized studies and small randomized controlled trials showed that rifaximin may be effective at preventing infections in patients with cirrhosis[46,47] However, whether rifaximin could replace quinolones in the prevention of SBP should be proven in well-designed clinical trials.

Nonantibiotic Prophylaxis

Use of proton pump inhibitors in patients with cirrhosis is frequently inappropriate and has been associated with a higher risk of developing SBP and non-SBP infections.[48] Therefore, their use should be restricted to patients with a clear indication. In patients with ACLF, the high level of instrumentation may favor nosocomial infections, therefore it is important to remove central venous catheters, bladder catheters, and stop mechanical ventilation as soon as possible.

Long-term human albumin administration has been shown to improve survival and reduce the incidence of SBP and non-SBP infections in stable patients with uncomplicated grade 2 and 3 ascites or in those with refractory ascites.[49,50] These effects are probably related to the immunomodulatory properties of albumin.[51] However, in the setting of AD, short-term albumin administration did not reduce the incidence of BIs and is associated with side effects such as pulmonary edema or fluid overload.[52] Therefore, there are not enough data to suggest the use of albumin to prevent infections in patients with ACLF.

Nonselective beta-blockers (NSBBs) were associated with a reduced risk of SBP.[53] NSBBs were also shown to decrease intestinal permeability, bacterial translocation, and level of inflammatory cytokines, independently from portal pressure reduction.[54] In patients with ACLF, the use of NSBBs was associated with better survival,[55] therefore their use should not be discontinued in ACLF unless in case of circulatory failure or severe acute kidney injury with hypotension.

By reversing gut dysbiosis and creating a health microbiome,[56] fecal microbiota transplantation may represent a promising strategy in the prevention of BIs and decompensation but must be evaluated in further clinical trials.

MANAGEMENT OF BACTERIAL INFECTIONS IN ACUTE-ON-CHRONIC LIVER FAILURE

Early diagnosis and prompt antibiotic treatment of BIs are paramount in the management of patients with AD and ACLF. Indeed, each hour delay in performing a diagnostic paracentesis and starting an effective antimicrobial therapy has been associated with an increased risk of mortality in patients with SBP.[57,58] Any patient with proven BI should be assessed for the presence of sepsis/septic shock and organ failures, through sepsis-3 criteria[59] and CLIF-SOFA score,[1] respectively, in order to identify patients at higher risk of mortality that need more intensive management.

Diagnosis of Bacterial Infections

Since the clinical presentation of BIs may be subtle and the onset of AD and/or organ dysfunction and failure can be the sole sign of infection, diagnosis of BIs in patients with cirrhosis is challenging and requires a high index of suspicion. Therefore, every patient with ACLF should be considered potentially infected until proven otherwise and a complete work-up (blood cell count and culture; diagnostic paracentesis with ascites fluid culture; urinary sediment and culture; chest X-ray) should be carried out at admission and whenever a hospitalized patient deteriorates in order to detect and treat a possible infection.[37]

Acute-phase proteins, such as CRP and procalcitonin (PCT) have been proven to be useful in predicting BIs in patients with cirrhosis, especially when used in combination.[60] However, although BIs-related ACLF is associated with higher levels of inflammatory markers,[2] systemic inflammation is a typical feature in all patients with ACLF and is not restricted to patients with active infections.[1] For this reason, the distinction between patients with ongoing BIs and those with sterile inflammation is challenging and novel diagnostic biomarkers are urgently needed at this purpose.

Screening for colonization by MDR bacteria should be considered in patients admitted to the intensive care unit (ICU), in particular in centers with a high prevalence of MDR bacteria. In fact, rectal colonization by MDR bacteria has been associated with a higher risk of infection by MDR bacteria in cirrhosis.[61]

Antibiotic Treatment

An appropriate empirical antibiotic treatment is the cornerstone in the management of BIs since it improves survival in patients with both AD and ACLF and prevents ACLF development.[2,3,5,9,10] However, the spread of antimicrobial resistance challenges the selection of the proper empirical therapy. Worldwide prevalence of infections sustained by MDR and XDR pathogens is 34% and 8%, respectively, and they are associated with a higher incidence of septic shock and ACLF and a worse outcome.[2,3,5,9,10] Nosocomial and healthcare-associated infections and recent exposure to systemic antibiotics, frequently encountered in patients with decompensated cirrhosis, are the main risk factors for their acquisition.[9]

Considering the high risk of mortality in patients with ACLF, a broad-spectrum antibiotic treatment is recommended for these patients. In fact, data from the CANONIC and PREDICT studies show that in Europe classic antibiotic schemes, based on third-generation cephalosporins, amoxicilliin/clavulanate, and quinolones, have unacceptable efficacy (<40%) in nosocomial infections and in those triggering ACLF whereas empirical MDR-covering strategies (carbapenems ± glycopeptides or daptomycin/linezolid in areas with a high prevalence of vancomycin-resistant *Enterococci*) are associated with higher rates of infection resolution and improved survival.[3,10] The empirical antibiotic treatment should be the one suggested for nosocomial infections or healthcare-associated infections in centers with a high prevalence of MDR (eg, carbapenems ± glycopeptides or daptomycin for SBP).[62,63] Piperacillin/tazobactam is an alternative to carbapenems in centers with lower prevalence of ESBL-producing *Enterobacteriaceae*, while ceftolozane/tazobactam could be considered as a potential "carbapenem-sparing" strategy. Whenever microbiological cultures allow the identification of bacteria responsible for infections, antibiotic therapy should be narrowed according to antimicrobial susceptibility tests.[37] Data from the GLOBAL study confirmed that adherence to these recommendations is associated with higher microbiological efficacy and lower mortality rates.[9]

Empirical use of novel antibiotics active against carbapenem-resistant Gram-negative bacteria (ceftazidime/avibactam, meropenem/vaborbactam, imipenem/relebactam, cefiderocol) should be reserved for colonized patients.[61,64] In carbapenem-resistant bacteria the type of gene conferring resistance should be identified and

Table 2
Recommended empirical antibiotic treatment for the most frequent bacterial infections in patients with ACLF

Type of Infection	Empirical Antibiotic Treatment		
	Gram Negative Coverage[f]	**Gram Positive Coverage**	**Antifungal Agents**
SBP, SBE and spontaneous bacteremia	Piperacillin/tazobactam[a] or Carbapenems or Ceftolozane/tazobactam[b]	Glycopeptides or Daptomycin or Linezolid[c]	Consider empirical echinocandin in patients with risk factors for invasive fungal infections[d]
UTI	Piperacillin/tazobactam[a] or Carbapenems or Ceftolozane/tazobactam[b]	Glycopeptides[e]	Candiduria can be a contaminant in patients with urinary catheter and catheter removal/substitution can be sufficient. Fluconazole for symptomatic infections
Pneumonia	Piperacillin/tazobactam[a] or Carbapenems or Ceftolozane/tazobactam[b]	Linezolid or Glycopeptides	Consider empirical echinocandin in patients with risk factors for invasive fungal infections[d] Isavuconazole or liposomal amphotericin B in case of aspergillosis
SSTI	Piperacillin/tazobactam or Carbapenems	Daptomycin or Glycopeptides[e] or Linezolid	

Legend: SBP, spontaneous bacterial peritonitis; SBE, spontaneous bacterial empyema; UTI, urinary tract infection, SSTI, skin and soft tissue infection.
[a] In areas with a low prevalence of ESBL-producing Enterobacteriaceae.
[b] Carbapenem-sparing strategy in areas with a high prevalence of ESBL-producing Enterobacteriaceae.
[c] Glycopeptides in areas with a high prevalence MRSA and vancomycin-susceptible *Enterococci*. Daptomycin should be preferred if MRSA MIC for vancomycin is > 1 mg/L. Linezolid should be preferred in areas with a high prevalence of vancomycin-resistant *Enterococci*.
[d] Central venous catheter, parenteral nutrition, recent endoscopy, and antibiotic exposure, in-hospital stay greater than 15 d, diabetes, AKI, second infections.
[e] IV vancomycin or teicoplanin in areas with a high prevalence MRSA and vancomycin-susceptible *Enterococci*. Vancomycin must be replaced by linezolid in areas with a high prevalence of vancomycin-resistant *Enterococci*.
[f] Consider empirical treatment with ceftazidime/avibactam or meropenem/varbobactam or imipenem/relebactam in patients colonized by carbapenem-resistant *Enterobacteriaceae/Pseudomonas aeruginosa*. In patients with colonization by carbapenem-resistant *Acinetobacter baumannii* or metallobetalactamases producers consider empirical treatment with cefiderocol.

cefiderocol should be used in case of metallobetalactamases producing strains (not susceptible against other novel antibiotics). Empirical antifungal therapy should be considered in patients with risk factors for invasive fungal infections (central venous catheter, parenteral nutrition, recent endoscopy, and antibiotic exposure, in-hospital stay>15 days, diabetes, AKI) and in those not improving after 48 to 72 hours on broad-spectrum antibiotics.[21,64,65] Due to emergence of fluconazole-resistant organisms, echinocandins are the treatment of choice in this scenario.[11] Details about empirical antibiotic treatment strategies have been reported in **Table 2** and **Fig. 2**.

Pharmacokinetic Optimization of Antibiotic Schedules

Beyond the microbiological activity of drugs, the optimization of antibiotics' dosage is a major contributor to their effectiveness. Critically ill patients with cirrhosis frequently present hypoalbuminemia and third space expansion resulting in increased volume of distribution and potentially sub-therapeutic concentration of hydrophilic antibiotics, when standard approved dosages are administered.[11] Therefore, high antibiotic doses should be considered within the first 48 hours after the diagnosis of severe infections. Moreover, a continuous or extended infusion should be considered for the administration of time-dependent antibiotics (eg, beta-lactams, glycopeptides).[11] Indeed, continuous infusion of beta-lactams was associated with better 30-day survival than intermittent infusion in patients with cirrhosis and bloodstream infections.[66] Five to 7 days of antibiotic treatment are sufficient in most cases.

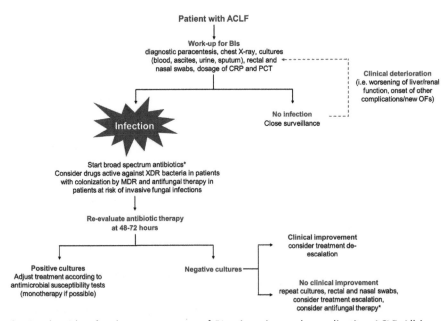

Fig. 2. Algorithm for the management of BIs triggering and complicating ACLF. All inpatients with ACLF should undergo a thorough diagnostic work-up for infections at admission or anytime clinical deterioration occurs. In case of proven or suspected BIs, broad-spectrum antibiotics should be administered. After 48 to 72 hours of therapy antibiotic schedules should be re-evaluated according to results of microbiology/susceptibility tests, and clinical course. *, See **Table 2**. ACLF, acute-on-chronic liver failure; BIs, bacterial infections; CRP, C-reactive protein; PCT, procalcitonin; OFs, organ failures; XDR, extensively drug resistant.

Nonantibiotic Management of Bacterial Infections in Acute-On-Chronic Liver Failure

The management of patients with BIs and ACLF involve also the management and prevention of organ failures as well as the bridging strategies to liver transplant (LT). The management of organ failures has been discussed in another section of this issue of Clinics in Liver Disease. As far as the prevention of organ failures is concerned, the use of albumin in patients with SBP has been shown to reduce the incidence of renal failure and mortality.[67] Controversial results have been shown in patients with infections other than SBP.[68–70] Although in the INFECIR-2 trial, the administration of albumin was associated with higher rates of ACLF resolution and lower rates of nosocomial infections, no difference in survival was found.[70] Therefore, there is no evidence to support albumin use in non-SBP infections. LT is certainly the most effective treatment of severe ACLF,[71] however, BIs are associated with a high risk of death and/or of permanent delisting.[72] In fact, BIs requires temporary suspension from the waiting list and the LT can be delayed due to the fear of poor outcomes. Although the post-LT course is more complex in patients with pretransplant infections than those without, the survival is excellent and therefore transplant should not be delayed as soon as patients are resolving infections.[73] However, it should be highlighted that an MDR bacterial infection before transplant is an independent risk factor of post-LT mortality in ACLF.[74]

SUMMARY

BIs are by far the most frequent precipitating event and complication of ACLF. Patients with ACLF and BIs are at higher risk of mortality than noninfected ones. For this reason, BIs triggering and complicating ACLF should be promptly diagnosed and treated. The administration of broad-spectrum antibiotics is associated with higher rates of infection resolution and better survival than classic antibiotic schemes in ACLF. New strategies for preventing BIs in patients with ACLF are urgently needed. Finally, in patients surviving ACLF and BIs, liver transplant should not be delayed.

CLINICS CARE POINTS

- Bacterial infections should be ruled out in all patients with ACLF

- A complete work-up for BIs (paracentesis with PMN count, blood, ascitic fluid, and urine cultures, Chest X-ray) is recommended in patients ACLF.

- An early and appropriate empirical antibiotic treatment improves survival in patients with ACLF and BIs.

- Due to the spread of MDR bacteria empirical broad-spectrum antibiotic treatment should be used in patients with BIs either triggering or complicating ACLF.

- Extended/continuous infusion of time-dependent antibiotics (eg, beta-lactams) should be considered in patients with BIs and ACLF

FINANCIAL STATEMENT

No specific funding supported this study.

DISCLOSURE

The authors have nothing to disclose regarding the work under consideration for publication.

AUTHORS' CONTRIBUTION

S. Incicco, P. Angeli, and S. Piano reviewed the literature and drafted of the article

REFERENCES

1. Moureau R, Jalan R, Gines P, et al. Acute-on-Chronic Liver Failure is a distinct syndrome that develops in patients with acute decompensation of Cirrhosis. Gastroenterology 2013;144:1426–37.
2. Fernandez J, Acevedo J, Weist R, et al. Bacterial and fungal infections in acute-on-chronic liver failure: prevalence, characteristics and impact on prognosis. Gut 2018;67:1870–80.
3. Trebicka J, Fernandez J, Papp M, et al. PREDICT identifies precipitating events associated with the clinical course of acutely decompensated cirrhosis. J Hepatol 2021;74:1097–108.
4. Bajaj JS, O'Leary JG, Reddy KR, et al. Survival in infection-related acute-on-chronic liver failure is defined by extrahepatic organ failures. Hepatology 2014; 60:250–6.
5. Wong F, Piano S, Singh V, et al. Clinical features and evolution of bacterial infection-related acute-on-chronic liver failure. J Hepatol 2021;74:1330–9.
6. Mücke MM, Rumyantseva T, Mücke VT, et al. Bacterial infection-triggered acute-on-chronic liver failure is associated with increased mortality. Liver Int 2018;38: 645–53.
7. Martin-Mateos R, Alvarez-Mon M, Albillos A. Dysfunctional immune response in acute-on-chronic liver failure: it Takes two to Tango. Front Immunol 2019;10:973.
8. Wasmuth HE, Kunz D, Yagmur E, et al. Patients with acute on chronic liver failure display "sepsis-like" immune paralysis. J Hepatol 2005;42:195–201.
9. Piano S, Singh V, Caraceni P, et al. Epidemiology and effects of bacterial infections in patients with cirrhosis worldwide. Gatsroenterology 2019;156:1368–80.
10. Fernandez J, Prado V, Trebicka J, et al. Multidrug-resistant bacterial infections in patients with decompensated cirrhosis and with acute-on-chronic liver failure in Europe. J Hepatol 2019;70:398–411.
11. Fernandez J, Piano S, Bartoletti M, et al. Management of bacterial and fungal infections in cirrhosis: the MDRO challenge. J Hepatol 2021;75:S101–17.
12. Clària J, Stauber RE, Coenraad MJ, et al. Systemic inflammation in decompensated cirrhosis: Characterization and role in acute-on-chronic liver failure. Hepatology 2016;64:1249–64.
13. Bernardi M, Moreau R, Angeli P, et al. Mechanisms of decompensation and organ failure in cirrhosis: from peripheral arterial vasodilation to systemic inflammation hypothesis. J Hepatol 2015;65:1272–84.
14. Casulleras M, Zhang IW, López-Vicario C, et al. Leukocytes, systemic inflammation and immunopathology in acute-on-chronic liver failure. Cells 2020;9:2632.
15. Moreau R, Clària J, Aguilar F, et al. Blood metabolomics uncovers inflammation-associated mitochondrial dysfunction as a potential mechanism underlying ACLF. J Hepatol 2020;72:688–701.
16. Kumar H, Kawai T, Akira S. Pathogen recognition by the innate immune system. Int Rev Immunol 2011;30:16–34.
17. Byl B, Roucloux I, Crusiaux A, et al. Tumor necrosis factor alpha and interleukin 6 plasma levels in infected cirrhotic patients. Gastroenterology 1993;104:1492–7.
18. Navasa M, Follo A, Filella X, et al. Tumor necrosis factor and interleukin-6 in spontaneous bacterial peritonitis in cirrhosis: relationship with the development of renal impairment and mortality. Hepatology 1998;27:1227–32.

19. Arroyo V, Moreau R, Kamath PS, et al. Acute-on-chronic liver failure in cirrhosis. Nat Rev Dis Primers 2016;2:16041.

20. Gustot T, Fernandez J, Garcia E, et al. Clinical Course of acute-on-chronic liver failure syndrome and effects on prognosis. Hepatology 2015;62:243–52.

21. Bartoletti M, Rinaldi M, Pasquini Z, et al. Risk factors for Candidaemia in hospitalized patients with liver cirrhosis: a multicentre case–control–control study. Clin Microbiol Infect 2020;27:276–82.

22. Wiest R, Lawson M, Geukin M. Pathological bacterial translocation in liver cirrhosis. J Hepatol 2014;60:197–209.

23. Taylor CT, Dzus AL, Colgan SP. Autocrine regulation of epithelial permeability by hypoxia: role for polarized release of tumor necrosis factor alpha. Gastroenterology 1998;114:657–68.

24. Suzuki T, Yoshinaga N, Tanabe S. Inter leukin-6 (IL-6) regulates claudin-2 expression and tight junction permeability in intestinal epithelium. J Biol Chem 2011;286: 31263–71.

25. Clark E, Hoare C, Tanianis-Hughes J, et al. Interferon gamma induces translocation of commensal Escherichia coli across gut epithelial cells via a lipid raft-mediated process. Gastroenterology 2005;128:1258–67.

26. Freestone PP, Williams PH, Haigh RD, et al. Growth stimulation of intestinal commensal Escherichia coli by catecholamines: a possible contributory factor in trauma-induced sepsis. Shock 2002;18:465–70.

27. Worlicek M, Knebel K, Linde HJ, et al. Splanchnic sympathectomy prevents translocation and spreading of E. coli but not S. aureus in liver cirrhosis. Gut 2010;59:1127–34.

28. Solé C, Guilly S, Da Silva K, et al. Alterations in gut microbiome in cirrhosis as assessed by quantitative metagenomics: relationship with acute-on-chronic liver failure and prognosis. Gatroenterology 2021;160:206–18.

29. Bajaj JS, Vargas HE, Reddy KR, et al. Association between intestinal microbiota collected at hospital admission and outcomes of patients with cirrhosis. Clin Gastroenterol Hepatol 2019;17:756–65.

30. Munoz L, Borrero M-J, Ubeda M, et al. Intestinal immune dyregulation driven by dysbiosis promotes barrier disruption and bacterial translocation in rats with cirrhosis. Hepatology 2019;70:925–38.

31. Lin CY, Tsai IF, Ho YP, et al. Endotoxemia contributes to the immune paralysis in patients with cirrhosis. J Hepatol 2007;46:816–26.

32. Antoniades CG, Wendon J, Vergani D. Paralysed monocytes in acute on chronic liver disease. J Hepatol 2005;42:163–5.

33. Bernsmeier C, Pop OT, Singanayagam A, et al. Patients with acute-on-chronic liver failure have increased numbers of regulatory immune cells expressing the receptor tyrosine kinase MERTK. Gastroenterology 2015;148:603–15.

34. Bernsmeier C, Triantafyllou E, Brenig R, et al. CD14(+) CD15(-) HLA-DR(-) myeloid-derived suppressor cells impair antimicrobial response in patients with acute-on-chronic liver failure. Gut 2018;67:1155–67.

35. Korf H, du Plessis J, van Pelt J, et al. Inhibition of glutamine synthetase in monocytes from patients with acute-on-chronic liver failure resuscitates their antibacterial and inflammatory capacity. Gut 2019;68:1872–83.

36. Fernandez J, Acevedo J, Castro M, et al. Prevalence and risk factors of infections by multiresistant bacteria in cirrhosis: a prospective study. Hepatology 2012;55: 1551–61.

37. Angeli P, Bernardi M, Villanueva C, et al. EASL clinical practice guidelines for the management of patients with decompensated cirrhosis. J Hepatol 2018;69: 406–60.

38. Fernandez J, Tandon P, Mensa J, et al. Antibiotic prophylaxis in cirrhosis: good and bad. Hepatology 2016;63:2019–31.

39. Kutmutia R, Tittanegro T, China L, et al. Evaluating the role of antibiotics in aptients admitted to hospital with decompensated cirrhosis: lessons from the ATTIRE trial. Am J Gastroenterol 2022;12. https://doi.org/10.14309/ajg. 0000000000001937.

40. Chavez-Tapia NC, Barrientos-Gutierrez T, Tellez-Avila F, et al. Meta-analysis: antibiotic prophylaxis for cirrhotic patients with upper gastrointestinal bleeding – an updated Cochrane review. Aliment Pharmacol Ther 2011;34:509–18.

41. De Franchis R, Bosh J, Garcia-Tsao G, et al. Baveno VII – Renewing consensus in portal hypertension. J Hepatol 2022;76:959–74.

42. Fernandez J, del Arbol LR, Gomez C, et al. Norfloxacin vs ceftriaxone in the prophylaxis of infections in patients with advanced cirrhosis and hemorrhage. Gastroenterology 2006;131:1049–56.

43. Gines P, Rimola A, Planas R, et al. Norfloxacin prevents spontaneous bacterial peritonitis recurrence in cirrhosis: results of a double-blind, placebo-controlled trial. Hepatology 1990;12:716–24.

44. Fernandez J, Navasa M, Planas R, et al. Primary prophylaxis of spontaneous bacterial peritonitis delays hepatorenal syndrome and improves survival in cirrhosis. Gastroenterology 2007;133:818–24.

45. Moreau R, Elkrief L, Bureau C, et al. Effects of long-term norfloxacin therapy in patients with advanced cirrhosis. Gastroenterology 2018;155:1816–27.

46. Caraceni P, Vargas V, Solà E, et al. The use of rifaximin in patients with cirrhosis. Hepatology 2021;74:1660–73.

47. Patel VC, Lee S, McPhail MJW, et al. Rifaximin-α reduces gut-derived inflammation and mucin degradation in cirrhosis and encephalopathy: RIFSYS randomised controlled trial. J Hepatol 2022;76:332–42.

48. Wang J, Wu Y, Bi Q, et al. Adverse outcomes of proton pump inhibitors in chronic liver disease: a systematic review and meta-analysis. Hepatol Int 2020;14: 385–98.

49. Caraceni P, Riggio O, Angeli P, et al. Long-term albumin administration in decompensated cirrhosis (ANSWER): an open-label randomised trial. Lancet 2018;391: 2417–29.

50. Di Pascoli M, Fasolato S, Piano S, et al. Long-term administration of human albumin improves survival in patients with cirrhosis and refractory ascites. Liver Int 2019;39:98–105.

51. Bernardi M, Angeli P, Claria J, et al. Albumin in decompensated cirrhosis: new concepts and perspectives. Gut 2020;69:1127–38.

52. China L, Freemantle N, Forrest E, et al. A randomized trial of albumin infusions in hospitalized patients with cirrhosis. N Eng J Med 2021;384:808–17.

53. Senzolo M, Cholongitas E, Burra P, et al. b-Blockers protect against spontaneous bacterial peritonitis in cirrhotic patients: a meta-analysis. Liver Int 2009;29: 1189–93.

54. Reiberger T, Ferlitsch A, Payer BA, et al. Non-selective betablocker therapy decreases intestinal permeability and serum levels of LBP and IL-6 in patients with cirrhosis. J Hepatol 2013;58:911–21.

55. Mookerjee RP, Pavesi M, Thomsen KL, et al. Treatment with non-selective beta blockers is associated with reduced severity of systemic inflammation and

improved survival of patients with acute-on-chronic liver failure. J Hepatol 2016; 64:574–82.

56. Bajaj JS, Kassam Z, Fagan A, et al. Fecal microbiota transplant from a rational stool donor improves hepatic encephalopathy: a randomized clinical trial. Hepatology 2017;66:1727–38.

57. Kim JJ, Tsukamoto MM, Mathur AK. et al., Delayed paracentesis is associated with increased in-hospital mortality in patients with spontaneous bacterial peritonitis. Am J Gastroenterol 2014;109:1436–42.

58. Karvellas CJ, Abraldes JG, Arabi YM, et al. Appropriate and timely antimicrobial therapy in cirrhotic patients with spontaneous bacterial peritonitis-associated septic shock: a retrospective cohort study. Aliment Pharmacol Ther 2015;41: 747–57.

59. Piano S, Bartoletti M, Tonon M, et al. Assessment of Sepsis-3 criteria and quick SOFA in patients with cirrhosis and bacterial infections. Gut 2018;67:1892–9.

60. Papp M, Vitalis Z, Altorjay I, et al. Acute phase proteins in the diagnosis and prediction of cirrhosis associated bacterial infections. Liver Int 2012;32:603–11.

61. Prado V., Hernández-Tejero M., Mücke M.M., et al., Rectal colonization by resistant bacteria increases the risk of infection by the colonizing strain in critically ill patients with cirrhosis, J Hepatol, 76, 2022,1079–1089.

62. Piano S, Fasolato S, Salinas F, et al. The empirical antibiotic treatment of nosocomial spontaneous bacterial peritonitis: results of a randomized, controlled clinical trial. Hepatology 2016;63:1299–309.

63. Merli M, Lucidi C, Di Gregorio V, et al. An empirical broad spectrum antibiotic therapy in health-care–associated infections improves survival in patients with cirrhosis: a randomized trial. Hepatology 2016;63:1632–9.

64. Piano S, Tonon M, Angeli P. Changes in the epidemiology and management of bacterial infections in cirrhosis. Clin Mol Hepatol 2021;27:437–45.

65. Bajaj JS, Reddy RK, Tandon P, et al. Prediction of fungal infection development and their impact on survival using the NACSELD cohort. Am J Gastroenterol 2018;113:556–63.

66. Bartoletti M, Giannella M, Lewis RE, et al. Extended infusion of beta-lactams for bloodstream infection in patients with liver cirrhosis: an observational multicenter study. Clin Infect Dis 2019;69:1731–9.

67. Sort P, Navasa M, Arroyo V, et al. Effect of intravenous albumin on renal impairment and mortality in patients with cirrhosis and spontaneous bacterial peritonitis. N Engl J Med 1999;341:403–9.

68. Guevara M, Terra C, Nazar A, et al. Albumin for bacterial infections other than spontaneous bacterial peritonitis in cirrhosis. A randomized, controlled study. J Hepatol 2012;57:759–65.

69. Thévenot T, Bureau C, Oberti F, et al. Effect of albumin in cirrhotic patients with infection other than spontaneous bacterial peritonitis. A randomized trial. J Hepatol 2015;62:822–30.

70. Fernández J, Angeli P, Trebicka J, et al. Efficacy of albumin treatment for patients with cirrhosis and infections Unrelated to spontaneous bacterial peritonitis. Clin Gastroenterol Hepatol 2020;18:963–73.e14.

71. Sundaram V, Jalan R, Wu T, et al. Factors associated with survival of patients with severe acute-on-chronic liver failure before and after liver transplantation. Gastroenterology 2019;156:1381–91.e3.

72. Reddy KR, O'Leary JG, Kamath PS, et al. High risk of delisting or death in liver transplant candidates following infections: results from the North American Consortium for the Study of End-Stage Liver Disease. Liver Transpl 2015;21:881–8.

73. Piano S, Incicco S, Tonon M, et al. Impact of bacterial infections prior liver transplantation on post-transplant outcomes in patients with cirrhosis. Hepatology 2021;74(S1):1222A (abstract).

74. Belli LS, Duvoux C, Artzner T, et al. Liver transplantation for patients with acute-on-chronic liver failure (ACLF) in Europe: results of the ELITA/EF-CLIF collaborative study (ECLIS). J Hepatol 2021;75:610–22.

Management of Portal Hypertension in Patients with Acute-on-Chronic Liver Disease

Florence Wong, MBBS, MD, FRACP, FRCPC, FAASLD*

KEYWORDS

- Acute-on-chronic liver failure • Cirrhosis • Nonselective beta-blockers
- Portal hypertension • Vasoconstrictors

KEY POINTS

- Portal hypertension is intricately involved in the development of acute-on-chronic liver failure (ACLF) and some of the precipitating events of ACLF.
- Lowering portal pressure potentially could reduce the likelihood for the development of ACLF.
- Kidney failure is the most common organ failure in patients with ACLF, and it can be treated with terlipressin, which lowers portal pressure with reversal of kidney failure in approximately 36% to 44% of patients.
- Careful patient selection is key to the successful use of terlipressin to treat kidney failure.

INTRODUCTION

The progression in the natural history of chronic liver disease to cirrhosis is associated with the development of portal hypertension, which has been recognized as the pivotal pathogenetic mechanism responsible for the multiple complications of cirrhosis.[1] As the cirrhotic process advances, there is a general progression of portal hypertension, and worsening of the attendant hemodynamic abnormalities. It is the splanchnic and systemic vasodilatation with its consequent effective arterial underfilling that triggers the compensatory activation of systemic vasoconstrictor systems, leading to renal sodium and water retention, as well as renal vasoconstriction that predisposes these patients to the development of renal failure that forms part of the acute-on-chronic liver failure (ACLF) syndrome.[2] Portal hypertension is also involved in the pathological process of bacterial translocation, which has been implicated in the development of

Department of Medicine, Division of Gastroenterology & Hepatology, University Health Network, University of Toronto, Toronto, Ontario, Canada
* Toronto General Hospital, Room 222, 9th floor, Eaton Wing, 200 Elizabeth Street, Toronto, Ontario M5G2C4, Canada.
E-mail address: florence.wong@utoronto.ca

Clin Liver Dis 27 (2023) 717–733
https://doi.org/10.1016/j.cld.2023.03.014   liver.theclinics.com
1089-3261/23/© 2023 Elsevier Inc. All rights reserved.

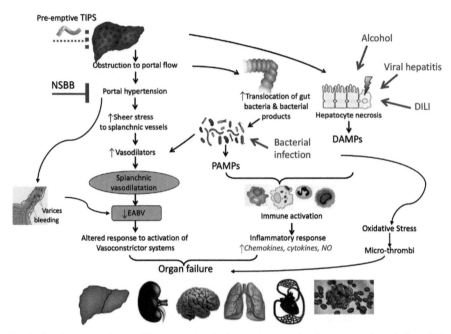

Fig. 1. Involvement of portal hypertension in the pathogenesis of acute-on-chronic liver failure, with possible precipitating events and sites of action of potential portal pressure lowering agents. DAMP, damage associated molecular pattern; DILI, drug-induced liver injury; EABV, effective arterial blood volume; NO, nitric oxide; NSBB, nonselective beta-blocker; PAMP, pathogen-associated molecular pattern; TIPS, transjugular intrahepatic portal systemic stent shunt.

various bacterial infections that are commonly observed in cirrhosis.[3] These infections can themselves worsen the aforementioned hemodynamic changes and, therefore, significantly increase the likelihood of developing ACLF.[4] The presence of bacterial infections can exaggerate the inflammatory milieu of cirrhosis, accompanied by increased oxidative stress, which can induce changes in organ microcirculation, leading to the formation of microthrombi, further compromising the microcirculation of various organs,[5] contributing to organ failures that is pathognomonic of the ACLF syndrome. In addition, a direct consequence of portal hypertension, such as a variceal bleeding, can result in volume contraction, further upsetting the precarious hemodynamic state of advanced cirrhosis, and has been recognized as a trigger for ACLF (**Fig. 1**). Therefore, portal hypertension is intricately involved in the pathogenesis of ACLF, and managing portal hypertension can potentially reduce the risk for the development of ACLF.[6] Once ACLF develops, and there is organ failure, then the management is to treat the various organ failures themselves (**Fig. 2**). This review will focus on effects of various measures that lower portal pressure on ACLF development and patient outcomes, and the management of the most common organ failure of ACLF, namely, renal failure.

THE EFFECTS OF NONSELECTIVE BETA-BLOCKERS ON ACUTE-ON-CHRONIC LIVER FAILURE

Because portal hypertension plays a central role in the pathogenesis of many events that either directly or indirectly lead to the development of ACLF, it stands to reason

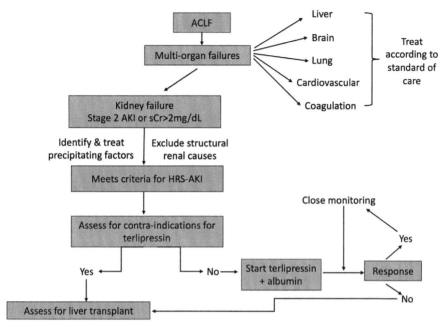

Fig. 2. Suggested algorithm for the management of kidney failure in the context of acute-on-chronic liver failure. ACLF, acute-on-chronic liver failure; AKI, acute kidney injury; HRS-AKI, hepatorenal syndrome-acute kidney injury; sCr, serum creatinine. The International Club of ASCITES recommends treating kidney failure when patient has developed stage 2 (reference 29). The EASL-CLIF consortium does not specify at what severity of renal dysfunction to start treatment, but has defined kidney failure as a serum creatinine of greater than 2 mg/dL.

that lowering the portal pressure could potentially be beneficial to the at-risk patients. Nonselective beta-blockers (NSBBs) have been the mainstay of treatment of lowering portal hypertension by reducing portal inflow and splanchnic resistance in cirrhosis for several decades. In addition, NSBBs have been shown to increase gut motility and to reduce bacterial translocation. Therefore, they have been effective in the primary and secondary prophylaxis against variceal bleeding[7,8] and in reducing the occurrence of spontaneous bacterial peritonitis (SBP) and other infections,[9] events that could trigger ACLF. However, in patients with advanced cirrhosis, the use of NSBBs has been controversial, with some citing benefits, whereas others reporting deleterious effects.[10] Indeed, the use of NSBBs in patients with hemodynamic abnormalities such as those with decompensated cirrhosis and ascites could lower the systemic blood pressure even further, putting patients at risk for the development of acute kidney injury (AKI).[11] Furthermore, the use of NSBBs in patients with underlying cardiac dysfunction was associated with an increased waitlist mortality.[12] Therefore, there are cautionary recommendations against the use of NSBBs in patients with advanced cirrhosis[13] and by extension in patients with ACLF.[14]

Further analyses of the data showed that the use of high doses of NSBBs was associated with increased mortality.[15,16] This led to the reevaluation of the CANONIC study data, and this showed that the continuation of NSBBs in patients admitted with ACLF was associated with improved 28-day survival, perhaps via a reduction in the extent of inflammation because there was a significant decrease in the total white cell count.[6] A further retrospective study showed that the preadmission use of NSBBs was associated with an increased 28-day survival, irrespective of whether the patient developed ACLF or not,[16] once again setting the scene that the use of NSBBs in patients with ACLF could be beneficial. However, the survival advantage was attenuated in patients with a mean arterial blood pressure of 82 mm Hg or lesser and completely lost in those with mean arterial blood pressure less than 65 mm Hg. In a prospective randomized controlled trial (RCT) from India, enrolling patients with ACLF according to the definition of the Asian Pacific Association for the Study of the Liver (APASL)[17] all with a hepatic venous pressure gradient of greater than 12 mm Hg, the use of carvedilol resulted in improved transplant-free survival, a reduction in the incidence of AKI and SBP at 28 days but these beneficial effects were lost at 90 days. This loss of beneficial effects beyond 28 days is intriguing. The authors proposed that carvedilol mainly exerts its effects through a reduction in intestinal permeability and consequently reduction in bacterial translocation but why carvedilol's effects on the decrease in intestinal permeability are lost beyond few weeks in the setting of ACLF remains a mystery.

Clearly, lowering the portal pressure such as using an NSBB to improve outcomes in patients with ACLF makes sense mechanistically, and is an attractive treatment strategy. However, it seems that we must tread a fine line because too high a dose may lead to deleterious results. Identifying the appropriate patient population for an NSBB use is also essential. Future investigations will need to clarify these issues before we can recommend NSBBs as the standard of care for patients with ACLF.

PREEMPTIVE TRANSJUGULAR PORTAL-SYSTEMIC STENT SHUNT AND ACUTE-ON-CHRONIC LIVER FAILURE

Another means of lowering portal pressure is to create a direct connection between the portal venous and hepatic venous systems by inserting a portal-systemic stent shunt via the transjugular route, the so-called transjugular portal-systemic stent shunt (TIPS) insertion. It is the recommended treatment of patients with variceal bleeding that is refractory to endoscopic and pharmacological treatments.[18] However, TIPS insertion at the stage of refractory variceal bleeding is usually met with adverse outcomes because these patients are usually ill from hemodynamic instability. The prevalence of variceal bleeding as the precipitant of ACLF ranges from 13% to 28%,[19] through the mechanisms of hepatic ischemia, increased bacterial translocation, and increased risk for bacterial infections. In turn, the presence of ACLF increases the rebleeding risks and mortality.[20] Therefore, the concept of early or preemptive TIPS has been advocated in these patients to prevent their deterioration into ACLF.[21] In the retrospective analysis of a database containing results of 34 international, prospective observational studies conducted under the auspices of the BAVENO Corporation, 22 patients with ACLF who received a preemptive TIPS was compared with 147 patients with ACLF who did not.[20] It was noted that despite the presence of ACLF, those who received a preemptive TIPS had significantly improved survival at 42 days and at 1 year. However, there were plenty of skeptics who pointed out that patients who underwent preemptive TIPS insertion had lower pre-TIPS model for end-stage liver disease (MELD) scores and lower ACLF grades than those who did not undergo TIPS insertion.[22–24] Clearly, the number of patients who received a preemptive TIPS with ACLF was too small for any conclusions to be made but this has certainly stimulated the interest to further investigate the use of preemptive TIPS in patients with ACLF to determine its possible benefits.

MANAGEMENT OF PORTAL HYPERTENSION-RELATED ORGAN FAILURE IN ACUTE-ON-CHRONIC LIVER FAILURE

The development of ACLF is characterized by the presence of multiorgan failures. The single organ failure that is most closely attributed to portal hypertension driven hemodynamic changes and increased inflammation from bacterial translocation (see **Fig. 1**) is kidney failure. It is also the most common organ failure in ACLF. A study in Europe reported that 92% of patients with ACLF had some form of renal dysfunction, with 42% of patients having stage 2 or 3 AKI[25]; although 50% to 80% of patients in a cohort of veterans from the United States developed kidney failure, the incidence varied depending on the grade of ACLF that the patient had as defined by the European Association for the Study of the Liver-Chronic Liver Failure Consortium (EASL-CLIF).[26] It must be mentioned the APASL does not recognize organ failure in their definition of ACLF, whereas the North American Consortium for the Study of End-Stage Liver Disease (NACSELD) defines kidney failure as the need for dialysis, and hence too late for any form of treatment that could reverse the kidney failure. The following section will be devoted to the management of kidney failure of ACLF (see **Fig. 2**).

Definition of Kidney Failure

Because the definition of kidney failure has undergone significant changes in the past decade, mostly led by another organization, The International Club of ASCITES (Ascites, Spontaneous bacterial peritonitis, Cardiac Involvement, Therapy, and End-Stage liver disease), it is becoming confusing when reading the literature as to what is the severity of the renal dysfunction the term "kidney failure" actually refers to. **Table 1** lists the various terms and their definitions when describing renal failure in cirrhosis, with type 1 hepatorenal syndrome (HRS1) being slowly phased out, because it describes the most severe form of renal failure that makes pharmacological treatment less effective.

Removal and Treatment of Precipitating Factors

The management of kidney failure in cirrhosis in the context of ACLF begins with identifying the precipitating factor(s) that have triggered its development. The most common precipitant is bacterial infection, estimated to be responsible for 28% to 33% of cases of ACLF.[19] The fact that cirrhosis is a relative immune-deficient state[31] that predisposes these patients to the development of bacterial infections. Once it occurs, it also has a negative impact on the outcome of ACLF.[32] The most common bacterial infection is SBP but no site is exempt including soft tissue and skin infections.[33,34] The next most common precipitant is excess alcohol, accounting for 6% to 25% of cases of ACLF, followed by acute gastrointestinal hemorrhage. In Asian countries where viral hepatitis and use of alternative medicines are more prevalent, a flare of viral hepatitis and drug-induced liver injury are much more common precipitants for ACLF.[35] Other less common precipitants include procedures such as TIPS insertion, endoscopic retrograde cholangio-pancreatogram, or surgery. Of course, in a significant number of cases, no precipitant can be identified.

Therefore, it is imperative that a full septic workup including culturing samples from all possible sites is done as soon as possible. Empirical antibiotics need to be started promptly, considering the local antibiotic resistance profile because every hour of delay in initiating antibiotic is associated with a 3.3% increase in mortality.[36] Patients with a history of previous colonization, antibiotic treatment for 5 days or greater in the last 3 months, or hospitalization for 5 days or greater in the last 3 months, or those from nursing home/long-term care facilities are at high risk for having infections

Table 1
Various definitions of renal dysfunction in cirrhosis with ascites

Name	Defining Organization	sCr for Definition	Other Criteria
Type 1 hepatorenal syndrome (HRS1)[27]	International Ascites Club	2.5 mg/dL (233 µmol/L)	• No improvement in sCr after diuretic withdrawal or fluid challenge with albumin at a dose of 1 gm/kg of body weight for 2 d • Absence of shock or untreated infection needing vasopressor support • No recent nephrotoxic drug use • No evidence of structural renal damage in the form of hematuria (>50RBC/mL) or proteinuria (>500 mg/d) or casts
Acute kidney injury (Ref:[28])	International Club of ASCITES[a]	Increase in sCr by 0.3 mg/dL (26.4 µmol/L) from baseline	• Severity is defined by stages • Stage 1: Increase in sCr by 0.3 mg/dL (26.4 µmol/L) or from 1.5 to 2 times from baseline • Stage 2: Increase in sCr from >2–3 times from baseline • Stage 3: Increase in sCr from >3 times from baseline, or sCr of >4 mg/dL (352 µmol/L) with an acute increase of >0.3 mg/dL (26.4 µmol/L), or initiation of renal replacement therapy
HRS-AKI[29]	International Club of ASCITES[a]	Increase in sCr by 0.3 mg/dL (26.4 µmol/L) from baseline	Patient has to fulfill all other diagnostic criteria of HRS1 with the exception of the sCr threshold of 2.5 mg/dL (233 µmol/L)
Kidney Failure[30]	EASL-CLIF consortium	sCr ≥2 mg/dL	Part of EASL-CLIF organ failure scoring system

Abbreviations: AKI, acute kidney injury; EASL-CLIF, European Association for the Study of the Liver-Chronic Liver Failure Consortium; HRS1, type 1 hepatorenal syndrome; HRS-AKI, hepatorenal syndrome-acute kidney injury; RBC, red blood cell; sCr, serum creatinine.
[a] The International Ascites Club changed its name in 2007 to the Internal Club of Ascites, Spontaneous bacterial peritonitis, Cardiac Involvement, Therapy, and End-Stage liver disease.

from multidrug-resistant organisms, and therefore should receive broader spectrum antibiotic coverage,[37] as are patients who have nosocomial infections[38] and higher grades of ACLF.[39]

Other precipitants of ACLF such as alcoholic hepatitis are usually self-evident from the medical history and the hospitalization precludes further alcohol use. These patients are at high risk for bacterial infections because alcohol adds to the immunosuppression in these patients. Viral hepatitis flare requires the institution of antiviral therapy, whereas selected patients with autoimmune hepatitis may benefit from corticosteroid therapy, especially those with MELD score of 27 or less and without grade 3 or greater hepatic encephalopathy (brain failure).[40]

The other important general measure is to replenish the intravascular volume. Patients with gastrointestinal blood loss should be resuscitated with packed red blood cells. Otherwise, resuscitation with colloid solutions such as albumin should be initiated in patients with intravascular volume loss, especially if the kidney failure occurs after excessive fluid shifts such as overzealous diuretic or lactulose use or large volume paracentesis. Nonselective beta-blockers if already prescribed, should be withheld if there is systemic hypotension.[41]

It is imperative that other organ failures, if present, will need to be treated simultaneously. Patients who only have kidney failure will need to be treated promptly because it has been shown that the presence of grade 1 ACLF or 1 organ failure such as kidney failure is a predictor of subsequent grade 3 ACLF or multiorgan failure.[42]

Albumin

Albumin is a molecule that has pluripotent properties including volume expanding, anti-inflammatory, antioxidant, and immune regulatory functions. The ACLF syndrome is an intensely inflammatory state; therefore, it would be appropriate to provide albumin to patients with ACLF and kidney failure. Various academic societies have recommended the use of albumin in kidney failure irrespective of whether it is part of the ACLF syndrome or not.[43,44] Indeed, high dose of albumin has been shown to reduce the levels of various inflammatory cytokines in patients with bacterial infections.[45] In patients with HRS1, a meta-analysis found that a total of 600 gm of albumin given during the course of HRS treatment provided patients a significant survival benefit compared with patients who received a total dose of 200 gm of albumin.[46] However, it must be emphasized that albumin alone seems to be ineffective in reversing kidney failure,[47] and yet it seems to enhance the beneficial effects of vasoconstrictors.[48] The International Club of ASCITES recommends a dose of 20 to 40gm albumin per day to be used with vasoconstrictors,[27] although no formal dose response study with albumin has ever been done.

Vasoconstrictors

Vasoconstrictors are the mainstay of treatment of renal failure in cirrhosis. Worldwide, terlipressin is the most used vasoconstrictor,[49] followed by norepinephrine. With the recent approval of terlipressin by the Food and Drug Administration in the United States, the use of midodrine and octreotide for kidney failure in cirrhosis will diminish. To date, all the studies reported on the use of these vasoconstrictors in patients with HRS1 (see **Table 1**), a more severe form kidney failure. In accordance with various treatment guidelines,[27,43,44] albumin is recommended to be given with vasoconstrictors.

Terlipressin

Terlipressin is a vasopressin analog, which predominantly acts on vasopressin type 1 receptors located at vascular smooth muscle cells. In the splanchnic vessels, it attaches onto the V1 receptors located on the arterial side of the splanchnic vessels and causes splanchnic vasoconstriction, thereby reduces portal inflow by about 30%.[50] There is some evidence that terlipressin also dilates intrahepatic vessels, thereby reducing intrahepatic resistance to portal flow.[51] The overall result is lowering of the portal pressure by at least 20%.[52] Some of the splanchnic volume is then transferred to the central circulation, improving the overall effective arterial blood volume. Terlipressin also has a vasoconstrictive effect on the systemic circulation, thereby increasing the peripheral vascular resistance and mean arterial pressure. This can improve the renal perfusion pressure. In the renal circulation, terlipressin also causes a reduction in the resistive index, related to an improved effective arterial blood volume, leading to a reduction in the activities of the renin-angiotensin system. Thus, the renal circulation improves, potentially leading to improvement in renal function. Furthermore, terlipressin has also been shown to ameliorate systemic inflammation by reducing bacterial translocation in decompensated cirrhosis,[53] thus reducing the inflammatory burden to help improve renal function.

There are 4 RCTs comparing terlipressin versus placebo, both with albumin for the treatment of HRS1, 1 from Spain and 3 from North America, totaling 654 patients, with 375 patients randomized to receive terlipressin and the remaining 279 patients receiving placebo[46,54–56] **(Table 2)**. All the studies showed that terlipressin was more effective than placebo in reversing HRS1 defined as a sustained reduction of the serum creatinine (sCr) to less than 1.5 mg/dL (133 μmol/L), with 3 of the 4 studies showing a statistical significance. The overall response rate was 36% to 44%.[57] Despite improvement in renal function with terlipressin, there was no difference in the overall or transplant-free survival up to 90 days after completion of treatment. However, in those patients who responded with a reduction in their sCr to less than 1.5 mg/dL irrespective of the treatment arm, there was a significant improvement in survival. In fact, even a partial response with a greater than 20% reduction in sCr was associated with an improved survival.[58] A meta-analysis showed that a fall in creatinine of 1 mg/dL while on treatment resulted in a 27% reduction in relative risk for mortality when compared with placebo.[59]

Because terlipressin is a vasoconstrictor, its use is associated with ischemic side effects. V1 receptors are also present in the heart, aorta, and the peripheral circulation, and therefore, it potentially can cause coronary and peripheral ischemia in addition to splanchnic ischemia.[60] The use of a continuous infusion of terlipressin, which allows for a lower total daily dose (2–4 mg/d) rather than bolus injections seems to mitigate some of these ischemic side effects.[61] However, in the latest RCT from North America, an unexpected severe adverse event of respiratory failure appeared[46] only in patients who received terlipressin and not in those who received placebo. Further dissection of the data showed that respiratory failure was only observed in patients with at least grade 3 ACLF as defined by the EASL-CLIF consortium.[62] It seems that terlipressin, independent of its vasoconstrictive effects, also has a cardiac depressant effect. In a physiological study involving 20 patients with cirrhosis and ascites, a 2-mg acute dose of terlipressin induced a reduction of the ejection fraction by 16%. Consequently, the cardiac output fell by 17%. The end-diastolic volume increased by 18% with all these changes occurring without any changes in myocardial perfusion.[60] It was thought that an increase in cardiac afterload was responsible for these hemodynamic changes.[63] Why did it only occur in patients with grade 3 or higher ACLF is not clear. It is possible that the intense inflammation observed in patients with high-grade ACLF may have induced an increase in pulmonary vascular permeability.[64] Indeed, in the latest terlipressin versus placebo RCT, patients with at least grade 3 ACLF had more evidence of inflammation, including a higher proportion of patients with systemic

Table 2
Randomized controlled trials involving terlipressin versus placebo, both with albumin for hepatorenal syndrome type 1

Author, Year	Trial Design	Primary End Point(s)	Primary End Point Results: n/N (%)	Comments
Sanyal et al,[55] 2008	Multicenter double-blind randomized controlled	Treatment success (decrease in sCr to ≤1.5 mg/dL for at least 48 h by day 14 without dialysis, death or relapse of HRS)	Terlipressin: 19/56 (33.9%) vs Placebo: 7/56 (12.5%) (P = .093)	Terlipressin was superior to placebo for HRS reversal (34% vs 13%, P = .008)
Martin-Llahi et al,[54] 2008	Multicenter open label	1. Decrease in sCr <1.5 mg/dL 2. survival for 3 M	1. Terlipressin: 10/23 (43.5%) vs Controls: 2/23 (8.7%) (P = .017) 2. Terlipressin: 6/23 (27%) vs Controls: 4/23 (19%) (P = .70)	11 of the 46 enrolled patients had type 2 HRS
Boyer et al,[56] 2016	Multicenter double-blind randomized controlled	Confirmed HRS reversal (2 consecutive sCr ≤1.5 mg/dL ≥ 40 h apart)	Terlipressin: 19/97 (19.6%) vs Placebo: 13/99 (13.1%) (P = .13)	Terlipressin group had greater improvement in renal function but it was not statistically significant
Wong et al,[47] 2021	Multicenter double-blind randomized controlled	Verified HRS reversal (2 consecutive sCr of ≤1.5 mg/dL ≥ 2 h apart) + no RRT and alive for 10 d after Rx completion	Terlipressin: 63/199 (32%) vs Placebo: 17/101 (17%) (P = .006)	Patients in terlipressin group who had grade 3 ACLF had more cases of respiratory failure

Abbreviations: ACLF, acute-on-chronic liver failure; HRS, hepatorenal syndrome; M, months; RRT, renal replacement therapy; Rx, treatment; sCr, serum creatinine.

Table 3
Recommendations for patient selection for terlipressin treatment in patients with cirrhosis and kidney failure

	Patient Characteristics	Reason
Appropriate	Patients with alcoholic hepatitis, SIRS, sepsis	Better response to terlipressin treatment
Warning and precautions	ACLF ≥ grade 3 sCr≥ 5 mg/dL (170 µmol/L)	Less likely to respond Increased likelihood for adverse events
Contraindications	Patients with ongoing coronary, peripheral, or mesenteric ischemia	Risk for ischemic side effects
	Patients experiencing hypoxia or worsening respiratory symptoms	Risk for respiratory failure

Abbreviations: ACLF, acute-on-chronic liver failure; sCr, serum creatinine; SIRS, systemic inflammatory response syndrome; SpO$_2$, pulse oximeter oxygen saturation.

inflammatory response syndrome or alcoholic hepatitis, a higher white cell count, and tachycardia,[47] when compared with patients with lower grades of ACLF. Predictors of respiratory failure include a high international normalized ratio, a high mean arterial blood pressure, and a low oxygen saturation of less than 90% as measured on a pulse oximeter on room air.[62]

Because patients with HRS1 do not universally respond to terlipressin with a reduction in sCr, various investigators have sought predictors of response. Lower grade of ACLF pretreatment,[65] a baseline bilirubin of less than 10 mg/dL (170 µmol/L) and sCr of less than 5 mg/dL (440 µmol/L),[66,67] as well as a sustained increase in the mean arterial pressure by 5 to 10 mm Hg with treatment[68] have been identified as predictors of response. Patients with inflammatory conditions such as alcoholic hepatitis or sepsis also seem to respond better to terlipressin, and those with systemic inflammatory response syndrome.[46,53]

Now that terlipressin is approved for commercial use in the United States, how do we choose the appropriate patient with kidney failure for terlipressin use? **Table 3** lists the contraindications for terlipressin and the reasons why. In general, cirrhotic patients with ascites who develop stage 2 or higher of AKI in the absence of any evidence of structural renal disease should be considered for terlipressin. Patients with a history of coronary, peripheral, or mesenteric ischemia should not receive terlipressin, as are patients with advanced liver or renal dysfunction (see **Table 3**). By definition, all patients with kidney failure have at least grade 1 ACLF and, therefore, can only have one additional organ failure when they receive terlipressin. Otherwise, they will run a high risk of developing respiratory failure and will be better served by being referred for liver transplant assessment.

Terlipressin is approved in the United States to be given as bolus injections. Terlipressin is packaged as 1 mg of terlipressin acetate per vial, which contains 0.85 mg of free terlipressin. The starting dose is 1 mg every 6 hours. Because terlipressin is recommended to be given with albumin, patients need to be monitored for volume overload, in addition to ischemic side effects. Patients should be inspected for signs of peripheral ischemia such as cyanosis and skin discoloration and queried for chest or abdominal pain. Because patients with multiorgan failure such as those with grade 3 or higher ACLF are not recommended to receive terlipressin, respiratory failure should not occur but it is advisable to monitor for tissue oxygenation regularly as

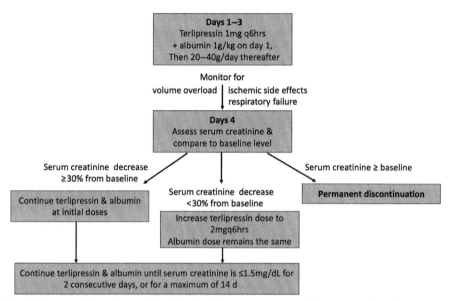

Fig. 3. Suggested treatment algorithm for the management of hepatorenal syndrome type 1 using terlipressin in patients with cirrhosis and ascites. (*Adapted from* Wong F, Kwo P. Practical management of HRS-AKI in the era of terlipressin: what the gastroenterologist needs to know. Am J Gastroenterol 2023 (in press).)

well as daily auscultation of the chest. Assessment of response should be done at day 4. If the sCr is unchanged or higher than at pretreatment level, the patient is a nonresponder and terlipressin should be stopped. If the sCr has decreased but less than 30% from baseline, then the terlipressin dose can be increased to 2 mg every 6 hours, with the same monitoring regimen for side effects. If the sCr has reduced to more than 30% from baseline, then terlipressin should be continued at the same dose. In the last 2 scenarios, terlipressin should be continued until the sCr has declined to less than 1.5 mg/dL (133 μmol/L) for 2 consecutive days, or until a maximum of 14 days (**Fig. 3**).[69]

Norepinephrine

Norepinephrine is a systemic vasoconstrictor and does not affect the portal circulation per se. It has been compared with terlipressin as a treatment of HRS1 in several small trials. Its mechanism of action is to improve the systemic hemodynamics, and hence to improve the renal perfusion pressure. Norepinephrine has been shown to be equally efficacious as terlipressin in reversing HRS1.[70,71] However, in the context of ACLF as defined by the APASL which does not include kidney failure in its definition, the use of terlipressin was superior to norepinephrine in reversing HRS1.[72]

Future development in modulation of portal hypertension in acute-on-chronic liver failure

Because terlipressin is a drug that is associated with significant side effects, manipulation of the V1 agonist molecule has led to the development of a partial agonist, which is a ligand that has both agonist and antagonist actions. Therefore, it competes with itself for the V1 receptor, which will reduce its ischemic side effects without losing too much of its portal hypotensive effects. One such V1 receptor partial agonist is

FE204038. In an animal model of cirrhosis, the use of FE204038 was able to induce a significant reduction of portal pressure 90 minutes after subcutaneous bolus injection, magnitude of which was much greater than that induced by an intravenous injection of terlipressin.[73] Unlike terlipressin, which induced a significant increase in systemic vascular resistance and mean arterial pressure, no systemic hemodynamic effects were observed with FE204038. Despite this, there was a significant increase in renal sodium and water excretion with FE204038. Long-term administration of FE204038 also reduced the pressor effects to terlipressin. These animals did not have baseline renal dysfunction and no change in renal function was observed with FE204038.

Because of the potential advantage of a partial agonist over terlipressin on lowering the portal pressure and hence may have a beneficial effect on renal function in patients with kidney failure, there is now a clinical trial (NCT05309200), which assesses the effects of another V1 partial agonist on the renal function in patients with kidney failure in cirrhosis. It will be interesting to learn whether lowering the portal pressure alone without altering the systemic hemodynamics will be sufficient to improve renal function in cirrhosis with renal failure.

SUMMARY

The presence of portal hypertension is intricately linked to the development of ACLF in cirrhosis. Therefore, lowering the portal pressure either with NSBBs or with a preemptive TIPS in the appropriate patients could potentially reduce the likelihood of developing ACLF. However, once ACLF has developed, it is imperative to assess whether these means of lowering portal pressure are still beneficial. For example, NSBBs will cause systemic hypotension and TIPS will cause hepatic ischemia, either of these would be detrimental to patient outcomes. However, once ACLF develops, especially with kidney failure, lowering the portal pressure with a splanchnic vasoconstrictor is beneficial, especially if it also improves systemic hemodynamics, but one needs to exercise caution as such a generalized vasoconstrictor can also cause ischemia. The future is exciting as we develop other portal hypotensive agents that will provide the appropriate amount of portal pressure reduction without significant side effects to manage the organ failures of ACLF.

CLINICS CARE POINTS

- The use of NSBB in patients without systemic hypotension could potentially improve survival.
- The use of pre-emptove TIPS in patients with low grade ACLF could improve survival from preliminary data, but this needs to be confirmed before it can be recommended as standard of care.
- Kidney failure is the most common organ failure in patients with ACLF. Diagnose it early as per the International Club of ASCITES diagnostic criteria, and treat promptly for better results.
- Terlipressin with albumin can reverse renal failure in approximately 36-44% of patients. Monitor for side effects, and no not use in patients with ACLF $\geq$ grade 3 or serum creatinine $\geq$5mg/dL.

CONFLICTS OF INTEREST

Consultants for Mallinckrodt Pharmaceutical Inc, Ocelot Bio, and River 2 Renal. Grant support provided to institution by Mallinckrodt Pharmaceutical Inc, and Ocelot Bio.

REFERENCES

1. Iwakiri Y, Trebicka J. Portal hypertension in cirrhosis: pathophysiological mechanisms and therapy. JHEP Rep 2021;3:100316.
2. Gustot T, Stadlbauer V, Laleman W, et al. Transition to decompensation and acute-on-chronic liver failure: role of predisposing factors and precipitating events. J Hepatol 2021;75(Suppl 1):S36–48.
3. Ponziani FR, Zocco MA, Cerrito L, et al. Bacterial translocation in patients with liver cirrhosis: physiology, clinical consequences, and practical implications. Expert Rev Gastroenterol Hepatol 2018;12:641–56.
4. Trebicka J, Macnaughtan J, Schnabl B, et al. The microbiota in cirrhosis and its role in hepatic decompensation. J Hepatol 2021;75(Suppl 1):S67–81.
5. Lisman T, Stravitz RT. Rebalanced hemostasis in patients with acute liver failure. Semin Thromb Hemost 2015;41:468–73.
6. Mookerjee RP, Pavesi M, Thomsen KL, et al. CANONIC Study Investigators of the EASL-CLIF Consortium. Treatment with non-selective beta blockers is associated with reduced severity of systemic inflammation and improved survival of patients with acute-on-chronic liver failure. J Hepatol 2016;64:574–82.
7. Sharma M, Singh S, Desai V, et al. Comparison of therapies for primary prevention of esophageal variceal bleeding: a systematic review and network meta-analysis. Hepatology 2019;69:1657–75.
8. Bernard B, Lebrec D, Mathurin P, et al. Beta-adrenergic antagonists in the prevention of gastrointestinal rebleeding in patients with cirrhosis: a meta-analysis. Hepatology 1997;25:63–70.
9. Sasso R, Rockey DC. Non-selective beta-blocker use in cirrhotic patients is associated with a reduced likelihood of hospitalisation for infection. Aliment Pharmacol Ther 2021;53:418–25.
10. Rodrigues SG, Mendoza YP, Bosch J. Beta-blockers in cirrhosis: evidence-based indications and limitations. JHEP Rep 2019;2:100063.
11. Kim SG, Larson JJ, Lee JS, et al. Beneficial and harmful effects of nonselective beta blockade on acute kidney injury in liver transplant candidates. Liver Transplant 2017;23:733–40.
12. Giannelli V, Roux O, Laouénan C, et al. Impact of cardiac function, refractory ascites and beta blockers on the outcome of patients with cirrhosis listed for liver transplantation. J Hepatol 2020;72:463–71.
13. Krag A, Wiest R, Albillos A, et al. The window hypothesis: haemodynamic and non-haemodynamic effects of β-blockers improve survival of patients with cirrhosis during a window in the disease. Gut 2012;61:967–9.
14. Gananandan K, Mookerjee R, Jalan R. Use of Non-selective beta blockers in decompensated cirrhosis and ACLF. Curr Hepat Rep 2022;21:29–36.
15. Bang UC, Benfield T, Hyldstrup L, et al. Effect of propranolol on survival in patients with decompensated cirrhosis: a nationwide study based Danish patient registers. Liver Int 2016;36:1304–12.
16. Tergast TL, Kimmann M, Laser H, et al. Systemic arterial blood pressure determines the therapeutic window of non-selective beta blockers in decompensated cirrhosis. Aliment Pharmacol Ther 2019;50:696–706.
17. Kumar M, Kainth S, Choudhury A, et al. Treatment with carvedilol improves survival of patients with acute-on-chronic liver failure: a randomized controlled trial. Hepatol Int 2019;13:800–13.
18. Garcia-Tsao G, Abraldes JG, Berzigotti A, et al. Portal hypertensive bleeding in cirrhosis: risk stratification, diagnosis, and management: 2016 practice guidance

by the American Association for the Study of Liver Diseases. Hepatology 2017; 65:310–35.

19. Cullaro G, Sharma R, Trebicka J, et al. Precipitants of acute-on-chronic liver failure: an opportunity for preventative measures to improve outcomes. Liver Transplant 2020;26:283–93.

20. Trebicka J, Gu W, Ibáñez-Samaniego L, et al. Rebleeding and mortality risk are increased by ACLF but reduced by pre-emptive TIPS. J Hepatol 2020;73: 1082–91.

21. García-Pagán JC, Caca K, Bureau C, et al. For early TIPS (Transjugular intrahepatic portosystemic shunt) Cooperative study Group. Early use of TIPS in patients with cirrhosis and variceal bleeding. N Engl J Med 2010;362:2370–9.

22. Wong YJ, Ho WLD, Abraldes JG. Pre-emptive TIPSS in acute variceal bleeding: current status, controversies, and future directions. J Clin Transl Hepatol 2022;10: 1223–8.

23. Cornman-Homonoff J, Madoff DC. Commentary on: " Rebleeding and mortality risk are increased by ACLF but reduced by pre-emptive TIPS. Am J Roentgenol 2021;216:878.

24. Elhence A, Kumar R, Shalimar. Pre-emptive TIPS for acute variceal bleeding in acute-on-chronic liver failure: is there enough evidence for a routine recommendation? J Hepatol 2020;73:976–7.

25. Napoleone L, Solé C, Juanola A, et al. Patterns of kidney dysfunction in acute-on-chronic liver failure: relationship with kidney and patients' outcome. Hepatol Commun 2022;6:2121–31.

26. Mahmud N, Kaplan DE, Taddei TH, et al. Incidence and mortality of acute-on-chronic liver failure using two definitions in patients with compensated cirrhosis. Hepatology 2019;69:2150–63.

27. Salerno F, Gerbes A, Ginès P, et al. Diagnosis, prevention and treatment of hepatorenal syndrome in cirrhosis. Gut 2007;56:1310–8.

28. Wong F, Nadim MK, Kellum JA, et al. Working Party proposal for a revised classification system of renal dysfunction in patients with cirrhosis. Gut 2011;60: 702–9.

29. Angeli P, Gines P, Wong F, et al. International Club of Ascites. Diagnosis and management of acute kidney injury in patients with cirrhosis: revised consensus recommendations of the International Club of Ascites. Gut 2015;64:531–7.

30. Moreau R, Jalan R, Ginès P, et al. Acute-on-chronic liver failure is a distinct syndrome that develops in patients with acute decompensation of cirrhosis. Gastroenterology 2013;144:1426–37.

31. Van der Merwe S, Chokshi S, Bernsmeier C, et al. The multifactorial mechanisms of bacterial infection in decompensated cirrhosis. J Hepatol 2021 Jul;75(Suppl 1):S82–100.

32. Arvaniti V, D'Amico G, Fede G, et al. Infections in patients with cirrhosis increase mortality four-fold and should be used in determining prognosis. Gastroenterology 2010;139:1246–56.

33. Bajaj JS, O'Leary JG, Wong F, et al. Bacterial infections in end-stage liver disease: current challenges and future directions. Gut 2012;61:1219–25.

34. Wong F, Piano S, Singh V, et al. International Club of Ascites Global Study Group. Clinical features and evolution of bacterial infection-related acute-on-chronic liver failure. J Hepatol 2021;74:330–9.

35. Cao Z, Liu Y, Cai M, et al. The use of NACSELD and EASL-CLIF classification systems of ACLF in the prediction of prognosis in hospitalized patients with cirrhosis. Am J Gastroenterol 2020;115:2026–35.

36. Kim JJ, Tsukamoto MM, Mathur AK, et al. Delayed paracentesis is associated with increased in-hospital mortality in patients with spontaneous bacterial peritonitis. Am J Gastroenterol 2014;109:1436–42.
37. Fernandez J, Tandon P, Mensa J, et al. Antibiotic prophylaxis in cirrhosis: good and bad. Hepatology 2016;63:2019–31.
38. Piano S, Fasolato S, Salinas F, et al. The empirical antibiotic treatment of nosocomial spontaneous bacterial peritonitis: results of a randomized, controlled clinical trial. Hepatology 2016;63:1299–309.
39. Wieser A, Li H, Zhang J, et al. Evaluating the best empirical antibiotic therapy in patients with acute-on-chronic liver failure and spontaneous bacterial peritonitis. Dig Liver Dis 2019;51:1300–7.
40. Anand L, Choudhury A, Bihari C, et al. Flare of autoimmune hepatitis causing acute on chronic liver failure: diagnosis and response to corticosteroid therapy. Hepatology 2019;70:587–96.
41. Moctezuma-Velazquez C, Kalainy S, Abraldes JG. Beta-blockers in patients with advanced liver disease: has the dust settled? Liver Transplant 2017;23:1058–69.
42. Mahmud N, Sundaram V, Kaplan DE, et al. Grade 1 acute on chronic liver failure is a predictor for subsequent grade 3 failure. Hepatology 2020;72:230–9.
43. European Association for the Study of the Liver. EASL Clinical Practice Guidelines for the management of patients with decompensated cirrhosis. J Hepatol 2018;69:406–60.
44. Biggins SW, Angeli P, Garcia-Tsao G, et al. Diagnosis, evaluation, and management of ascites, spontaneous bacterial peritonitis and hepatorenal syndrome: 2021 Practice Guidance by the American Association for the Study of Liver Diseases. Hepatology 2021;74:1014–48.
45. Fernández J, Clària J, Amorós A, et al. Effects of albumin treatment on systemic and portal hemodynamics and systemic inflammation in patients with decompensated cirrhosis. Gastroenterology 2019;157:149–62.
46. Salerno F, Navickis RJ, Wilkes MM. Albumin treatment regimen for type 1 hepatorenal syndrome: a dose-response meta-analysis. BMC Gastroenterol 2015;15:167.
47. Wong F, Pappas SC, Curry MP, et al. Terlipressin plus albumin for the treatment of type 1 hepatorenal syndrome. N Engl J Med 2021;384:818–28.
48. Ortega R, Ginès P, Uriz J, et al. Terlipressin therapy with and without albumin for patients with hepatorenal syndrome: results of a prospective, nonrandomized study. Hepatology 2002;36:941–8.
49. Facciorusso A, Chandar AK, Murad MH, et al. Comparative efficacy of pharmacological strategies for management of type 1 hepatorenal syndrome: a systematic review and network meta-analysis. Lancet Gastroenterol Hepatol 2017;2:94–102.
50. Møller S, Hansen EF, Becker U, et al. Central and systemic haemodynamic effects of terlipressin in portal hypertensive patients. Liver 2000;20:51–9.
51. Kiszka-Kanewitz M, Henricksen JH, Hansen EF, et al. Effect of terlipressin on blood volume distribution in patients with cirrhosis. Scand J Gastroenterol 2004;39:486–92.
52. Villanueva C, Planella M, Aracil C, et al. Hemodynamic effects of terlipressin and high somatostatin dose during acute variceal bleeding in non-responders to the usual somatostatin dose. Am J Gastroenterol 2005;100:624–30.
53. Wong F, Pappas SC, Boyer TD, et al. Terlipressin improves renal function and reverses hepatorenal syndrome in patients with systemic inflammatory response syndrome. Clin Gastroenterol Hepatol 2017;15:266–672.

54. Martín-Llahí M, Pépin MN, Guevara M, et al. Terlipressin and albumin vs albumin in patients with cirrhosis and hepatorenal syndrome: a randomized study. Gastro-enterology 2008;134:1352–9.

55. Sanyal AJ, Boyer T, Garcia-Tsao G, et al. A randomized, prospective, double-blind, placebo-controlled trial of terlipressin for type 1 hepatorenal syndrome. Gastroenterology 2008;134:1360–8.

56. Boyer TD, Sanyal AJ, Wong F, et al. Terlipressin plus albumin is more effective than albumin alone in improving renal function in patients with cirrhosis and hep-atorenal syndrome type 1. Gastroenterology 2016;150:1579–1589 e2.

57. Wong F. Latest treatment of acute kidney injury in cirrhosis. Curr Treat Options Gastroenterol 2020;18:281–94.

58. Boyer TD, Wong F, Sanyal AJ, et al. Time for a new, more inclusive endpoint for treatment of type 1 hepatorenal syndrome (HRS-1)? Small changes in serum creatinine of >20% are equivalent to HRS reversal in predicting survival and need for renal replacement therapy during treatment of HRS-1 with terlipressin and albumin. [Abstract]. Hepatology 2016;64:1030A–10311A.

59. Belcher JM, Coca SG, Parikh CR. Creatinine change on vasoconstrictors as mor-tality surrogate in hepatorenal syndrome: systematic review & meta-analysis. PLoS One 2015;10:e0135625.

60. Krag A, Bendtsen F, Mortensen C, et al. Effects of a single terlipressin administra-tion on cardiac function and perfusion in cirrhosis. Eur J Gastroenterol Hepatol 2010;22:1085–92.

61. Cavallin M, Piano S, Romano A, et al. Terlipressin given by continuous intrave-nous infusion versus intravenous boluses in the treatment of hepatorenal syn-drome: a randomized controlled study. Hepatology 2016;63:983–92.

62. Wong F, Pappas SC, Reddy KR, et al. Terlipressin use and respiratory failure in patients with hepatorenal syndrome type 1 and severe acute-on-chronic liver fail-ure. Aliment Pharmacol Ther 2022;56:1284–93.

63. Allegretti AS, Subramanian RM, Francoz C, et al. Respiratory events with terli-pressin and albumin in hepatorenal syndrome: a review and clinical guidance. Liver Int 2022;42:2124–30.

64. Kaku S, Nguyen CD, Htet NN, et al. Acute respiratory distress syndrome: etiology, pathogenesis, and summary on management. J Intensive Care Med 2020;35:723–37.

65. Piano S, Schmidt HH, Ariza X, et al. Association between grade of acute on chronic liver failure and response to terlipressin and albumin in patients with hep-atorenal syndrome. Clin Gastroenterol Hepatol 2018;16:1792–800.e3.

66. Boyer TD, Sanyal AJ, Garcia-Tsao G, et al. Predictors of response to terlipressin plus albumin in hepatorenal syndrome (HRS) type 1: relationship of serum creat-inine to hemodynamics. J Hepatol 2011;55:315–21.

67. Nazar A, Pereira GH, Guevara M, et al. Predictors of response to therapy with ter-lipressin and albumin in patients with cirrhosis and type 1 hepatorenal syndrome. Hepatology 2010;51:219–26.

68. Sanyal AJ, Boyer TD, Frederick RT, et al. Reversal of hepatorenal syndrome type 1 with terlipressin plus albumin vs. placebo plus albumin in a pooled analysis of the OT-0401 and REVERSE randomised clinical studies. Aliment Pharmacol Ther 2017;45:1390–402.

69. Wong F, Kwo P. Practical management of HRS-AKI in the era of terlipressin: what the gastroenterologist needs to know. Am J Gastroenterol 2023. https://doi.org/10.14309/ajg.0000000000002115.

70. Gilford FJ, Morling JR, Fallowfield JA. Systematic review with meta-analysis: vasoactive drugs for the treatment of hepatorenal syndrome type 1. Aliment Pharmacol Ther 2017;45:593–603.
71. Best LM, Freeman SC, Sutton AJ, et al. Treatment for hepatorenal syndrome in people with decompensated liver cirrhosis: a network meta-analysis. Cochrane Database Syst Rev 2019;9:CD013103.
72. Arora V, Maiwall R, Rajan V, et al. Terlipressin is superior to noradrenaline in the management of acute kidney injury in acute on chronic liver failure. Hepatology 2020;71:600–10.
73. Fernández-Varo G, Oró D, Cable EE, et al. Vasopressin 1a receptor partial agonism increases sodium excretion and reduces portal hypertension and ascites in cirrhotic rats. Hepatology 2016;63:207–16.

Liver Transplantation in Acute-on-Chronic Liver Failure

Anand V. Kulkarni, MD[a], K. Rajender Reddy, MD[b],*

KEYWORDS

- Liver transplantation • ACLF • Severity scores • Predictors of post-LT outcomes
- Share 35

KEY POINTS

- Liver transplantation (LT) is the best and ultimate treatment option for patients with acute-on-chronic liver failure (ACLF).
- Regular assessment of the need for LT and early listing and LT are the key to a successful outcome in patients with ACLF.
- Patients with advanced grades of ACLF and those with multiorgan failure are not likely to benefit from LT; thus it is essential to identify such patients in whom it is futile to pursue LT.
- Patients with ACLF are at higher risk of developing surgical and infectious complications post-LT.
- Patients who survive the initial period of 1 year have excellent long-term outcomes post-LT.

INTRODUCTION

Acute-on-chronic liver failure (ACLF) is a form of acute and advanced liver failure in patients with underlying chronic liver disease and is associated with nonhepatic organ failures and high mortality.[1–4] The incidence of ACLF has significantly increased in recent years.[5] The 3 major definitions of ACLF, that is, the European Association for Study of Liver, the Asian Pacific Association for Study of the Liver (APASL), and the North American Consortium for Study of End-Stage Liver Disease conclude that

Author contributions: A.V. Kulkarni prepared the initial draft. K.R. Reddy critically assessed and edited the article. Both authors approved the final version.
Financial support: None.
Supporting foundations: None.
Potential conflicts of interest: None.
[a] Department of Hepatology, Asian Institute of Gastroenterology, Hyderabad-500032, India;
[b] Division of Gastroenterology and Hepatology, University of Pennsylvania, 2 Dulles, Liver Transplant Office 3400 Spruce Street, Philadelphia, PA 19104, USA
* Corresponding author.
E-mail address: reddyr@pennmedicine.upenn.edu

Clin Liver Dis 27 (2023) 735–762
https://doi.org/10.1016/j.cld.2023.03.015
1089-3261/23/© 2023 Elsevier Inc. All rights reserved.

ACLF is associated with high short-term mortality despite several differences among them in defining the syndrome (**Table 1**). Mortality depends on the grade of ACLF and can range between 50% and 75% in advanced grades.[1] Although several advances have been made in the management of these very ill patients, the outcomes remain poor in the absence of liver transplantation (LT). However, most patients cannot undergo timely LT due to organ shortages, the presence and severity of extrahepatic organ failures, and the development of sepsis. In Asian settings, apart from the avenue of living healthy donors, the lack of uniform national health care policies, lack of expertise, and lack of financial support preclude timely LT. It is well known that patients with grade 3 ACLF have higher waitlist mortality at day 14 than patients with status 1a acute liver failure.[6] Recent studies have reported excellent outcomes following LT for patients with ACLF.[7] The timing of LT and the selection of candidates after the onset of organ failures is debatable. However, an early LT (<30 days) may prolong the survival of these sick patients. This review discusses the need, challenges, optimization of candidates, and outcomes of LT, along with predictors of survival and futility of LT in patients with ACLF.

IS ACUTE-ON-CHRONIC LIVER FAILURE REVERSIBLE? OR IS LIVER TRANSPLANTATION INVARIABLY NECESSARY?

The mortality in patients with ACLF is high in the absence of a transplant. Transplant-free mortality in a large cohort of patients with ACLF was 23%, 32%, and 75% in grades 1, 2, and 3 at day 28, respectively.[2] On the contrary, it is well known that the liver has a regenerative capacity, and as such, the course of patients with ACLF is dynamic.[8] ACLF may resolve in 55% of patients with ACLF-1, 35% of patients with ACLF-2, and 15% of patients with ACLF-3.[8] However, at least 5% of those who achieve resolution of ACLF die within 28 days. Furthermore, the mortality is 18%, 42%, and 92% in patients with ACLF-1, -2, and -3, respectively, at day 28, who remain in the same grades.[8] The grade of ACLF on days 3 to 7 determines the outcomes of patients, and as such, patients, particularly those patients with advanced grades, merit early transplant consideration and listing of potentially viable candidates. However, such an early listing (<7 days) is impractical in resource-limited settings, although LT remains the therapy of choice because nontransplanted patients with ACLF have dismal survival of 8% at 1 year compared with 80% in those who undergo LT.[9]

CAUSE OF ACUTE-ON-CHRONIC LIVER FAILURE AND LIVER TRANSPLANTATION

Common causes of ACLF include alcohol, hepatitis B, and infection, which can be easily controlled/suppressed. The outcome of alcohol-induced ACLF is poor compared with that of non-alcohol-induced ACLF.[10–12] However, the survival and outcomes posttransplant for alcohol-induced ACLF are excellent even when transplanted within 3 months of the last alcohol intake.[13] There has been a significant increase in the incidence of nonalcoholic fatty liver disease in recent years.[14] Although the development of ACLF is less frequent in patients with non-alcoholic steatohepatitis (NASH) and hepatitis C, the waitlist mortality is high, meriting early LT.[15] Similarly, patients with hepatitis B virus (HBV)-related ACLF merit urgent LT.[16]

Infections are more common in patients with ACLF than in those with decompensated cirrhosis.[17] Nearly 40% to 50% of patients with ACLF present with infections at baseline, and 42% to 60% develop infections by 4 weeks.[17–19] Furthermore, fungal infections are also frequent in patients with ACLF and are reported between 4% and 15%.[17,20,21] Infections can either be a precipitant or a consequence of ACLF.[3,4] Active infection is a contraindication for LT and is associated with poorer survival post-LT.[9,22] However, a

Table 1
Differences between the 3 major definitions of acute-on-chronic liver failure

	EASL-CLIF	APASL	NACSELD
Definition	Acute decompensation presenting with extrahepatic organ failure in a patient with cirrhosis	Jaundice (>5 mg/dL) and coagulopathy (INR>1.5) followed by ascites and/or hepatic encephalopathy within 4 wk in a patient with known or unknown liver disease	Often infection-related extrahepatic organ failure in a patient with cirrhosis
Liver involvement	Not required (bilirubin >12 mg/dL is considered as organ failure)	Bilirubin > 5 mg/dL is must	Not required
Coagulopathy	Not required (INR >2.5 is considered as organ failure)	INR >1.5 is must	Not required
Renal involvement	Must (serum creatinine level should be > 1.5 mg/dL to identify ACLF and > 2 to define organ failure)	Not required	Renal replacement therapy required
Infection	Most often is a precipitant	Can be a precipitant but usually considered as a consequence	Most often is a precipitant
Reversibility	Unlikely	Possible	Unlikely
Data on liver transplantation	Robust	Few studies	Few studies
Severity scores to predict transplant free-survival	CLIF-C ACLF; CLIF-C OF	AARC	-
Validation of TAM score to predict post-LT outcomes	Yes	No	No
TIPS for variceal bleed	Possible	Not applicable (variceal bleed is not considered as a precipitant unless the bleed leads to increase in bilirubin level and INR)	Possible

Abbreviations: AARC, APASL ACLF research consortium; APASL, Asian Pacific Association for Study of the Liver; CLIF-C, chronic liver failure-consortium organ failure; CLIF-C ACLF, chronic liver failure-consortium ACLF; EASL-CLIF, European Association for Study of Liver-Consortium for Liver Failure; INR, international normalized ratio; NACSELD, North American Consortium for Study of End-Stage Liver Disease; TAM, transplantation for ACLF-3 model; TIPS, transjugular intrahepatic portosystemic shunt.

patient with a controlled infection can undergo LT for ACLF as early as 2 days.[9] Last, patients with primary biliary cholangitis who develop ACLF have higher waitlist mortality but excellent post-LT survival.[23] Therefore, all patients with ACLF, irrespective of the cause, should be given consideration for early LT to improve survival.

CHALLENGES WITH EARLY LIVER TRANSPLANTATION UNDER MODEL FOR END-STAGE LIVER DISEASE SCORE–BASED ORGAN ALLOCATION SYSTEM

The clinical characterization of ACLF includes extrahepatic organ failures, which is not captured in the model for end-stage liver disease (MELD) scoring system, the gold-standard organ allocation method. In a retrospective study of 18,979 admitted patients with ACLF, 48.5% had grade 1, 38.2% had grade 2, and 13.3% had grade 3 ACLF.[24] Precipitants of ACLF were variceal bleeding, bacterial infections, and alcohol abuse. The median model for end-stage liver disease sodium (MELD Na) score was 24, 27, and 32 in ACLF-1, -2, and -3 grades, respectively. The 90-day mortality was significantly higher in patients with ACLF than the expected mortality based on the MELD Na scores. The disparity was more apparent in patients with MELD Na between 10 and 30. The lower the MELD Na score, higher was the disparity. At a score of 10 to 19, the mortality was 5 to 10 times higher than expected in ACLF. At a MELD Na score of 20 to 29, the mortality was 2 to 4 times higher than expected in patients with ACLF. The disparity remained significant across various definitions, that is, consortium of acute-on-chronic liver failure in cirrhosis (CANONIC), the North American Consortium for Study of End-Stage Liver Disease, and APASL.[24] This underestimation by MELD Na score led to a significantly lower number of patients with ACLF being listed for LT. Despite having a higher median MELD Na score, during the index admission, only 0.7% of patients with ACLF-1, 1.9% with ACLF-2, and 2.7% with ACLF-3 were considered for LT, and this increased by merely 3.5%, 7.3%, and 4.2% at 6 months.[24] A similar study reported higher waitlist mortality (33%–40%) in patients with ACLF and low MELD (<25) compared with only less than 10% in patients with MELD score less than 25 and no ACLF.[7,25]

Most of the patients with ACLF have been noted to have MELD Na scores between 30 and 35, which disadvantages these patients from "Share 35" eligibility.[24,26] Share 35 is a rule implemented in 2013 to prioritize critically ill patients for LT and reduce the waitlist mortality of these sick patients.[27] Share 35 is associated with reduced waitlist mortality among patients with ACLF and MELD-Na score greater than or equal to 35.[28,29] Furthermore, the number of transplants for patients with ACLF and MELD Na score greater than or equal to 35 have significantly increased due to increased regional sharing.[29] However, several patients with ACLF have score less than 35 and may be disadvantaged from Share 35 eligibility.[24] Thus, it has been suggested that the MELD-based allocation system may disadvantage those patients with ACLF.[28] Such inference, however, is largely based on the UNOS database, which inherently has issues with proper coding and missing data elements.[30,31] The validity of MELD score allocation system in patients with ACLF is limited. However, MELD scoring may be more valuable in patients with ACLF identified by the APASL criteria, which largely depends on liver failure.[29,32,33] An increase in MELD score by greater than or equal to 2 points at 2 weeks can predict survival at 60 days, which may be more useful in Asian settings where living donor LT (LDLT) is commonly performed.[32,34]

PREDICTORS OF WAITLIST MORTALITY

The waitlist mortality is directly proportional to the number of organ failures. Approximately 10% of patients without any organ failure, 80% of those with 2 organ failures, and 98% with of those with 3 or more organ failures are delisted within 30 days.[35,36]

Abdallah and colleagues[37] developed a novel score based on age, sex, year of listing, listing MELD score, ACLF grade, race, obesity, performance status, and cause of liver disease to predict the waitlist mortality among patients with ACLF. The score ranged from −0.06 to 27.6. The score was divided into 4 quartiles (<10.42, 10.42–12.82, 12.82–15.5, and >15.5), and the waitlist mortality increased linearly from 13% in Q1 to 36.3% in Q4.[37] The major strength of the study was the derivation and validation of the score from a large UNOS database; however, the study included only alcohol and NASH as causes limiting its universal utility.[37]

In recent years, the global threat of multidrug-resistant organisms (MDROs) has become a significant concern. Belli and colleagues[38] reported that age greater than 60 years, a higher number of organ failures, and infections with MDROs increased the risk of waitlist mortality. Goudsmit and colleagues[39] developed a dynamic model to assess the need for urgent LT in patients with ACLF. The dynamic model named as ACLF-JM (Joint Model) includes the age, grade of ACLF, gender, the requirement of life support, spontaneous bacterial peritonitis, MELD Na, and the change in MELD Na (slope) over 2, 7, and 14 days. The investigators reported accurate prediction of 28-day and 90-day waitlist mortality in patients with ACLF.[39]

WHO WOULD BENEFIT FROM LIVER TRANSPLANTATION?

Several severity scores, including MELD, chronic liver failure-consortium (CLIF-C) ACLF, chronic liver failure consortium organ failure (CLIF-C OF), and APASL ACLF research consortium (AARC) scores, have been developed to predict transplant-free survival in patients with ACLF.[40,41] However, these scores cannot predict the post-LT survival. The long-term survival (post-LT) of patients depends on recipient and donor factors.[42–45] Few scores have been developed to identify those who would benefit from LT. Various variables and scores that predict post-LT outcomes are high-lighted in **Tables 2** and **3**.

To predict post-LT survival in patients with ACLF grade 3, Artzner and colleagues developed a score based on 4 important pre-LT factors, which included age (≥53 years), pre-LT arterial lactate level (≥4 mmol/L), mechanical ventilation with Pao_2/Fio_2 (fraction of inspired oxygen) (P/F) ratio less than or equal to 200 mm Hg, and pre-LT leukocyte counts (≤10 G/L).[46] A score greater than 2 predicted survival of 8% at 1 year compared with 84% in those with score less than or equal to 2. Transplantation for ACLF-3 model score within 48 hours before LT better predicted survival than intensive care unit (ICU) admission score. It has been demonstrated that optimization of patients and downstaging the score before LT was associated with improved survival in patients with ACLF-3.[47] Similarly, Huebener and colleagues[48] proposed an *OLT-Survival Score* based on CLIF-C ACLF score at LT and clinical improvement (defined as recovery of at least previously failed organ) before LT. The OLT-Survival Score accurately predicts 90-day post-LT survival. The score is calculated as 0.03 × CLIF-C score-Clinical improvement (yes: 1; no: 0).

Another model to predict post-LT survival for patients with ACLF-3 was developed by Singal and colleagues[49] using the UNOS data. The model included the recipient's age, alcohol as cause, pulmonary failure, brain failure, and cardiovascular failure. LT recipients were stratified for 1-year survival to low risk (score <7.55; survival 89%), medium risk (score between 7.55 and 11.57; survival 82%), and high risk (score >11.57; survival 80%) based on the tertiles of this score. The investigators also reported that patients with high-risk scores who received good-quality grafts (defined as donor risk index [DRI]<1.5) had better survival at 1 year (83% vs 78%) than those who received poor-quality grafts (DRI≥1.5).

Table 2
Variables associated with poor outcomes posttransplantation for patients with acute-on-chronic liver failure

Recipient Factors	Operative Factors	Donor-Related Factors
Age > 53 y[42]	Cold ischemia time > 8.5 h[45]	DRI ≥ 1.7[7,36,57]
WBC counts	Time to transplant <30 d from listing[7,8]	Male donor[50]
Infection in the previous month		Donor BMI[93]
ALT>100 U/l[43]		Hepatic macrosteatosis >15%[49]
Mechanical ventilation at LT[7]		
Respiratory failure with P/F ratio <200 mm Hg[16,43,67]		
Hepatitis C infection[7,36]		
Cerebral failure[16,43]		
CLIF-C ACLF score >64		
>3 OF[16]		
ACLF, MELD score and serum creatinine at LT[76]		
Arterial lactate > 4 mmol/L[38,46,68]		
Need of RRT[38]		
MDROs[38]		
Number of OFs		
Pre-transplant ICU care (shorter stay better outcomes)[85]		
Transplantation from ICU[48]		
TAM score >2		
Portal vein thrombosis[69]		
Futility risk score >8[7,71]		
Clinical frailty score ≥7[22]		

Abbreviations: ALT, alanine transaminase; BMI, body mass index; DRI, donor risk index; FiO_2, fraction of inspired oxygen; ICU, intensive care unit; OFs, organ failures; P/F ratio, PaO_2; FiO_2; RRT, renal replacement therapy; TAM, transplantation for ACLF-3 model; WBC, white blood cell;.

Table 3
Scores and models to predict posttransplant outcomes

Score Name/Author Name	Components of Score	Comments
Transplantation for ACLF-3 model (TAM score) by Artzener et al,[46]	Recipient age ≥53 y Pre-LT arterial lactate level ≥4 mml/L Mechanical ventilation with Pao₂/Fio₂ ≤ 200 mm Hg Pre-LT leukocyte count ≤10 G/L	Predicts 1 y survival post-LT (>2: 8.3% survival versus 84% in ≤2)
OLT-Survival Score by Huebener et al.[48]	CLIF-C score Clinical improvement	90-d post-LT survival Applicable for all grades of ACLF
Model by Singal et al.[49]	Recipient age Pulmonary failure Brain failure Cardiovascular failure Alcohol etiology	1-y post-LT survival Applicable for ACLF grade 3 Score >9.7 inversely related to survival
Model by Levsque et al.[50]	Recipient age (>57.2 y) and gender (male) Male donor Indication for LT (ESLD or HCC) Infection Presence of ACLF	90-d post-LT mortality
Nomogram by Chen et al.[16]	White cell counts ALT/AST ratio Number of organ failures	Predicts 1-y post-LT survival Applicable for HBV-related ACLF diagnosed either by APASL or EASL criteria
Computed tomography based score by Wackenthaler et al.[51]	Splenomegaly (>500 cm³): 5 points Liver atrophy (>20% smaller than the expected liver volume): 5 points Inferior vena cava diameters ratio (VCR≤0.2): 12 points	Applicable for patients with ACLF-3 Vena cava diameter 1 cm above (VC supra) and below (VC infra) the left renal vein was calculated first. VCR = VC supra-VC infra VC supra

Abbreviations: ALT, alanine transaminase; AST, aspartate transaminase; CLIF-C ACLF, chronic liver failure-consortium ACLF; ESLD, end-stage liver disease; Fio₂, fraction of inspired oxygen; HBV, hepatitis B virus; HCC, hepatocellular carcinoma; OLT, orthotopic liver transplantation; TAM, Transplantation for ACLF-3 model; VCR, vena cava diameters.

A nomogram based on white cell counts, alanine transaminase/aspartate transaminase ratio, and the number of organ failures can predict the survival till 1 year for patients with HBV-related ACLF undergoing LT.[16] Similarly, Levesque and colleagues[50] developed a model to predict 90-day mortality. This complex model included age (57.2 years), gender of recipient and donor, indication for LT (hepatocellular carcinoma or end-stage cirrhosis), infection in the month before LT, and ACLF at LT. A male recipient with end-stage liver cirrhosis (indication) reduced the risk of mortality, whereas the other variables (infection, ACLF at LT, age, male donor) increased the risk of 90-day mortality.[50]

A recent study also reported on pre-LT computed tomographic scan features to predict 1-year survival post-LT.[51] The score was based on three parameters: splenomegaly (>500 cm^3), liver atrophy (>20% smaller than the expected liver volume), and inferior vena cava diameters ratio ($\leq$0.2). A total score greater than 10 predicted poorer survival post-LT.[51] However, such scores and models need further validation in prospective studies.

BRIDGING A PATIENT WITH ACUTE-ON-CHRONIC LIVER FAILURE TO LIVER TRANSPLANTATION

There is a critical need to prevent ACLF through the prevention of infection or by modulating the course of liver disease through the timely use of antivirals for hepatitis B and C infections, vaccinations, and beta-blocker as indicated.[52–54] More than 60% of patients with ACLF are ineligible for LT due to sepsis, organ failures, or being too sick to transplant, contributing to the high waitlist mortality.[55] Clinical improvement before LT is associated with better survival post-LT.[48,56] It is well known that downgrading ACLF grade before LT improves the survival post-LT.[57] Improvement in circulatory and brain failure, improving respiratory status, and eliminating the need for mechanical ventilation have been associated with reduced mortality post-LT.[57] Therefore, measures to favorably modify the course, support the failing organs, and bridge a patient with ACLF to LT are required.[52,58–62] Thus, for optimal outcomes in a patient with ACLF and organ failure, it is essential that the care be multidisciplinary, requiring the involvement of a pulmonologist, intensivist, anesthetist, transfusion medicine specialist, nephrologist, and nutritionist for adequate optimization of the patient with organ failure.[63,64] Furthermore, an experienced hepatologist and a well-equipped medical center are the keys to optimizing and bridging a patient with ACLF to LT and then eventually achieving good outcomes. **Fig. 1** highlights some measures to bridge a patient with ACLF to LT.

WHO WOULD NOT BENEFIT FROM LIVER TRANSPLANTATION OR THE FUTILITY OF LIVER TRANSPLANTATION IN ACUTE-ON-CHRONIC LIVER FAILURE?

Although LT is associated with survival benefits in patients with ACLF, identifying an appropriate candidate and the timing of LT determines the outcomes in these patients. It is to be recognized that LT would be futile considering the low survival post-LT in advanced grades of ACLF.[65] LT in a patient with ACLF who has a high probability of mortality early after LT or has an unacceptable quality of life and or/multiple complications post-LT is a "potentially inappropriate candidate," and in such patients, LT is a futile exercise.[45] Patients with ACLF may become too sick for LT, and identifying those who are inappropriate candidates is valuable. A post-LT survival of less than 3 months (or in-hospital mortality) is considered as a futile LT.[44] Artru and colleagues evaluated Preallocation Survival Outcomes Following Liver Transplantation score, Balance of Risk Score, and University of California, Los Angeles (UCLA) score and reported

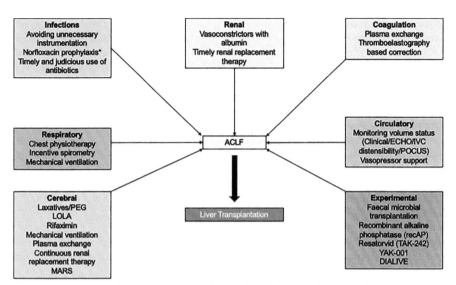

Fig. 1. Optimization of care in acute-on-chronic liver failure to bridge to liver transplantation. ECHO, echocardiography; IVC, inferior vena cava; LOLA, L-ornithine L-aspartate; MARS, molecular adsorbent recirculating system; PEG, polyethylene glycol; POCUS, point-of-care ultrasonography. *Norfloxacin is not available universally.

that none of the scores could identify survival accurately.[9] However, the UCLA score was a (comparatively) better predictor of post-LT survival. The following are some of the indicators of futility (or conditions in which patients with ACLF were not found suitable for LT):

- Greater than or equal to 4 organ failures[8]
- CLIF-C score greater than 64 at day 3 to 7[8]
- Respiratory failure [37,43,66,67]
- Mechanical ventilation[36]
- MELD Na greater than 30 with advanced hepatic encephalopathy (HE) at baseline[55]
- High lactate levels[22,66–68]
- Development of hepatic encephalopathy, increase in creatinine levels, and white cell counts in 7 days[55]
- Patients with ACLF grade 2/3 patients with either active gastrointestinal bleed, controlled sepsis for less than 24 hours, high vasopressor support (3 mg/h), and/or P/F ratio less than 150.[9]
- Active drug abuse, infections by MDROs or invasive fungal infections, high cardiac risk, significant comorbidities[44,69]
- Clinical frailty score greater than or equal to 7[22]
- Futility risk score greater than 8[7,70]

OPTIMAL DONOR AND TRANSPLANT CENTER

For good outcomes following LT, it is essential that we target high-quality grafts for those with ACLF, particularly those of a higher grade.[49,71] High-risk patients with ACLF who receive a liver from donors with age less than 60 years, macrosteatosis of less than 15%, and those with a lower DRI have an excellent survival advantage.[49] In LDLT settings, a graft-to-recipient weight ratio of 0.8 to 1 would provide more benefit to a sicker patient.[72–74] Despite getting a liver from a young, healthy donor with a lower body mass index, patients with ACLF may have poorer graft survival, and such outcome depends on multiple recipient factors, including the presence of ACLF itself, pre-LT severity scores, and organ failures.[75] In a large LT center in China where 100 patients with ACLF underwent LT, there was a reported 20% mortality irrespective of the type of transplant, that is, deceased donor or living donor.[76] Recent studies have also reported comparable outcomes with LDLT and deceased donor liver transplantation (DDLT) in patients with high MELD scores.[56,77] Conversely, Toshima and colleagues[71] reported a dismal survival rate of 33% in patients with ACLF-3 who underwent LDLT. This heterogeneity in outcomes may depend on the experience of the transplant team and may be center dependent apart from the quality of the graft.[69]

Organ availability has improved over the past decade. However, the acceptance of an organ has decreased and is center based, is selective, and biased on the DRI.[78,79] Waitlist mortality is inversely related to the number of organ failures.[36] Therefore, the timely availability of an organ is of utmost importance in cadaveric LT settings. On the contrary, the time to transplantation would be shorter in LDLT settings.[77,80,81] However, the acceptance of LT in settings of LDLT is poor.[82,83] Furthermore, the lack of national policies and poor participation in the organ donation and transplantation process by public hospitals preclude a successful DDLT in patients with ACLF and organ failures.[82] Last, with a survival of approximately 50% in patients with advanced ACLF, convincing a family for such an expensive surgery and liver donation is challenging.[71,84]

WHAT IS THE IDEAL TIMING OF LIVER TRANSPLANTATION IN ACUTE-ON-CHRONIC LIVER FAILURE?

Identifying those who require an LT is the key to prolonged survival. The seminal research on emergent LT reported survival in 75% of patients with ACLF who underwent early LT (<28 days).[8] Day 3 to 7 grades of ACLF determined the outcomes. A total of 35 patients underwent LT, and of them, 10 had resolution of ACLF at the time of LT. Of the 25 patients with ACLF at the time of LT, 22% had cerebral failure, 36% had circulatory failure, 65% had renal failure (40% on renal replacement therapy), 50% to 60% had liver and coagulation failure, and none had respiratory failure. Of these, 28% of patients were on mechanical ventilation. The time to transplant was 11 (1–28) days. The type of organ failure determines the time to LT, with cerebral failure having the longest waiting time (15 days).[36] Survival of patients with ACLF grades 2 and 3 (on days 3–7) undergoing LT within 28 days was 81% at 6 months compared with 10% in those who did not undergo LT. Mortality in those with 4 or more organ failures and/or CLIF-C score greater than 64 and not undergoing LT was 100% at 90 days. A similar study from Asia reported that the transplant eligibility of an ACLF candidate increased from 35% to 60% within 7 days.[55] However, only 4% of patients with ACLF underwent LT in a large multicenter study of 1021 patients assessed for LT suitability. Furthermore, the investigators reported that the development of hepatic encephalopathy, increase in white cell counts, and increase in creatinine levels within 7 days increased the risk of 28-day mortality.[55] LT also improved a patient's performance status within 1 year if performed within 30 days of listing, thus highlighting the need for early listing and timely LT.[85]

LONG-TERM OUTCOMES OF LIVER TRANSPLANTATION IN ACUTE-ON-CHRONIC TRANSPLANTATION

There have been multiple studies evaluating the results following LT in patients with ACLF. Initial studies reported poorer outcomes in patients with ACLF and multiorgan failures.[50,84] However, several retrospective and national database-based studies have demonstrated excellent outcomes with LT in ACLF (**Table 4**). The survival in patients with ACLF and non-ACLF undergoing LT is comparable with respect to survival.[8,9,86,87] However, posttransplant survival depends on the grade of ACLF.[8,88] Survival post-LT for ACLF grade 1 is 90% compared with 70% to 80% in patients with ACLF grades 2 and 3 at 1 year.[8] The long-term survival of patients with ACLF undergoing LT is greater than 80% compared with only less than 40% in nontransplanted patients with ACLF.[9,89]

The complications of LT are frequent in the early post-LT period (initial 6–12 months), and patients surviving the early period have excellent long-term outcomes.[88,90] It is well known that patients with ACLF have higher morbidity post-LT requiring higher health care utilization due to prolonged hospitalization, ICU care, renal replacement therapy, and recurrent readmissions for infections.[9,38,75] Posttransplant vascular and biliary complications, re-explorations, pulmonary, neurologic, and cardiovascular complications are significantly higher in patients with ACLF grade 3 who undergo LT.[9,75] The prevalence of infections post-LT increases with the grade of ACLF at LT.[91] Common sites of infection include the urinary tract, lung, and spontaneous bacteremia. Patients with ACLF grade 3 are prone to develop multisite infections.[91] Kidney dysfunction is frequent in patients with ACLF. The incidence of chronic kidney disease post-LT is slightly higher in patients with ACLF than non-ACLF, although renal recovery is similar.[86,88,92,93] However, the development of other comorbidities, including diabetes mellitus, dyslipidemia, systemic hypertension, and obesity, are similar among patients with ACLF and those without ACLF post-LT.

Goosmann and colleagues[88] compared the quality of life (QoL) post-LT among patients with ACLF and non-ACLF. The median follow-up in the whole cohort was 8.7 years. Approximately 60% of patients responded to the QoL questionnaire survey. Patients with ACLF reported an inability to perform usual activities and had a higher incidence of anxiety/depression, and less than 50% of patients reported "optimal" health. Patients with ACLF reported poorer physical and psychological health. The QoL was inversely related to the duration of ICU hospitalization following LT, indicating a measurable and significant impact of liver disease severity on long-term outcomes.[88]

POST-LIVER TRANSPLANTATION IMMUNOSUPPRESSION

Renal dysfunction is common in patients with ACLF. Renal-sparing regimens are suggested to protect the kidneys. Strategies to prevent renal dysfunction include maintaining a lower trough level of calcineurin inhibitors (CNIs, tacrolimus, and cyclosporine), delayed introduction of CNIs by using an anti-IL-2-receptor antibody (basiliximab), and early introduction of mammalian target of rapamycin inhibitors (mTORi).[50,94] Any ongoing surgical complication is a strict contraindication for mTORi, whereas the development of anasarca, significant proteinuria, and dyslipidemia can lead to withdrawal of mTORi. Tacrolimus trough levels between 4 and 8 mg/mL during the first month with intrapatient variability of tacrolimus levels less than 40%, use of basiliximab, and early introduction of mycophenolate mofetil (day 1) can prolong the survival in patients with ACLF.[95] Conversely, lower immunosuppression to protect kidneys may increase the risk of acute cellular rejection, especially in patients with ACLF-3.[91] Last, as the risk of infections is high in patients with ACLF, surveillance cultures may help identify infections early and aid in modifying the immunosuppression regimen.

FUTURE DIRECTIONS

Although LT is a definitive therapy for patients with ACLF, they may not have equitable access to LT due to the current allocation policies in Western countries.[96] The health

Table 4
Current literature on liver transplantation in acute-on-chronic liver failure

Serial No.	Author Name, Country, Definition Used, Ref.	Total Number of Transplants	Grade of ACLF at LT (MELD Score)	Organ Failures at LT	Time to LT	Survival	Comments
1	Umgelter et al,[84] 2011	13	MELD: 38	Renal: 38.5% RRT: 77%	—	46% Survival at 1 y	Reduction in MELD within 48 h of ICU admission by 2 points improved survival
2	Bahirwani et al,[86] 2011	ACLF: 156 No ACLF: 175	MELD: 28.77 in ACLF vs 21.23 in no ACLF	Renal: 76%	—	74.5% Survival in ACLF vs 83.4% in non-ACLF group	Renal recovery, death, and retransplantation were similar among ACLF and non-ACLF groups
3	Finkenstedt et al,[87] 2013, APASL	33 ACLF (MELD Na-30) vs 356 non-ACLF (MELD Na-18)	—		24 (5–115) d	85% Survival vs 84% in non-ACLF group at 29 mo	Waitlist mortality 54%
4	Gustot et al,[8] 2015 CANONIC	35	10: No ACLF ACLF: 1–5 ACLF: 2–11 ACLF: 3–9	Liver: 56% Coagulation: 60% Renal: 64% (RRT: 40%) Circulatory: 36% Cerebral: 22% (mechanical ventilation: 28%) Respiratory: 0%	11 (1–28) d	Survival at 1 y No ACLF: 90% (71.4–100) ACLF-1: 80% (71.4–100) ACLF-2: 71.6% (44.2–99) ACLF-3: 77.8% (50.6–100)	Grade of ACLF at day 3–7 determined the outcome Early LT (<28 d) for patients with ACLF had excellent survival benefit

#	Study					
5	Levesque et al,[50] 2017 CANONIC	ACLF: 140 (MELD: 29.5) Non-ACLF: 210 (MELD: 14.3)	ACLF-1: 48.57% ACLF-2: 30% ACLF-3: 21.42%	—	70% Survival at 1 y in ACLF compared with 91.4% in those without ACLF	Survival of 43.3% in ACLF-3 at 1 y compared with ~80% in ACLF-1 and -2
6	Artru et al,[9] 2017 CANONIC	1303	No ACLF: 292 (MELD: 16) ACLF-1: 133 (MELD: 29) ACLF-2: 181 (MELD: 35) ACLF-3: 73 (MELD: 38)	8 (3–24) d	Survival at 1 y: No ACLF: 90%; ACLF-1: 82.3%; ACLF-2: 86.2%; ACLF-3: 83% Nontransplanted controls: 8%	Bacterial infections in 80% of ACLF-3 post-LT. Higher morbidity (cardiac, neurologic, renal, and pulmonary complications) in ACLF-3 post-LT
7	Moon et al,[73] 2017 CANONIC	Non-ACLF: 137 (MELD: 33.7) ACLF-1: 90 (MELD: 38.4)	ACLF-1: 50.5% ACLF-2: 22.63% ACLF-3: 26.8%	Kidney failure most common followed by brain	Survival in ACLF: 79.5% vs 90.5% at 1 y	ACLF associated with poorer graft survival
8	Huebener et al,[48] 2018 CANONIC	ACLF: 98 (MELD: 34.5) Non-ACLF: 152 (MELD: 23.5)	ACLF-1: 24 ACLF-2: 45 ACLF-3: 29	Liver: 57% Coagulation: 46% Renal: 92% Circulatory: 29.6% Brain: 39.8% Lung: 16.3%	86.8% Survival in non-ACLF group compared with 60.2% in the ACLF group	Higher transfusion; more interventions post-LT. Pretransplant clinical improvement predicted post-LT survival

(continued on next page)

Table 4
(continued)

Serial No.	Author Name, Country, Definition Used, Ref.	Total Number of Transplants	Grade of ACLF at LT (MELD Score)	Organ Failures at LT	Time to LT	Survival	Comments
9	Bhatti et al,[81] 2018 CANONIC	119; Transplanted ACLF: 60 (MELD: 29); Nontransplanted ACLF: 59 (MELD: 36)	ACLF-1: 43 vs 15 not transplanted ACLF-2: 15 transplanted vs 19 in nontransplanted ACLF-3: 2 transplanted vs 25 in nontransplanted	Liver: 73% Coagulation: 36% Renal: 20% Circulatory: 0% Brain: 1.6% Lung: 0%	—	1-y Survival: 91% in transplanted patients vs 11% in nontransplanted ACLF	Survival better with LT. However, the baseline characteristics were not evenly distributed. More number of ACLF-3 in nontransplanted group
10	Thuluvath et al,[36] 2018, CANONIC	19,375 transplanted within 30 d	MELD: 25.3	0 OF: 42.6% 1 OF: 24.7% 2 OF: 19.5% 3 OF: 8.6% 4 OF: 3% 5/6 OF: 1.7%	No OF: 156 d 1 OF: 26 d 2 OF: 8 d 3–4 OF: 5 d 5–6 OFs: 4 d	90% survival in no OF vs 81% in those with 5/6 OFs	Patients with MOFs died on waitlist. Post-LT survival was not dependent on OF. Poor survival in patients with respiratory failure and those requiring life-support systems
11	O'Leary et al,[92] 2019, NACSELD	ACLF: 57 No ACLF: 208	MELD-ACLF: 31.1 No ACLF: 27.3	—	CLF: 27 ± 60 d No ACLF: 43.5 ± 94	93% Survival among ACLF and no ACLF group at 1 y	Despite higher creatinine levels and RRT in ACLF group renal recovery was similar among patients with ACLF and no ACLF

#	Study	Sample	ACLF grade (MELD)	Organ failures	Days	Survival	Comments
12	Sundaram et al,[7] 2019	No ACLF: 29,283 vs 21,269 in ACLF group	ACLF-1: 7375 (MELD Na: 28.8) ACLF-2: 7513 (MELD: 34.2) ACLF-3: 6381 (MELD: 37.4)	—	No ACLF: 106 (32–291) d ACLF-1: 48 (12–175) d ACLF-2: 23 (7–120) d ACLF-3: 12 (4–62) d	Survival at 1 y: ACLF-1/2: 90% ACLF-3: 82%	Mechanical ventilation at LT associated with reduced survival post-LT. High mortality among patients with ACLF-3 with MELD <25
13	Artzner et al,[46] 2019 CANONIC	152	All ACLF-3 (MELD: 40)	Liver: 81.6% Coagulation: 80.3% Renal: 73% (RRT: 65.1%) Circulatory: 69.7% Cerebral: 55.6% (mechanical ventilation: 73%) Respiratory: 50.7%	8 (4–15) d	67.1% Survival at 1 y	Developed TAM score to predict post-LT survival
14	Yadav et al,[72] 2019 CANONIC	117: LDLT (MELD: 30.6) vs 101 no LDLT (MELD: 31.3)	ACLF-1: 80% ACLF-2: 72.7% ACLF-3: 35%	Liver: 59% Coagulation: 0% Renal: 0% Circulatory: 0% Cerebral: 1.7% Respiratory: 0%	—	ACLF-1: 93% ACLF-2: 85.4% ACLF-3: 75.6%	High mortality in first 3 mo post-LT
15	Marciano et al,[93] 2019 CANONIC	ACLF: 60 (MELD Na: 28.7) No ACLF: 125 (MELD Na: 20.5)	ACLF-1: 56.7%; ACLF-2: 30% ACLF-3: 13.3%	—	—	85% Survival at 1 y in ACLF vs 91.2% in those without ACLF	No association between ACLF and post-LT CKD

(continued on next page)

Table 4
(continued)

Serial No.	Author Name, Country, Definition Used, Ref.	Total Number of Transplants	Grade of ACLF at LT (MELD Score)	Organ Failures at LT	Time to LT	Survival	Comments
16	Sundaram et al,[57] 2020 CANONIC	All ACLF-3 (3925 underwent LT and 2256 died pre-LT)	75% Remained in ACLF-3 (MELD: 41) at LT. 25% improved (ACLF-0-2; MELD: 34.3)	—	<28 d	82.43% Survival at 1 y vs 88%–90% in those who improved to ACLF-0-2	Optimization and downgrading ACLF grade improved survival Improvement in circulatory and brain failure and removal from mechanical ventilation improved survival
17	Abgim et al,[75] 2020 CANONIC	ACLF: 101 (MELD: 31) No ACLF: 589 (MELD: 16)	Grade 1: 49.5% Grade 2: 31.7% Grade 3: 19%	Liver: 45.5% Coagulation: 41.6% Renal: 64.4% Circulatory: 4% Cerebral: 13% Respiratory: 10%	—	92% Survival in non-ACLF group compared with 82% in ACLF (grade 1: 86%; grade 2: 81%; grade 3: 74%)	Prolonged hospitalization and ICU care for patients with ACLF. Early surgical re-explorations (26.7% in ACLF group vs 14.6% in non-ACLF group Graft loss dependent on ACLF grade (6%, 19%, and 21% respectively) Higher need for RRT post-LT. Delayed renal recovery in ACLF

	Study	Patients / MELD	ACLF grades / MELD Na	Organ failures	Time	Survival	Comments
18	Goosmann et al,[88] 2020 CANONIC	ACLF: 98 (MELD: 31.5) Non-ACLF: 152 (MELD: 12.5)	ACLF grade 1: 21 Grade 2: 30 Grade 3: 38	Liver: 57% Coagulation: 46% Renal: 91.8% Circulatory: 29.6% Cerebral: 39.8% Respiratory: 16.3%	—	68.4% Survival in non-ACLF patients compared with 49% in patients with ACLF at 10 y	ACLF grade 3 at LT had poorest post-LT prognosis. Higher incidence of infections (34%) in ACLF group
19	Sundaram et al,[90] 2020 CANONIC	56,801	No ACLF: 31,024 (MELD Na: 20.7) ACLF-1: 8757 (MELD Na: 29) ACLF-2: 9039 (MELD Na: 34.8) ACLF-3: 7981 (MELD Na: 40.1)	3 OFs in 54.8% and rest of the patients with ACLF had $\geq$4 OFs	No ACLF-1: 3 (29–303) d ACLF-1: 48 (12–181) d ACLF-2: 22 (7–119) d ACLF-3: 12 (4–60) d	5-y survival ACLF-3: 67.7% vs 75%–79% in no ACLF, ACLF-1 and ACLF-2	Infection commonest cause of mortality. High mortality in first year. OFs predicted long-term mortality
20	Choudhury et al,[55] 2021 APASL	41	—		18 (5–90) days	—	4% (41/565) underwent LT
21	Chen et al,[16] 2021, APASL	290 Patients with HBV ACLF	MELD: 35	Liver: 75% Coagulation: 61% Renal: 24.5% Circulatory: 5.2% Brain: 23.4% Lung: 29.3% >3 OF: 35.5%	—	77% Survival at 1 y	Patients with circulatory, brain, and respiratory failure had high post-LT mortality
22	Goussous et al,[98] 2021 CANONIC	Transplanted ACLF: 86 (MELD: 33.6) vs nontransplanted ACLF: 58 (MELD: 31.7)	ACLF-1: 2.3% ACLF-2: 21% ACLF-3: 76.7%	Liver: 68.6% Coagulation: 72.1% Renal: 82.6% Circulatory: 48.4% Cerebral: 72% Respiratory: 55.8%	—	86% In LT group vs 12% in non-LT group at 1 y	Cost for LT group was $2,27,886 vs $88,900 in non-LT group

(continued on next page)

Table 4
(continued)

Serial No.	Author Name, Country, Definition Used, Ref.	Total Number of Transplants	Grade of ACLF at LT (MELD Score)	Organ Failures at LT	Time to LT	Survival	Comments
23	Belli et al,[38] 2021, CANONIC	308	ACLF-1: 68 ACLF-2: 109 ACLF-3: 131	Liver: 82% Coagulation: 47% Renal: 46% Circulatory: 20% Brain: 24% Lung: 15%	8 (3–19.5) d	84% Survival (ACLF-1: 88.6% and ACLF-3-79%)	Waitlist mortality: 24% Infections by MDROs increased the risk of waitlist mortality and also predicted post-LT survival
24	Kim et al,[56] 2021 CANONIC	76 (59 DDLT, 17 LDLT)	ACLF-1: 13.2% ACLF-2: 44.7% ACLF-3: 42%	Liver: 77.6% Coagulation: 60.5% Renal: 34.2% Circulatory: 40.8% Cerebral: 26.3% Respiratory: 5.3%	12 (5–20) d	83% Survival in LT vs 17.6% in nontransplanted ACLF	ACLF grade progression before LT and MELD scores predicted post-LT mortality
25	Wang et al,[74] 2021 APASL	112	ACLF-1: 32.1% (MELD: 25.8) ACLF-2: 26.8% (MELD: 31.5) ACLF-3: 18% (MELD: 34.8)	Liver: 74.1% Coagulation: 28.6% Renal: 10.7% Circulatory: 7.1% Cerebral: 22.3% Respiratory: 14.3%	—	95.5% And 93% survival at 3 and 5 y, respectively	More frequent portal vein complications in ACLF group

26	Sundaram et al,[68,91] 2022, CANONIC	318	No ACLF: 33.3% (MELD Na: 18) ACLF-1: 67.6% (MELD Na: 26) ACLF-2: 23.2% (MELD Na: 28) ACLF-3: 24.2% (MELD Na: 31)	—	Liver: 50.3% Coagulation: 33.2% Renal: 36.2% Circulatory: 20.7% Cerebral: 36.7% Respiratory: 5.3%	Length of stay post-LT: No ACLF: 9 d ACLF-1: 16 d ACLF-2: 24 d ACLF-3: 39 d	Higher ACR in ACLF-3 (13%) More infections in ACLF-2 and 3 High resource utilization in ACLF 2 and 3 PVT increased the risk of post-LT within 1 y Comparable outcomes between those with and without circulatory failure
27	Chen et al,[89] 2022, APASL	Transplanted ACLF: 29 (MELD: 25) vs nontransplanted ACLF: 110 (MELD: 25) Decompensated cirrhosis (matched population: 32)	—	—		1-y Survival 87% in transplanted group vs 42.7% in nontransplanted group vs 78.1% in patients with decompensated cirrhosis	LT for ACLF was associated with survival benefit but had higher morbidity and risk of pulmonary infections
28	Laici et al,[67] 2022, CANONIC	19 Transplanted ACLF 45 Nontransplanted ACLF	ACLF-1: 21% ACLF-2: 32% ACLF-3: 47%	—	Liver: 84% Coagulation: 32% Renal: 58% Circulatory: 32% Cerebral: 53% Respiratory: 16%	84.2% Survival in LT vs 13.3% in those who did not undergo LT	Respiratory failure, CLIF-C ACLF score, lactate levels predicted mortality

(continued on next page)

Table 4
(continued)

Serial No.	Author Name, Country, Definition Used, Ref.	Total Number of Transplants	Grade of ACLF at LT (MELD Score)	Organ Failures at LT	Time to LT	Survival	Comments
29	Chang et al,[25] 2022, CANONIC	ACLF: 25 Non-ACLF: 28	Grade 1–14 (MELD: 30.5) Grade 2/3: 11 (MELD: 32) Non-ACLF: 27	Renal (RRT): 44% Circulatory: 4% Cerebral (encephalopathy): 56% Respiratory: 4% None in non-ACLF group had respiratory, renal, or circulatory failure	—	71% Survival in ACLF group and 83% in non-ACLF group at 1 y	18% Waitlist mortality Waitlist mortality high in patients with ACLF and low MELD (<25) Survival of patients with ACLF and non-ACLF post-LT was similar
30	Xia et al,[43] 2022, CANONIC and APASL	330 No ACLF 162 EASL-CLIF 230 APASL	ACLF-1: 3.2% ACLF-2: 17.2% ACLF-3: 8.3% AARC-1: 8%; AARC-2: 21% AARC-3: 12%	—	—	Similar transplant-free survival in each grade/class	APASL and EASL-CLIF had similar accuracy in predicting outcomes
31	Toshima et al,[71] 2022, Japanese criteria	31	ACLF-0: 19.4% ACLF-1: 22.6% ACLF-2: 29% ACLF-3: 29%	Liver: 74.2% Coagulation: 16.1% Renal: 22.6%	—	ACLF-0-2: 80%– 100% survival at 5 y vs 33.3% in ACLF-3	ACLF-3 had poor outcome post-LDLT

Abbreviations: AARC, APASL ACLF research consortium; ACR, acute cellular rejection; CKD, chronic kidney disease; CLIF-C ACLF, Chronic Liver Failure-Consortium ACLF; DDLT, deceased donor liver transplantation; EASL, European Association for Study of Liver; HBV, hepatitis B virus; ICU, intensive care unit; MOF, multiorgan failure; NA, sodium; NACSELD, North American Consortium for Study of End-Stage Liver Disease; OF, organ failure; PVT, portal vein thrombosis; RRT, renal replacement therapy; TAM, transplantation for ACLF-3 model.

care utilization and costs for LT for a patient with ACLF have gradually increased in recent years and now exceed the expenses for patients with alcohol-associated hepatitis undergoing early LT.[5,97,98] Resource utilization (due to prolonged hospital stay, recurrent infections, and postoperative complications) and expenditures proportionately increase with the grade of ACLF.[91] Patients with ACLF have higher morbidity post-LT than matched patients with decompensated cirrhosis who undergo LT.[89] Measures to reduce resource utilization and expenses are required.

The role of intraoperative continuous renal replacement therapy in preventing hemodynamic alterations and managing electrolyte and acid-base disturbances needs to be evaluated in patients with ACLF.[99] Decision to list a patient with ACLF can be made in the first week of diagnosis; however, the time to transplant is debatable given the high risk of organ failures in the early period. Prospective studies in LDLT settings are required to assess both the feasibility and futility of early LDLT for patients with ACLF. Most of the studies on LT in ACLF are based on registry data and/or are retrospective studies. Such registry-based data do not capture appropriate data and are prone to bias due to a lack of proper coding.[30,100] Thus, prospective studies are required to identify patients with ACLF requiring early LT and also assess the role of noninvasive biomarkers in correlating with outcomes following LT. Last, the role of ABO-incompatible LT and simultaneous liver-kidney transplants needs to be evaluated in patients with ACLF.

In conclusion, LT in ACLF is feasible in an appropriately selected candidate, provided a quality graft is available timely. Furthermore, it is most important to invoke the futility rule when the potential outcomes are suboptimal. If survival is the only goal, LT seems reasonable, but if we were to consider resource utilization, including the use of a graft, a society resource, well, it is important that we carefully select the candidates for LT with the expectation of a good outcome. **Fig. 2** summarizes LT in ACLF.

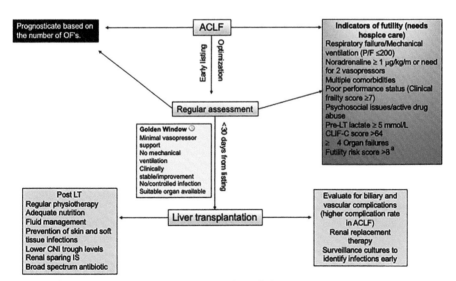

Fig. 2. LT for patients with ACLF. CLIF, chronic liver failure-consortium; IS, immunosuppression; OF, organ failure. [a]Futility risk score is based on ventilator support (5 points), recipient age greater than 60 years (3 points), preoperative dialysis (3 points), preoperative diabetes (2 points), and preoperative creatinine levels greater than or equal to 1.5 mg/dL but no dialysis (2 points). A score greater than 8 is associated with poor graft survival.

CLINICS CARE POINTS

- Identifying patients with ACLF meriting LT early (<30 days) is critical in the management of ACLF.
- More than 3 organ failures is an indicator of futility.
- Individuals with donor risk index ≥1.7 and hepatic macrosteatosis (>15%) are not ideal candidates for donation.
- Survival post-LT for ACLF grade 1 is 90% compared with 70% to 80% in patients with ACLF grades 2 and 3 at 1 year.

DISCLOSURES

None in relation to this article.

REFERENCES

1. Hernaez R, Solà E, Moreau R, et al. Acute-on-chronic liver failure: an update. Gut 2017;66(3):541–53.
2. Moreau R, Jalan R, Gines P, et al. Acute-on-chronic liver failure is a distinct syndrome that develops in patients with acute decompensation of cirrhosis. Gastroenterology 2013;144(7):1426–37, 1437.e1-1437.
3. Bajaj JS, O'Leary JG, Reddy KR, et al. Survival in infection-related acute-on-chronic liver failure is defined by extrahepatic organ failures. Hepatology 2014;60(1):250–6.
4. Sarin SK, Choudhury A, Sharma MK, et al. Acute-on-chronic liver failure: consensus recommendations of the Asian Pacific association for the study of the liver (APASL): an update. Hepatol Int 2019;13(4):353–90.
5. Allen AM, Kim WR, Moriarty JP, et al. Time trends in the health care burden and mortality of acute on chronic liver failure in the United States. Hepatology 2016; 64(6):2165–72.
6. Sundaram V, Shah P, Wong RJ, et al. Patients with acute on chronic liver failure Grade 3 have Greater 14-day waitlist mortality than status-1a patients. Hepatology 2019;70(1):334–45.
7. Sundaram V, Jalan R, Wu T, et al. Factors associated with survival of patients with severe acute-on-chronic liver failure before and after liver transplantation. Gastroenterology 2019;156(5):1381–91.e3.
8. Gustot T, Fernandez J, Garcia E, et al. Clinical Course of acute-on-chronic liver failure syndrome and effects on prognosis. Hepatology 2015;62(1):243–52.
9. Artru F, Louvet A, Ruiz I, et al. Liver transplantation in the most severely ill cirrhotic patients: a multicenter study in acute-on-chronic liver failure grade 3. J Hepatol 2017;67(4):708–15.
10. Patidar KR, Peng JL, Kaur H, et al. Severe alcohol-associated hepatitis is associated with Worse survival in critically ill patients with acute on chronic liver failure. Hepatol Commun 2022;6(5):1090–9.
11. Kulkarni AV, Sharma M, Kumar P, et al. Adipocyte fatty acid-Binding Protein as a predictor of outcome in alcohol-induced acute-on-chronic liver failure. J Clin Exp Hepatol 2021;11(2):201–8.
12. Shalimar, Kumar D, Vadiraja PK, et al. Acute on chronic liver failure because of acute hepatic insults: etiologies, course, extrahepatic organ failure and predictors of mortality. J Gastroenterol Hepatol 2016;31(4):856–64.

13. Mathurin P, Moreno C, Samuel D, et al. Early liver transplantation for severe alcoholic hepatitis. N Engl J Med 2011;365(19):1790–800.
14. Idalsoaga F, Kulkarni AV, Mousa OY, et al. Non-alcoholic fatty liver disease and alcohol-related liver disease: two Intertwined Entities. Front Med 2020;7:448.
15. Mahmud N, Kaplan DE, Taddei TH, et al. Incidence and mortality of acute-on-chronic liver failure using two definitions in patients with Compensated cirrhosis. Hepatology 2019;69(5):2150–63.
16. Chen L, Zhang J, Lu T, et al. A nomogram to predict survival in patients with acute-on-chronic hepatitis B liver failure after liver transplantation. Ann Transl Med 2021;9(7):555.
17. Fernández J, Acevedo J, Wiest R, et al. Bacterial and fungal infections in acute-on-chronic liver failure: prevalence, characteristics and impact on prognosis. Gut 2018;67(10):1870–80.
18. Kulkarni AV, Anand L, Vyas AK, et al. Omega-3 fatty acid lipid emulsions are safe and effective in reducing endotoxemia and sepsis in acute-on-chronic liver failure: an open-label randomized controlled trial. J Gastroenterol Hepatol 2021;36(7):1953–61.
19. Fernández J, Prado V, Trebicka J, et al. Multidrug-resistant bacterial infections in patients with decompensated cirrhosis and with acute-on-chronic liver failure in Europe. J Hepatol 2019;70(3):398–411.
20. Bajaj JS, Reddy RK, Tandon P, et al. Prediction of fungal infection development and Their impact on survival using the NACSELD cohort. Am J Gastroenterol 2018;113(4):556–63.
21. Verma N, Singh S, Taneja S, et al. Invasive fungal infections amongst patients with acute-on-chronic liver failure at high risk for fungal infections. Liver Int 2019;39(3):503–13.
22. Weiss E, Saner F, Asrani SK, et al. When is a critically ill cirrhotic patient too sick to transplant? Development of consensus criteria by a multidisciplinary Panel of 35 international Experts. Transplantation 2021;105(3):561–8.
23. Singal AK, Wong RJ, Jalan R, et al. Primary biliary cholangitis has the highest waitlist mortality in patients with cirrhosis and acute on chronic liver failure awaiting liver transplant. Clin Transplant 2021;35(12):e14479.
24. Hernaez R, Liu Y, Kramer JR, et al. Model for end-stage liver disease-sodium underestimates 90-day mortality risk in patients with acute-on-chronic liver failure. J Hepatol 2020;73(6):1425–33.
25. Chang J, Matheja A, Krzycki S, et al. Model for end-stage liver disease underestimates mortality of patients with acute-on-chronic liver failure waiting for liver transplantation. Dig Liver Dis 2022;54(6):784–90.
26. Martin P, DiMartini A, Feng S, et al. Evaluation for liver transplantation in adults: 2013 practice guideline by the American association for the study of liver diseases and the American society of transplantation. Hepatology 2014;59(3):1144–65.
27. Sharma P, Schaubel DE, Gong Q, et al. End-stage liver disease candidates at the highest model for end-stage liver disease scores have higher wait-list mortality than status-1A candidates. Hepatology 2012;55(1):192–8.
28. Sundaram V, Shah P, Mahmud N, et al. Patients with severe acute-on-chronic liver failure are disadvantaged by model for end-stage liver disease-based organ allocation policy. Aliment Pharmacol Ther 2020;52(7):1204–13.
29. Laique SN, Zhang N, Hewitt WR, et al. Increased access to liver transplantation for patients with acute on chronic liver failure after implementation of Share 35 Rule: an analysis from the UNOS database. Ann Hepatol 2021;23:100288.

30. Mahmud N, Reddy KR. Con: patients with acute-on-chronic liver failure should not receive priority on the waiting list. Clinical Liver Disease 2022;19(5):207–12.

31. Lee BP, Cullaro G, Vosooghi A, et al. Discordance in categorization of acute-on-chronic liver failure in the United Network for Organ Sharing database. J Hepatol 2022;76(5):1122–6.

32. Kumar R, Krishnamoorthy TL, Tan HK, et al. Change in model for end-stage liver disease score at two weeks, as an indicator of mortality or liver transplantation at 60 days in acute-on-chronic liver failure. Gastroenterol Rep (Oxf). 2015;3(2):122–7.

33. Lin BY, Zhou L, Geng L, et al. High neutrophil-lymphocyte ratio indicates poor prognosis for acute-on-chronic liver failure after liver transplantation. World J Gastroenterol 2015;21(11):3317–24.

34. Choudhary NS, Saraf N, Saigal S, et al. Factors associated with survival of patients with severe acute-on-chronic liver failure before and after liver transplantation: Unanswered Questions. Gastroenterology 2019;157(4):1162–3.

35. Reddy KR, O'Leary JG, Kamath PS, et al. High risk of delisting or death in liver transplant candidates following infections: results from the North American Consortium for the Study of End-Stage Liver Disease. Liver Transpl 2015;21(7):881–8.

36. Thuluvath PJ, Thuluvath AJ, Hanish S, et al. Liver transplantation in patients with multiple organ failures: feasibility and outcomes. J Hepatol 2018;69(5):1047–56.

37. Abdallah MA, Kuo YF, Asrani S, et al. Validating a novel score based on interaction between ACLF grade and MELD score to predict waitlist mortality. J Hepatol 2021;74(6):1355–61.

38. Belli LS, Duvoux C, Artzner T, et al. Liver transplantation for patients with acute-on-chronic liver failure (ACLF) in Europe: results of the ELITA/EF-CLIF collaborative study (ECLIS). J Hepatol 2021;75(3):610–22.

39. Goudsmit BFJ, Braat AE, Tushuizen ME, et al. Development and validation of a dynamic survival prediction model for patients with acute-on-chronic liver failure. JHEP Rep 2021;3(6):100369.

40. Zheng YX, Zhong X, Li YJ, et al. Performance of scoring systems to predict mortality of patients with acute-on-chronic liver failure: a systematic review and meta-analysis. J Gastroenterol Hepatol 2017;32(10):1668–78.

41. Vipani A, Lindenmeyer CC, Sundaram V. Treatment of severe acute on chronic liver failure: management of organ failures, Investigational Therapeutics, and the role of liver transplantation. J Clin Gastroenterol 2021;55(8):667–76.

42. Zhou Z, Yi J, Li Q, et al. Factors Prognostic of survival in liver transplant recipients with hepatitis B Virus related acute-on-chronic liver failure. Can J Gastroenterol Hepatol 2022;2022:6390809.

43. Xia L, Qiao ZY, Zhang ZJ, et al. Transplantation for EASL-CLIF and APASL acute-on-chronic liver failure (ACLF) patients: the TEA cohort to evaluate long-term post-Transplant outcomes. EClinicalMedicine 2022;49:101476.

44. Petrowsky H, Rana A, Kaldas FM, et al. Liver transplantation in highest acuity recipients: identifying factors to avoid futility. Ann Surg 2014;259(6):1186–94.

45. Linecker M, Krones T, Berg T, et al. Potentially inappropriate liver transplantation in the era of the "sickest first" policy - a search for the upper limits. J Hepatol 2018;68(4):798–813.

46. Artzner T, Michard B, Weiss E, et al. Liver transplantation for critically ill cirrhotic patients: Stratifying utility based on pretransplant factors. Am J Transplant 2020;20(9):2437–48.

47. Michard B, Artzner T, Deridder M, et al. Pretransplant intensive care Unit management and selection of Grade 3 acute-on-chronic liver failure transplant candidates. Liver Transpl 2022;28(1):17–26.
48. Huebener P, Sterneck MR, Bangert K, et al. Stabilisation of acute-on-chronic liver failure patients before liver transplantation predicts post-transplant survival. Aliment Pharmacol Ther 2018;47(11):1502–10.
49. Singal AK, Kuo YF, Waleed M, et al. High-risk liver transplant recipients with grade 3 acute on chronic liver failure should receive the good quality graft. Liver Int 2022;42(7):1629–37.
50. Levesque E, Winter A, Noorah Z, et al. Impact of acute-on-chronic liver failure on 90-day mortality following a first liver transplantation. Liver Int 2017;37(5):684–93.
51. Wackenthaler A, Molière S, Artzner T, et al. Pre-operative CT scan helps predict outcome after liver transplantation for acute-on-chronic grade 3 liver failure. Eur Radiol 2022;32(1):12–21.
52. Kulkarni AV, Premkumar M, Arab JP, et al. Early diagnosis and prevention of infections in cirrhosis. Semin Liver Dis 2022;42(3):293–312.
53. Mahmud N, Chapin S, Goldberg DS, et al. Statin exposure is associated with reduced development of acute-on-chronic liver failure in a Veterans Affairs cohort. J Hepatol 2022;76(5):1100–8.
54. Kulkarni AV, Premkumar M, Kumar K, et al. Nonselective beta-blockers reduce mortality in patients with acute-on-chronic liver failure. Portal Hypertension & Cirrhosis 2022;1(1):15–22.
55. Choudhury A, Vijayaraghavan R, Maiwall R, et al. First week' is the crucial period for deciding living donor liver transplantation in patients with acute-on-chronic liver failure. Hepatol Int 2021;15(6):1376–88.
56. Kim JE, Sinn DH, Choi GS, et al. Predictors and outcome of emergent Liver transplantation for patients with acute-on-chronic liver failure. Dig Liver Dis 2021;53(8):1004–10.
57. Sundaram V, Kogachi S, Wong RJ, et al. Effect of the clinical course of acute-on-chronic liver failure prior to liver transplantation on post-transplant survival. J Hepatol 2020;72(3):481–8.
58. Larsen FS. Artificial liver support in acute and acute-on-chronic liver failure. Curr Opin Crit Care 2019;25(2):187–91.
59. Kulkarni AV, Tirumalle S, Premkumar M, et al. Primary Norfloxacin Prophylaxis for APASL-defined acute-on-chronic liver failure: a Placebo-controlled Double-Blind randomized trial. Am J Gastroenterol 2022;117(4):607–16.
60. Kulkarni AV, Ravikumar ST, Tevethia H, et al. Safety and efficacy of terlipressin in acute-on-chronic liver failure with hepatorenal syndrome-acute kidney injury (HRS-AKI): a prospective cohort study. Sci Rep 2022;12(1):5503.
61. Wong F, Pappas SC, Reddy KR, et al. Terlipressin use and respiratory failure in patients with hepatorenal syndrome type 1 and severe acute-on-chronic liver failure. Aliment Pharmacol Ther 2022;56(8):1284–93.
62. Abbas N, Rajoriya N, Elsharkawy AM, et al. Acute-on-chronic liver failure (ACLF) in 2022: have novel treatment paradigms already arrived? Expert Rev Gastroenterol Hepatol 2022;16(7):639–52.
63. Meersseman P, Langouche L, du Plessis J, et al. The intensive care unit course and outcome in acute-on-chronic liver failure are comparable to other populations. J Hepatol 2018;69(4):803–9.
64. Ngu NL, Saxby E, Worland T, et al. A home-based, multidisciplinary liver optimisation programme for the first 28 days after an admission for acute-on-chronic

liver failure (LivR well): a study protocol for a randomised controlled trial. Trials 2022;23(1):744.

65. Fernández J, Saliba F. Liver transplantation in patients with ACLF and multiple organ failure: time for priority after initial stabilization. J Hepatol 2018;69(5): 1004–6.

66. Michard B, Artzner T, Lebas B, et al. Liver transplantation in critically ill patients: Preoperative predictive factors of post-transplant mortality to avoid futility. Clin Transplant 2017;31(12). https://doi.org/10.1111/ctr.13115.

67. Laici C, Guizzardi C, Morelli MC, et al. Predictive factors of inhospital mortality for ICU patients with acute-on-chronic liver failure undergoing liver transplantation. Eur J Gastroenterol Hepatol 2022;34(9):967–74.

68. Sundaram V, Patel S, Shetty K, et al. Risk factors for posttransplantation mortality in recipients with Grade 3 acute-on-chronic liver failure: analysis of a North American consortium. Liver Transpl 2022;28(6):1078–89.

69. Artzner T, Bernal W, Belli LS, et al. Location and allocation: Inequity of access to liver transplantation for patients with severe acute-on-chronic liver failure in Europe. Liver Transpl 2022;28(9):1429–40.

70. Asrani SK, Saracino G, O'Leary JG, et al. Recipient characteristics and morbidity and mortality after liver transplantation. J Hepatol 2018;69(1): 43–50.

71. Toshima T, Harada N, Itoh S, et al. Outcomes of living-donor liver transplantation for acute-on-chronic liver failure based on newly proposed criteria in Japan. Clin Transplant 2022;36(8):e14739.

72. Yadav SK, Saraf N, Choudhary NS, et al. Living donor liver transplantation for acute-on-chronic liver failure. Liver Transpl 2019;25(3):459–68.

73. Moon DB, Lee SG, Kang WH, et al. Adult living donor liver transplantation for acute-on-chronic liver failure in high-model for end-stage liver disease score patients. Am J Transplant 2017;17(7):1833–42.

74. Wang YC, Yong CC, Lin CC, et al. Excellent outcome in living donor liver transplantation: Treating patients with acute-on-chronic liver failure. Liver Transpl 2021;27(11):1633–43.

75. Agbim U, Sharma A, Maliakkal B, et al. Outcomes of liver transplant recipients with acute-on-chronic liver failure based on EASL-CLIF consortium definition: a single-center study. Transplant Direct 2020;6(4):e544.

76. Duan BW, Lu SC, Wang ML, et al. Liver transplantation in acute-on-chronic liver failure patients with high model for end-stage liver disease (MELD) scores: a single center experience of 100 consecutive cases. J Surg Res 2013;183(2): 936–43.

77. Wong TC, Fung JY, Pang HH, et al. Analysis of survival benefits of living versus deceased donor liver transplant in high model for end-stage liver disease and hepatorenal syndrome. Hepatology 2021;73(6):2441–54.

78. Goldberg DS, Levine M, Karp S, et al. Share 35 changes in center-level liver acceptance practices. Liver Transpl 2017;23(5):604–13.

79. Washburn K, Harper A, Baker T, et al. Changes in liver acceptance patterns after implementation of Share 35. Liver Transpl 2016;22(2):171–7.

80. Kulkarni AV, Kumar P, Sharma M, et al. Letter to the editor: living donor liver transplantation or deceased donor liver transplantation in high model for end-stage liver disease score-which is better? Hepatology 2021;73(6): 2619–20.

81. Bhatti ABH, Dar FS, Butt MO, et al. Living donor liver transplantation for acute on chronic liver failure based on EASL-CLIF Diagnostic criteria. J Clin Exp Hepatol 2018;8(2):136–43.
82. Nagral S, Nanavati A, Nagral A. Liver transplantation in India: at the Crossroads. J Clin Exp Hepatol 2015;5(4):329–40.
83. Kulkarni AV, Premkumar M, Reddy DN, et al. The challenges of ascites management: an Indian perspective. Clin Liver Dis 2022;19(6):234–8.
84. Umgelter A, Lange K, Kornberg A, et al. Orthotopic liver transplantation in critically ill cirrhotic patients with multi-organ failure: a single-center experience. Transplant Proc 2011;43(10):3762–8.
85. Thuluvath PJ, Thuluvath AJ, Savva Y, et al. Karnofsky performance status following liver transplantation in patients with multiple organ failures and probable acute-on-chronic liver failure. Clin Gastroenterol Hepatol 2020;18(1):234–41.
86. Bahirwani R, Shaked O, Bewtra M, et al. Acute-on-chronic liver failure before liver transplantation: impact on posttransplant outcomes. Transplantation 2011;92(8):952–7.
87. Finkenstedt A, Nachbaur K, Zoller H, et al. Acute-on-chronic liver failure: excellent outcomes after liver transplantation but high mortality on the wait list. Liver Transpl 2013;19(8):879–86.
88. Goosmann L, Buchholz A, Bangert K, et al. Liver transplantation for acute-on-chronic liver failure predicts post-transplant mortality and impaired long-term quality of life. Liver Int 2021;41(3):574–84.
89. Chen GH, Wu RL, Huang F, et al. Liver transplantation in acute-on-chronic liver failure: excellent outcome and Difficult posttransplant course. Front Surg 2022;9:914611.
90. Sundaram V, Mahmud N, Perricone G, et al. Longterm outcomes of patients undergoing liver transplantation for acute-on-chronic liver failure. Liver Transpl 2020;26(12):1594–602.
91. Sundaram V, Lindenmeyer CC, Shetty K, et al. Patients with acute-on-chronic liver failure have Greater healthcare resource utilization after liver transplantation. Clin Gastroenterol Hepatol 2023;21(3):704–12.e3.
92. O'Leary JG, Bajaj JS, Tandon P, et al. Outcomes after listing for liver transplant in patients with acute-on-chronic liver failure: the multicenter North American consortium for the study of end-stage liver disease experience. Liver Transpl 2019;25(4):571–9.
93. Marciano S, Mauro E, Giunta D, et al. Impact of acute-on-chronic liver failure on post-transplant survival and on kidney outcomes. Eur J Gastroenterol Hepatol 2019;31(9):1157–64.
94. Karvellas CJ, Francoz C, Weiss E. Liver transplantation in acute-on-chronic liver failure. Transplantation 2021;105(7):1471–81.
95. Faitot F, Artzner T, Michard B, et al. Immunosuppression in patients with grade 3 acute-on-chronic liver failure at transplantation: a practice analysis study. Clin Transplant 2022;36(4):e14580.
96. Jalan R, Gustot T, Fernandez J, et al. Equity' and 'Justice' for patients with acute-on chronic liver failure: a call to action. J Hepatol 2021;75(5):1228–35.
97. Im GY, Vogel AS, Florman S, et al. Extensive health care utilization and costs of an early liver transplantation Program for alcoholic hepatitis. Liver Transpl 2022;28(1):27–38.
98. Goussous N, Xie W, Zhang T, et al. Acute on chronic liver failure: factors associated with transplantation. Transplant Direct 2021;7(12):e788.

99. Karvellas CJ, Taylor S, Bigam D, et al. Intraoperative continuous renal replacement therapy during liver transplantation: a pilot randomized-controlled trial (INCEPTION). Can J Anaesth 2019;66(10):1151–61. Traitement substitutif peropératoire continu de l'insuffisance rénale pendant une greffe hépatique: une étude randomisée contrôlée pilote (INCEPTION).

100. Goldberg DS, Bajaj JS. Acute-on-Chronic liver failure and liver transplantation: Putting the Cart before the Horse in data Analyses and Advocating for model for end-stage liver disease Exceptions. Liver Transpl 2022;28(4):535–8.

Maximizing the Donor Potential for Patients with Acute-on-Chronic Liver Failure Listed for Liver Transplant

Arpit Amin, MD, Guergana G. Panayotova, MD,
James V. Guarrera, MD*

KEYWORDS

- Static cold storage • Hypothermic machine perfusion
- Normothermic machine perfusion • Liver transplantation

KEY POINTS

- Liver grafts from donors after circulatory death and extended criteria donors after brain death are associated with an increased risk of early allograft dysfunction and ischemic cholangiopathy due to severe ischemia reperfusion injury when preserved with static cold storage.
- Marginal liver grafts preserved with hypothermic machine perfusion and normothermic machine perfusion have been found to have lower rates of early allograft dysfunction and ischemic cholangiopathy after liver transplantation.
- A broader application of hypothermic machine perfusion and normothermic machine perfusion in marginal liver graft preservation has the potential to increase overall number of liver grafts available for transplantation.

INTRODUCTION

In 2020, there were 24,936 adult candidates on the liver transplant (LT) waitlist in the United States[1]; 7979 adult deceased donor LTs (DDLTs) and 425 adult living donor LTs (LDLTs) were performed in the United States in 2020.[1] Allocation of deceased donor liver grafts in the United States is based on the model for end-stage liver disease-sodium (MELD-Na) score. However, the MELD-Na score tends to underestimate the mortality of patients with acute-on-chronic liver failure (ACLF).[2] It has been shown that only 9% of patients with ACLF exceeded median MELD-Na of 35 and only 35% of patients with ACLF exceeded respective transplant center-specific

Division of Transplant and HPB Surgery, Department of Surgery, Rutgers New Jersey Medical School, Newark, NJ, USA
* Corresponding author. 140 Bergen Street, Ambulatory Care Center, Suite E1766, Newark, NJ 07103.
E-mail address: jg1395@rutgers.edu

Clin Liver Dis 27 (2023) 763–775
https://doi.org/10.1016/j.cld.2023.03.016
1089-3261/23/© 2023 Elsevier Inc. All rights reserved.

median MELD-Na score at transplant.[2] Patients with ACLF have a 90-day mortality of 40% compared with 20% in patients without ACLF.[2] Hence, LT needs to be performed in a timely manner to rescue patients with ACLF despite the current limitations of MELD-Na score-based framework of liver organ allocation policy.

Currently, static cold storage (SCS) is the standard of care for liver graft preservation. There continues to be an increase in the number of patients on the LT waitlist annually. Conversely, the availability of donor livers preserved using SCS suitable for LT remains limited. To address this supply-demand mismatch, there needs to be an increase in the utilization of marginal liver grafts from donors after circulatory death (DCD) and donors after brain death (DBD) such as older donors (age > 70 years) and donors with liver macro steatosis greater than 30%.[3–5] However, there is an increased risk of ischemic type biliary lesions (ITBLs), early allograft dysfunction (EAD), and primary non-function (PNF) with the use of marginal liver grafts preserved with SCS due to severity of ischemia-reperfusion injury (IRI). Emerging ex vivo machine perfusion technology for liver graft preservation has the potential to safely expand the use of marginal liver grafts by overcoming the shortcomings of SCS preservation. To achieve optimal outcomes with marginal liver grafts preserved with ex vivo machine perfusion technology, appropriate recipients with lower MELD-Na score need to be selected from the waitlist. As many patients with ACLF are underserved by the current MELD-Na score-based organ allocation system, ex vivo machine perfusion preserved marginal liver grafts can be used to rescue these patients before they miss their therapeutic window for LT.

Hypothermic machine perfusion (HMP) and normothermic machine perfusion (NMP) are two major ex vivo machine perfusion technologies that have emerged as an alternative to SCS for liver graft preservation over the last decade. This review highlights the mechanism of IRI in liver grafts preserved with SCS and elaborates on the mechanistic benefits of ex vivo machine perfusion technology in mitigating IRI. In addition, the authors summarize current literature on HMP and NMP in clinical LT to highlight the potential of ex vivo machine perfusion technology in maximizing utilization of marginal liver grafts to expand the overall deceased donor pool available for LT.

ISCHEMIA-REPERFUSION INJURY WITH STATIC COLD STORAGE IN LIVER TRANSPLANTATION

IRI is a biphasic phenomenon that occurs initially during SCS liver graft preservation under hypoxic conditions causing both hepatocyte and cholangiocyte injury, which is further aggravated due to generation of reactive oxygen species (ROS) on restoration of oxygenated blood delivery during reperfusion of liver graft in LT.[6–8] Under SCS, cellular metabolism is significantly reduced within the liver graft resulting in decreased consumption of adenosine triphosphate (ATP).[3–5] However, as the cold ischemia time increases, the absence of oxygen during SCS leads to dysfunction of mitochondrial respiratory complex II component of the electron transport chain (ETC) and upstream accumulation of succinate.[9–13] This disruption of ETC leads to gradual ATP depletion and a switch to anaerobic glycolysis with resultant cellular acidosis due to gradual lactate accumulation.[3–5] ATP depletion leads to stunning of the ATP-dependent sodium–potassium pump, influx of sodium into the cytosol, cellular swelling, and death. This, in turn, causes the release of damage-associated molecular patterns (DAMPs), which perpetuate further cellular damage.[9–13]

Reperfusion of the liver graft in a succinate-rich environment leads to the dysfunction of mitochondrial respiratory complex I component of ETC resulting in further production of ROS and release of flavin mononucleotide (FMN), a signal of mitochondrial damage.[9–13] The combination of accumulated DAMPs during ischemia and mitochondrial ROS production during reperfusion of the liver graft leads to activation of innate inflammatory response and recruitment of Kupffer cells, T cells, and neutrophils resulting in IRI.[6–8] Severe IRI to hepatocytes during LT leads to EAD and PNF causing liver graft loss. Severe IRI to cholangiocytes during LT leads to formation of ITBL characterized by anastomotic and non-anastomotic biliary strictures. The phases of hypoxic injury and resulting IRI during SCS of liver grafts are shown in **Fig. 1**.[9–13]

Clinical experience has shown that marginal liver grafts preserved with SCS are prone to develop severe IRI resulting in an increased risk of ITBL, EAD, and PNF. Owing to current limitations of SCS in preservation for marginal liver grafts, there has been an increased interest within the transplant community to consider application of ex vivo machine perfusion technology with a goal to expand the overall available donor liver pool suitable for LT.

HYPOTHERMIC MACHINE PERFUSION IN LIVER TRANSPLANTATION

During HMP, liver grafts are preserved between 4°C and 10°C to maintain cellular hypometabolic state to decrease ATP consumption.[6–8] Liver grafts are continuously perfused with cooled preservation solution, which allows removal of toxic metabolic waste while maintaining delivery of critical substrates for ATP production.[14] The addition of oxygen to the HMP circuit avoids disruption of mitochondrial ETC and prevents buildup of succinate within the liver graft.[9,10] Owing to continued maintenance of low-flux ETC activity during HMP, there is continuous slow ATP upload, which, in turn, preserves sodium–potassium pump activity and osmotic cellular integrity, resulting in decreased injury and diminished release of DAMPs.[9,10] At subsequent reperfusion, mitochondrial respiratory complex I of the ETC is exposed to diminished levels of succinate and lactate leading to decreased production of ROS and dampened innate inflammatory responses.[9,10] In short, IRI severity is significantly reduced in liver grafts preserved with HMP due to these underlying mechanistic benefits. Also, in case of HMP pump failure, some systems revert to SCS, allowing continued liver graft preservation.

In 2010, Guarrera and colleagues reported the first clinical series of successful LT using end ischemic non-oxygenated HMP via cannulation of the portal vein and the hepatic artery.[15] This was a nonrandomized trial comprising 20 adult DBD liver grafts that underwent HMP.[15] Results of the study group were compared with a historical cohort of 20 patients transplanted using SCS-preserved liver grafts. The recipients

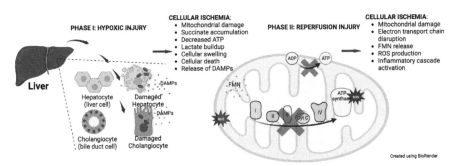

Fig. 1. Ischemia-reperfusion injury during static cold storage of liver grafts. ATP, adenosine triphosphate; DAMP, damage-associated molecular patterns; FMN, flavin mononucleotide; ROS, reactive oxygen species.

of HMP-preserved liver grafts showed lower peak aspartate aminotransferase (AST), lower peak alanine aminotransferase (ALT), and decreased biliary complications compared with SCS-preserved liver grafts.[15] This study was pivotal in establishing the safety and feasibility of HMP in clinical LT. Expanding on this experience, in 2015, Guarrera and colleagues reported results from end-ischemic HMP in 31 adult "orphan" extended criteria DBD liver grafts.[16] Liver grafts were defined as "orphan" in this study when all transplant centers within the United Network for Organ Sharing region declined these grafts. A control group of 30 adult SCS preserved DBD liver grafts matched for donor age, donor risk index, cold ischemia time, and recipient age was included in this study.[16] The HMP cohort had a significantly lower rate of biliary complications and similar 1-year patient survival compared with the matched SCS group.[16] This study further demonstrated that HMP can successfully salvage "orphan" extended criteria DBD liver grafts and expand the overall available donor liver pool for LT.

Concurrent to the pioneering work done by Guarrera's group on HMP for extended criteria DBD liver grafts in North America, there has been growing research on HMP for DCD liver grafts in Europe over the past decade. Biliary complications are the "Achilles heel" of DCD LT due to the increased susceptibility of cholangiocytes to hypoxic insult. This is further compounded by prolonged warm ischemia time during DCD liver procurement, which is frequently unavoidable due to underlying ethical concerns in many countries. Two modalities of HMP are currently used in clinical practice in Europe: hypothermic oxygenated perfusion (HOPE) of DCD liver grafts via single vessel (ie, portal vein only) perfusion and dual HOPE (dHOPE) of DCD liver grafts via dual vessel (ie, portal vein and hepatic artery) perfusion.

In 2014, Dutkowski and colleagues evaluated end-ischemic HOPE for a period of 1 to 2 hours in eight DCD liver grafts with median warm ischemia time of 38 minutes and compared with eight SCS-preserved DBD liver grafts.[17] Remarkably, the rate of EAD and biliary complications was similar in HOPE DCD study group compared with SCS DBD control group.[17] This pilot study paved the way for a subsequent larger multi-center trial in 2015 comparing 25 DCD livers preserved with HOPE to 50 case-matched DCD livers preserved with SCS.[18] The recipients of HOPE DCD liver grafts were found to have lower rates of EAD and biliary complications compared with the recipients of SCS DCD liver grafts.[18] In addition, actuarial 1-year graft survival of HOPE DCD liver grafts was noted to be significantly better than SCS DCD liver grafts.[18] Long-term outcomes after DCD LT are inferior to DBD LT due to the increased risk of ischemic cholangiopathy (IC) with DCD LT. Schlegel and colleagues focused on studying long-term outcomes of HOPE DCD LT in comparison to SCS DCD LT and SCS DBD LT.[19] Interestingly, Schlegel and colleagues found that 5-year graft survival of HOPE DCD liver grafts was equivalent to SCS DBD liver grafts and significantly superior to SCS DCD liver grafts.[19] As many patients with hepatocellular carcinoma (HCC) listed for LT are offered marginal liver grafts, there has been interest in evaluating the impact of HOPE in this subset of potential LT candidates. Mueller and colleagues found that 5-year tumor-free survival rate was higher in patients with HCC, who received HOPE-preserved DCD liver grafts compared with SCS-preserved DCD liver grafts.[20] Although HCC recurrence after LT is multifactorial, the investigators suggest that attenuated IRI after HOPE may be one potential protective mechanism that leads to decreased HCC recurrence in HOPE-treated liver grafts.[20] The findings of this study may lead to the increased use of HOPE-preserved liver grafts in LT recipients with HCC.

In 2017, Van Rijn and colleagues evaluated end-ischemic dHOPE for duration of 2 hours in 10 DCD liver grafts and compared with 20 SCS DCD liver grafts.[21] They found that DCD liver grafts preserved with dHOPE had an 11-fold increase in ATP content.[21] In addition, dHOPE DCD liver grafts were noted to have significantly lower peak ALT and bilirubin levels compared with SCS DCD liver grafts suggesting dampened cellular injury with dHOPE.[21] In 2019, Patrono and colleagues compared 25 dHOPE-preserved extended criteria DBD liver grafts to 50 SCS-preserved extended criteria DBD liver grafts.[22] They found that the incidence of postoperative acute kidney injury was significantly lower in the dHOPE DBD group compared with the SCS DBD group.[22] Most recently, Van Rijn and colleagues have published the first multicenter, randomized prospective trial in 2021 comparing 78 end-ischemic dHOPE-DCD liver grafts to 78 SCS-DCD liver grafts.[23] They reported that the incidence of non-anastomotic biliary strictures at 6 months post-LT was significantly lower in the dHOPE DCD cohort compared with the SCS DCD group.[23] Importantly, none of the LT recipients of dHOPE DCD liver grafts required re-transplantation, whereas two LT recipients of SCS DCD liver grafts required re-transplantation within 6 months of LT.[23] Results of this multicenter randomized prospective trial has further confirmed the beneficial effects of HMP in reducing IC rates after DCD LT. The results of all published clinical studies evaluating HMP in LT are summarized in **Table 1**. In addition, a North American multicenter RCT (NCT03484455) examining outcomes of portable HMP circuit with oxygen pre-charge for DCD and extended criteria DBD liver grafts has finished accrual, and the results are awaited. A portable circuit that can be transported via ground or air travel over large distances will allow transplant teams to apply HMP directly at the donor hospital.

Last, there is active interest in identifying viability parameters in HMP-preserved liver grafts that can help predict postoperative liver graft function. Guarrera and colleagues have shown that 2-h HMP pump effluent AST and lactate dehydrogenase (LDH) levels are strongly correlated with postoperative peak AST and LDH.[15] Patrono and colleagues have demonstrated that a liver perfusate ALT level greater than 537 IU/L after 90 minutes of HMP is predictive of postoperative EAD.[24] Muller and colleagues have identified perfusate FMN as a marker for mitochondrial injury that can be measured during HMP.[25] FMN trends during HMP of liver grafts have shown strong corelation to postoperative lactate clearance and coagulation profile.[25] A threshold perfusate FMN level greater than 10,000 AU during HMP has been strongly associated with early graft loss after LT in limited center data.[25] Multicenter validation of FMN as a biomarker of injury predictive of graft loss in HMP-treated LT is currently underway.

NORMOTHERMIC MACHINE PERFUSION IN LIVER TRANSPLANTATION

During NMP, liver grafts are preserved at near physiologic temperatures between 35°C and 38°C.[3–5] NMP involves continuous perfusion via dual cannulation (ie, hepatic artery and portal vein) of liver grafts with nutrients and oxygenated human packed red blood cells to maintain cellular metabolism.[3–5] Organ viability assessment using metabolic parameters such as lactate clearance, pH, and glucose production and bile production can be monitored during NMP.[3–5] In addition, the NMP provides a potential platform for the introduction of therapeutic agents for organ treatment.[3–5]

In 2015, initial case reports on successful application of NMP in clinical LT were reported by transplant teams at the University of Cambridge and the University of Birmingham. Watson and colleagues reported using NMP to resuscitate DCD liver graft with a warm ischemia time of 150 minutes.[26] After 5 hours of SCS, DCD liver graft underwent NMP for 132 minutes.[26] Decision was made to proceed with LT due to favorable organ viability indicators such as lactate clearance, glucose production, and bile production. The investigators reported that the recipient had a functioning

Table 1
Clinical studies of hypothermic machine perfusion in liver transplantation

Author, Year	Study Group (n)	Control Group (n)	Results
Guarrera et al,[15] 2010	Back-to-base HMP DBD (20)	SCS DBD (20)	EAD rate: 5% (HMP) vs 25% (SCS); Biliary complication rate: 10% (HMP) vs 20% (SCS); 1-y patient survival: 90% (HMP) vs 90% (SCS)
Dutkowski et al,[17] 2014	Back-to-base HOPE DCD (8)	SCS DBD (8)	EAD rate: 0% (HOPE) vs 0% (SCS); Biliary complication rate: 25% (HOPE) vs 25% (SCS); 1-y graft survival: 100% (HOPE) vs 100% (SCS)
Dutkowski et al,[18] 2015	Back-to-base HOPE DCD (25)	SCS DCD (50)	EAD rate: 20% (HOPE) vs 44% (SCS); Biliary complication rate: 20% (HOPE) vs 46% (SCS); 1-y graft survival: 90% (HOPE) vs 69% (SCS)
Guarrera et al,[16] 2015	Back-to-base HMP ECD-DBD (31)	SCS Extended criteria DBD (31)	EAD rate: 19% (HMP) vs 30% (SCS); Biliary complication rate: 19% (HMP) vs 43% (SCS); 1-y patient survival: 84% (HMP) vs 80% (SCS)
Van Rijn et al,[21] 2017	Back-to-base dHOPE DCD (10)	SCS DCD (20)	Peak ALT: 966 units/L (dHOPE) vs 1858 units/L (SCS); Biliary complication rate: 10% (dHOPE) vs 45% (SCS); 1-y graft survival: 100% (dHOPE) vs 85% (SCS)
Schlegel et al,[19] 2018	Back-to-base HOPE DCD (50)	SCS DCD (50)	Biliary complication rate: 40% (HOPE) vs 46% (SCS)

Patrono et al,[22] 2019	Back-to-base dHOPE DBD (25)	SCS DBD (269)	5-y graft survival: 94%(HOPE) vs 78% (SCS); EAD rate: 32% (dHOPE) vs 34% (SCS); Biliary complication rate: 24% (dHOPE) vs 18% (SCS); 1-y graft survival: 100% (dHOPE) vs 90% (SCS)
Mueller et al,[20] 2020	Back-to-base HOPE DCD in LT recipients with HCC (70)	SCS DCD in LT recipients with HCC (70)	5-year HCC recurrence rate: 8% (HOPE) vs 18% (SCS)
Van Rijn et al,[23] 2021	Back-to-base dHOPE DCD (78)	SCS DCD (78)	EAD rate: 26% (dHOPE) vs 40% (SCS); Biliary complication rate: 6% (dHOPE) vs 18% (SCS); 6-mo patient survival: 92% (dHOPE) vs 95% (SCS)

Abbreviations: ALT, alanine aminotransferase; DBD, donor after brain death; DCD, donor after circulatory death; dHOPE, dual hypothermic oxygenated machine perfusion; EAD, early allograft dysfunction; HCC, hepatocellular carcinoma; HMP, hypothermic machine perfusion; HOPE, hypothermic oxygenated machine perfusion; SCS, static cold storage.

liver graft without any biliary complications at 6 months post-LT.[26] Perera and colleagues reported using NMP in resuscitating a DCD liver graft with a warm ischemia time of 109 minutes.[27] After 7 hours of SCS, DCD liver graft underwent NMP for 416 minutes. At 2 hours after NMP, organ was noted to show favorable viability parameters such as normal lactate level and bile production. Decision was made to proceed with LT and recipient was noted to have a functioning liver graft at 15 months follow-up post-LT.[27]

In 2016, Ravikumar and colleagues published the first clinical series of successful LT in Europe using NMP.[28] This was a nonrandomized trial with a study group of 16 DBD liver grafts and 4 DCD liver grafts that underwent NMP at the donor hospital immediately after procurement.[28] Historical control group consisting of 32 DBD SCS liver grafts and 8 DCD SCS liver grafts was used.[28] The recipients of NMP-preserved liver grafts were found to have lower AST compared with the recipients of SCS-preserved liver grafts, suggesting decreased hepatocyte injury.[28] The investigators reported that the EAD rate and 6-month liver graft survival were similar between NMP and SCS groups.[28] Concurrently, Selzner and colleagues published the first North American clinical series of successful LT using NMP in 2016.[29] A study group consisted of 10 continuous NMP liver grafts, which demonstrated lactate clearance and bile production during NMP before liver graft implantation.[29] A historical control group of 30 SCS liver grafts was used in this study.[29] The investigators reported that there was no difference in 3-month graft and patient survival in both groups.[29] It must be noted that only donor offers within 2 hours of driving distance were eligible for consideration in this study.[29] These initial studies established the safety and feasibility of NMP utilization in clinical LT while highlighting logistical difficulties with transportation of NMP circuit over larger distances.

In 2018, Nasralla and colleagues published a pivotal randomized control trial comparing continuous NMP-preserved liver grafts ($n = 121$) to SCS-preserved liver grafts ($n = 101$).[30] The study showed peak AST level after LT was significantly lower in the NMP group compared with SCS group, suggesting that there is lower IRI with NMP use.[30] The investigators, also, reported significantly lower EAD rate in the NMP group compared with the SCS group.[30] There was no difference in biliary complication rates or in graft survival at 1-year post-LT between NMP and SCS groups.[30] The investigators reported that the organ discard rate was significantly lower within NMP group compared with SCS group and attributed it to the ability to perform viability assessment of marginal liver grafts with NMP.[30] Subsequently, a North American multicenter randomized control trial (NCT02775162) has been initiated to further evaluate outcomes of continuous NMP-preserved liver grafts to SCS-preserved liver grafts.

Owing to logistical difficulties with the transport of NMP circuit, there has been interest in evaluating "back-to-base" NMP at the recipient center after initial transport using SCS. In 2019, Ghinolfi and colleagues published a randomized trial comparing 10 "back-to-base" NMP resuscitated liver grafts to 10 SCS liver grafts procured from extended criteria DBD donors (age $\geq$ 70 years).[31] There were no differences in EAD rate, graft survival, or patient survival between the two groups.[31] Subsequently, in 2021, Bral and colleagues published results of a nonrandomized trial comparing outcomes of continuous NMP resuscitated liver grafts ($n = 17$) to "back-to-base" NMP resuscitated liver grafts ($n = 26$).[32] The investigators reported no difference in EAD rate, biliary complication rate, graft survival, or patient survival at 6 months between the two groups.[32] The results of this study suggest that "back-to-base" NMP resuscitation of liver grafts may offer a practical alternative to continuous NMP and help overcome the logistical drawback associated with continuous NMP. The results of all clinical studies evaluating NMP in clinical LT are summarized in **Table 2**.

Table 2
Clinical studies of normothermic machine perfusion in liver transplantation

Author, Year	Study Group (n)	Control Group (n)	Results
Ravikumar et al,[28] 2016	Continuous NMP DBD (16) and DCD (4)	SCS DBD (32) and SCS DCD (8)	EAD rate: 15% (NMP) vs 22% (SCS) 6-mo graft survival: 100% (HMP) vs 98% (SCS)
Selzner et al,[29] 2016	Continuous NMP DBD (8) and DCD (2)	SCS DBD (24) and SCS DBD (6)	Peak ALT: 619 units/L (NMP) vs 949 units/L (SCS) Biliary complication rate: 0% (NMP) vs 3% (SCS) 3-mo graft survival: 100% (NMP) vs 100% (SCS)
Nasralla et al,[30] 2018	Continuous NMP DBD (87) and DCD (34)	SCS DBD (80) and DCD (21)	EAD rate: 10% (NMP) vs 30% (SCS) Biliary complication rate: 8% (NMP) vs 11% (SCS) 1-y graft survival: 95% (NMP) vs 96% (SCS)
Ghinolfi et al,[31] 2019	Back-to-base NMP extended criteria DBD (10)	SCS extended criteria DBD (10)	EAD rate: 20% (NMP) vs 10% (SCS) Biliary complication rate: 10% (HMP) vs 0% (SCS) 1-y graft survival: 90% (NMP) vs 100% (SCS)
Bral et al,[32] 2021	Back-to-base NMP DBD (20) and DCD (6)	Continuous NMP DBD (13) and DCD (4)	EAD rate: 5% (back-to-base NMP) vs 6% (continuous NMP) Biliary complication rate: 15% (back-to-base NMP) vs 24% (continuous NMP) 6-mo graft survival: 100% (back-to-base NMP) vs 88% (continuous NMP)
Watson et al,[33] 2018	Back-to-base NMP for initially declined liver grafts (47)	Not applicable	22 out of 47 livers were able to be transplanted using following viability criteria: Bile pH > 7.5, bile glucose < 3 mmol/L,

(continued on next page)

Table 2
(continued)

Author, Year	Study Group (n)	Control Group (n)	Results
			perfusate pH > 7.2, peak lactate fall > 4.4 mmol/L/kg/h, ALT < 6000 units/L at 2 h
			EAD rate: 10%
			Biliary complication rate: 18%
			1-y graft survival: 82%
Mergental et al,[34] 2021	Back-to-base NMP for initially declined liver grafts (31)	Not applicable	22 out of 31 livers were able to be transplanted using viability criterion of lactate level <2.5 mmol/L within 4 h of NMP
			EAD rate: 7%
			Biliary complication rate: 27%
			1-y graft survival: 86%

Abbreviations: ALT, alanine aminotransferase; DBD, donor after brain death; DCD, donor after circulatory death; EAD, early allograft dysfunction; NMP, normothermic machine perfusion; SCS, static cold storage.

Last, the simultaneous progress has been made in identifying objective viability testing criteria for livers resuscitated with NMP. Watson and colleagues reported that hepatocyte viability criteria and cholangiocyte viability criteria based on a retrospective analysis of 47 NMP liver grafts out of which 22 liver grafts were eventually transplanted.[33] The investigators proposed that perfusate pH greater than 7.2, perfusate ALT less than 6000 IU/L at 2 hours, fall in lactate $\geq$ 4.4 mmol/L/kg/h, bile pH $\geq$ 7.5, and bile glucose $\leq$ 3 mmol/L are the predictive factors associated with favorable outcomes following LT.[33] Mergental and colleagues used lactate levels $\leq$ 2.5 mmol/L within 4 hours of NMP as a viability criterion.[34] Using this criterion, the investigators were able to successfully transplant 22 out of 31 liver grafts, which were initially deemed to be not suitable for LT.[34] One-year LT graft survival was reported to be 86%.[34] Re-transplant was eventually required in four patients due to biliary complications.[34] More research is required to continue to refine our understanding of viability testing criteria for liver grafts resuscitated with NMP.

CHALLENGES IN THE ERA OF EX VIVO LIVER MACHINE PERFUSION

There are regulatory, logistical, and financial challenges that need to be addressed for successful implementation of ex vivo liver machine perfusion in routine clinical practice.[35] Prospective multicenter randomized controlled trials evaluating HMP and NMP are currently in progress in United States. Regulatory approval from Food and Drug Administration agency for implementation of ex vivo liver machine perfusion is required before broader clinical application outside trials. In the interim, transplant centers and organ procurement organizations (OPO) will need to develop partnerships to allow broader implementation of HMP and NMP for marginal liver grafts once regulatory barriers are surmounted. This will require additional personnel training both at the individual transplant center level and at the OPO level. Cost associated with implementation of HMP and NMP technology for LT at individual transplant centers can be significant. Financial reimbursement models will need to be clarified between all stakeholders so that individual transplant centers can offer the benefit of ex vivo liver machine perfusion technology to patients on the LT waitlist.

Transplant teams may consider application of HMP or NMP for livers grafts from DCD and from extended criteria DBD such as older donors (age >70 years) and livers with greater than 30% macro steatosis. Once resuscitated with HMP or NMP, these marginal liver grafts can then be safely used to transplant underserved recipients, such as patients with ACLF or HCC. At the same time, recipients with high MELD-Na score and recipients with fulminant liver failure can continued to be transplanted using good quality SCS DBD liver grafts.

SUMMARY

The availability of ex vivo liver machine perfusion technology has expanded the armamentarium of transplant teams in increasing utilization of marginal liver grafts. Marginal liver grafts optimized by ex vivo liver machine perfusion technology can then be used to rescue patients with ACLF on the LT waitlist that are underserved by the current MELD-Na score allocation system.

DISCLOSURE

Dr J.V. Guarrera has received grants and consulting fees from Organ Recovery Systems (Itasca, IL, USA) and GATT technologies (Nijmegen, Netherlands) within the last 36 months. Dr A. Amin and Dr G. Panayotova have no conflicts of interest to report.

REFERENCES

1. Kwong AJ, Ebel NH, Kim WR, et al. OPTN/SRTR 2020 annual data report: liver. Am J Transplant 2022;22(Suppl 2):204–309.
2. Hernaez R, Liu Y, Kramer JR, et al. Model for end-stage liver disease-sodium underestimates 90-day mortality risk in patients with acute-on-chronic liver failure. J Hepatol 2020;73(6):1425–33.
3. Aufhauser DD Jr, Foley DP. Beyond Ice and the cooler: machine perfusion Strategies in liver transplantation. Clin Liver Dis 2021;25(1):179–94.
4. Bonaccorsi-Riani E, Bruggenwirth IMA, Buchwald JE, et al. Machine perfusion: cold versus warm versus neither. Update on clinical trials. Semin Liver Dis 2020;40(3):264–81.
5. Boteon YL, Afford SC. Machine perfusion of the liver: which is the best technique to mitigate ischaemia-reperfusion injury? World J Transplant 2019;9(1):14–20.
6. Peralta C, Jimenez-Castro MB, Gracia-Sancho J, et al. Hepatic ischemia and reperfusion: effects on the liver sinusoidal milieu. J Hepatol 2013;59(5):1094–106.
7. Zhai Y, Petrowsky H, Hong JC, et al. Ischaemia – reperfusion injury in liver transplantation – from bench to bedside. Nat Rev Gastroenterol Hepatol 2013;10(2):79–89.
8. Collard CD, Gelman S. Pathophysiology, clinical manifestations, and prevention of ischemia-reperfusion injury. Anesthesiology 2001;94(6):1133–8.
9. Schlegel A, Rougemont O, Graf R, et al. Protective mechanisms of end-ischemic cold machine perfusion in DCD liver grafts. J Hepatol 2013;58(2):278–86.
10. Schlegel A, Muller X, Dutkowski P, et al. Hypothermic liver perfusion. Curr Opin Organ Transplant 2017;22(6):563–70.
11. Karangwa S, Panayotova G, Dutkowski P, et al. Hypothermic machine perfusion in liver transplantation. Int J Surg 2020;82S:44–51.
12. Pell VR, Chouchani ET, Murphy MP, et al. Moving forwards by blocking backflow: the yin and yang of MI therapy. Circ Res 2016;118:898–906.
13. Amin A, Panayotova G, Guarrera JV. Hypothermic machine perfusion for liver graft preservation. Curr Opin Organ Transplant 2022;27(2):98–105.
14. Henry SD, Nachber E, Tulipan J, et al. Hypothermic machine preservation reduces molecular markers of ischemia/reperfusion injury in human liver transplantation. Am J Transplant 2012;12(9):2477–86.
15. Guarrera JV, Henry SD, Samstein B, et al. Hypothermic machine preservation in human liver transplantation: the first clinical series. Am J Transplant 2010;10(2):372–81.
16. Guarrera JV, Henry SD, Samstein B, et al. Hypothermic machine preservation facilitates successful transplantation of "orphan" extended criteria donor livers. Am J Transplant 2015;15(1):161–9.
17. Dutkowski P, Schlegel A, de Oliveira M, et al. HOPE for human liver grafts obtained from donors after cardiac death. J Hepatol 2014;60(4):765–72.
18. Dutkowski P, Polak WG, Muiesan P, et al. First comparison of hypothermic oxygenated perfusion versus static cold storage of human donation after cardiac death liver transplants. Ann Surg 2015;262(5):764–70.
19. Schlegel A, Muller X, Kalisvaart M, et al. Outcomes of DCD liver transplantation using organs treated by hypothermic oxygenated perfusion before implantation. J Hepatol 2019;70(1):50–7.
20. Mueller M, Kalisvaart M, O'Rourke J, et al. Hypothermic oxygenated liver perfusion (HOPE) prevents tumor recurrence in liver transplantation from donation after circulatory death. Ann Surg 2020;272(5):759–65.

21. van Rijn, Karimian N, Matton APM, et al. Dual hypothermic oxygenated machine perfusion in liver transplants donated after circulatory death. Br J Surg 2017; 104(7):907–17.
22. Patrono D, Surra A, Catalano G, et al. Hypothermic oxygenated machine perfusion of liver grafts from brain-dead donors. Sci Rep 2019;9(1):9337.
23. van Rijn, Schurink IJ, de Vries, et al. Hypothermic machine perfusion in liver transplantation – a randomized trial. N Engl J Med 2021;384(15):1391–401.
24. Patrono D, Catalano G, Rizza G, et al. Perfusate analysis during dual hypothermic oxygenated machine perfusion of liver grafts: Correlations with donor factors and early outcomes. Transplantation 2020;104(9):1929–42.
25. Muller X, Schlegel A, Kron P, et al. Novel real-time prediction of liver graft function during hypothermic oxygenated machine perfusion before liver transplantation. Ann Surg 2019;270(5):783–90.
26. Watson CJ, Kosmoliaptsis V, Randle LV, et al. Preimplant normothermic liver perfusion of a suboptimal liver donated after circulatory death. Am J Transplant 2016;16(1):353–7. https://doi.org/10.1111/ajt.13448d.
27. Perera T, Mergental H, Stephenson B, et al. First human liver transplantation using a marginal allograft resuscitated by normothermic machine perfusion. Liver Transpl 2016;22(1):120–4.
28. Ravikumar R, Jassem W, Mergental H, et al. Liver transplantation after ex vivo normothermic machine preservation: a Phase 1 (First-in-Man) clinical trial. Am J Transplant 2016;16(6):1779–87.
29. Selzner M, Goldaracena N, Echeverri J, et al. Normothermic ex vivo liver perfusion using steen solution as perfusate for human liver transplantation: first North American results. Liver Transpl 2016;22(11):1501–8.
30. Nasralla D, Coussios CC, Mergental H, et al. A randomized trial of normothermic preservation in liver transplantation. Nature 2018;557:50–6.
31. Ghinolfi D, Rreka E, de Tata V, et al. Pilot, open, randomized, prospective trial for normothermic machine perfusion evaluation in liver transplantation from older donors. Liver Transpl 2019;25:436–49.
32. Bral M, Dajani K, Leon Izquierdo D, et al. A back-to-base experience of human normothermic ex situ liver perfusion: Does the Chill Kill? Liver Transpl 2019;25: 848–58.
33. Watson CJ, Kosmoliaptsis V, Pley C, et al. Observations on the ex-situ perfusion of livers for transplantation. Am J Transplant 2018;18(8):2005–20.
34. Mergental H, Laing RW, Kirkham AJ, et al. Transplantation of discarded livers following viability testing with normothermic machine perfusion. Nat Commun 2020;11(1):2939.
35. Quintini C, Martins P, Shah S, et al. Implementing an innovated preservation technology: the American Society of Transplant Surgeons' (ASTS) Standards Committee White Paper on ex situ liver machine perfusion. Am J Transplant 2018;18(8): 1865–74.

Future Approaches and Therapeutic Modalities for Acute-on-Chronic Liver Failure

Ali Wakil, MD[a], Mumtaz Niazi, MD[a], Keri E. Lunsford, MD, PhD[b],
Nikolaos Pyrsopoulos, MD, PhD, MBA[a],*

KEYWORDS

- ACLF emerging therapies • Liver support devices • Liver stem cell transplant

KEY POINTS

- Several definitions for acute-on-chronic liver failure (ACLF) exist with the European Association for the Study of Liver-Chronic Liver Failure being most widely used in clinical practice.
- Artificial liver support devices have been emerging with varying outcomes, but till now there are no clear survival benefits from those devices in ACLF.
- Multiple promising medical therapies are emerging and being investigated for various ACLF etiologies such as granulocyte colony-stimulating factor, DUR 928, and albumin.
- Stem cell transplantation is an emerging therapy that can potentially alter the outcomes of ACLF in the future.

INTRODUCTION

Acute-on-chronic liver failure (ACLF) results from an acute decompensation of cirrhosis due to exogenous insult. The condition is characterized by a severe systemic inflammatory response, an inappropriate compensatory anti-inflammatory response, multisystem extrahepatic organ failure, and high short-term mortality.[1] Several organizations, including the Asian Pacific Association for the Study of the Liver and the European Association for the Study of Liver- Chronic Liver Failure (EASL- CLIF) have defined diagnostic criteria for ACLF,[2,3] with short-term (ie, 90-day) mortality rate approaching 50%.[4,5] Orthotopic liver transplantation (OLT) is the only curative therapy available for patients with ACLF, but due to limited organ availability, patients may expire from ACLF before an appropriate donor organ becoming available. There is a

[a] Division of Gastroenterology and Hepatology, Department of Medicine, Rutgers New Jersey Medical School, 185 South Orange Avenue, MSB H536, Newark, NJ 07103, USA; [b] Department of Surgery, Division of Liver Transplant and HPB Surgery, Rutgers New Jersey Medical School, 185 South Orange Avenue, MSB H536, Newark, NJ 07103, USA
* Corresponding author.
E-mail address: pyrsopni@njms.rutgers.edu

Clin Liver Dis 27 (2023) 777–790
https://doi.org/10.1016/j.cld.2023.03.017
1089-3261/23/© 2023 Elsevier Inc. All rights reserved.
liver.theclinics.com

dire need for effective bridging therapies to support until recovery or liver transplant. The emerging therapeutics can be categorized into the extrahepatic liver assist devices (eg, Molecular Adsorbent Recirculating System [MARS]), bioartificial liver support system, transplant of either isolated hepatocytes or mesenchymal stem cells (MSCs), and other emerging medical treatments. Here, the authors evaluate the current status of potential treatments for ACLF and assess their efficacy and therapeutic potential.

LIVER ARTIFICIAL ASSIST DEVICES

The liver artificial assist devices use the principles of dialysis to filter proteins and metabolites from the bloodstream. These devices share the basic mechanism of using a dialysate fluid and membrane system to filter toxic metabolites from the patient's bloodstream. Currently, there are at least four major liver assist devices under investigation. These include MARS, Prometheus, single-pass albumin dialysis (SPAD), and selective plasma filtrations therapy including the emerging double plasma molecular adsorption system (DPMAS). Multiple clinical studies have been performed evaluating the utility of artificial liver support systems (ALSS). Meta-analysis of 10 randomized and observational studies evaluating ALSS in ACLF demonstrates a 30% reduction in mortality risk at 1 and 3 months with suggestion of sustained long-term mortality benefit.[6] Thus, ALSS may have some benefit in ACLF treatment and bridge to transplant. Here, the authors review the currently available platforms for ALSS in ACLF.

Molecular Adsorbent Recirculating System

MARS was first introduced at the University of Rostock in Germany in the early 1990s and was made available for commercial use in 1998. It initially received Food and Drug Administration (FDA) approval for use in poisonings and overdose. Subsequently, MARS was approved for treatment of acute hepatic encephalopathy in patients with chronic liver disease[7]; however, it is not FDA-approved for use in the United States as a bridge to transplant in patients with ACLF.[8] The MARS has been tested in multiple clinical settings including acute liver failure (ALF) and ACLF, shock liver with elevated bilirubin, hepatorenal syndrome (HRS), progressive intrahepatic cholestasis, and severe hepatic encephalopathy.[9,10]

MARS is an extracorporeal absorbent support system, which uses an albumin dialysate with anion exchange, a standard dialysate circuit, and an activated charcoal absorber.[7] Venous bloodstream flows initially from the patient via continuous venovenous hemofiltration to the albumin dialysis filter containing 25% albumin. Here, the concentration gradient allows elimination of toxins due to the affinity of hydrophobic toxins for the free binding sites in albumin. The membrane is impermeable to proteins larger than 50 kDa; therefore, filtration of essential proteins, such as hormone transporters, is avoided. The albumin dialysate is then passed through sequential activated charcoal and anion exchange resins for removal of protein-bound toxins. The blood then passes through a standard hemodialysis filter for removal of water-soluble toxins[11] (Fig. 1).

Several clinical trials have evaluated the MARS for treatment or bridge to transplant in ACLF. Although improvement in bilirubin and creatinine was observed, no significant mortality benefits were demonstrated. The RELEIF trial was a prospective randomized control trial (RCT) in which 156 patients were randomized to either MARS ($n = 76$) or standard medical therapy (SMT, $n = 90$). No significant differences in 28-day survival was noted between groups on either an intent-to-treat or per protocol basis. The recipients of MARS therapy demonstrated greater reduction in serum

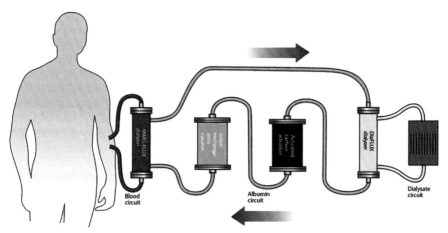

Fig. 1. The molecular adsorbent recirculating system. (Cheungpasitporn W, Thongprayoon C, Zoghby ZM, et al. MARS: Should I Use It?. Adv Chronic Kidney Dis. 2021;28(1):47-58. https://doi.org/10.1053/j.ackd.2021.02.004.)

creatinine and bilirubin and more frequent improvements in hepatic encephalopathy.[12] Gerth and colleagues performed retrospective analysis of 101 patients undergoing either MARS ($n = 47$) or SMT ($n = 54$) with organ failure liver sub-score of 3 by the ACLF-CLIF classification and without respiratory failure.[13] Short-term mortality up to 14 days was significantly improved in MARS recipients, with a tread toward improved mortality at 21 and 28 days, especially in patients with two or more organ failures. Of note, 34% of patients in the MARS group received successful liver transplant by 28 days compared with 9.3% of patients in the SMT group. The investigators additionally performed a secondary analysis of the RELIEF trials by ACLF-CLIFF grade. Although no overall mortality benefit was observed, they noted a similar trend toward 14-day survival improvement.

Although RCT data do not support for the use of MARS in ACLF, certain subsets of patients may obtain some benefit, but further prospective evidence is necessary to delineate this. The side effects reported from using MARS include bleeding, thrombocytopenia, and decreased fibrinogen levels. This raises a safety concern for the use of MARS in ACLF, given the baseline elevated bleeding risk of this patient population. In addition, the cost of use per patient is high and difficult to justify without clear mortality benefit.

Fractionated Plasma Separation and Adsorption (Prometheus)

Fractionated plasma separation and adsorption (FPSA) was first described by Falkenhagen and colleagues first in 1999, and this serves as the basis for the Prometheus system of ALSS.[14] Prometheus uses the patient plasma is passed through an AlbuFlow albumin-permeable polysulfon filter, which allows passage of large molecules up to 250 kDa into the secondary circuit. There, filtered plasma with albumin-bound toxins flow through resin absorbers (prometh01 and prometh02) where it is returned to the blood side of the albumin filter. The patients' blood then undergoes conventional hemodialysis to eliminate water-soluble toxins before being returned to the patient.

FPSA has been shown to significantly reduce metabolites, including ammonia, bilirubin, urea, aspartate aminotransferase, alanine aminotransferase, creatinine, glutamine, and tryptophan amino acids.[15,16] In addition, FPSA reduces cytokines concentration in plasma as well as inflammatory markers (C-reactive protein, erythrocyte sedimentation rate [ESR], and procalcitonin) and liver markers, such as hepatocyte growth factor.[17] However, only a handful of clinical studies have evaluated clinical endpoints following the use of FPSA in ACLF. In the HELIOS trial, a multicenter RCT of 145 patients with ACLF (FPSA, $n = 77$, SMT, $n = 68$), patients received 8 to 11 rounds of FPSA for 3 weeks. FSPA resulted in the significant reduction of serum bilirubin, and a slight but not statistically significant improvement in survival at 28-days (+3%) and 90-days (+9%). In addition, the incidence of transplant was similar between groups. Subgroup analysis demonstrated survival benefits among patients with MELD greater than 30 (HR 0.47 [CI 0.22–0.99] for FPSA vs SMT), suggesting potential utility of Prometheus in more patients with more severe ACLF, but conclusions are difficult due to the small sample size.[18]

Single-Pass Albumin Dialysis

SPAD is the simplest form of liver assist device and has been most recently established. For SPAD, blood passes through a high-flux hollow polysulfide filter, such as the one used in the MARS. Blood is cleaned via a simple human albumin (HA)-containing dialysate, which is discarded following passage. Conventional dialysis units may adapt to perform SPAD, unlike MARS and Prometheus. Because there are no additional adsorbent columns or circuits, and this device can be used in any intensive care unit with continuous dialysis capabilities and at a significantly lower cost than other forms of ALSS. Owing to the recency of its development, however, clinical data on the utility of SPAD are limited to case reports and retrospective studies, and no studies to date have compared SPAD with SMT. Only one randomized crossover study using SPAD and MARS has been described, which concluded similar efficacy for both devices on clinical parameters and the rate of bilirubin reduction.[19]

Therapeutic Plasma Exchange

Another relatively simple mechanism for treatment of both ALF and ACLF that has been explored is therapeutic plasma exchange (TPE). In theory, TPE removes toxins and inflammatory chemokines and cytokines which exacerbate immune dysfunction and cellular injury while replenishing the soluble proteins critical for hepatocytes recovery. TPE is more accessible than some of the other modalities, as it relies on widely available plasmapheresis equipment, which is available at most major medical centers. TPE has been shown to reduce of ammonia levels and total bilirubin in ACLF; however, it can worsen coagulopathy and hypocalcemia due to the striping of coagulation factors and binding of calcium by the instrument. It is therefore necessary to closely monitor components of the coagulation cascade via frequent prothrombin time/international normalised ratio (PT/INR), partial thromboplastin time (PTT), fibrinogen, and thromboelastography (TEG) measurements, with fresh frozen plasma or cryoprecipitate supplementation as necessary. In addition, pheresis with FFP or a combination of FFP and albumin may be considered to augment excessive coagulopathy. Calcium or ionized calcium levels should also be frequently monitored and aggressively supplemented.[20] One multicenter open-label RCT comparing high-volume plasma exchange (HVP) vs SMT has been reported for 183 patients with ACLF, in which HVP was administered for three consecutive days. There was a significant improvement in survival to hospital discharge as well as associated improvement in both the Sequential Organ Failure Assessment (SOFA) score and the CLIF-SOFA score in HVP recipients.[21] Although short-term efficacy of TPE is promising, this modality may not alter the long-term prognosis of patients with ACLF. In a retrospective propensity-matched analysis of 38 patients receiving TPE with SMT compared with 38 patients receiving SMT alone, TPE improved 30-day but not 90-day mortality.[22] Given promising short-term outcomes, however, RCTs will be critical for robust analysis.

Double Plasma Molecular Adsorption System

The DPMAS combines two extracorporeal hemoperfusion machines in series for absorption of both exogenous cytokines and bilirubin. Although the therapy is more expensive than TPE, the initial prospective evaluation suggests improved efficacy compared with TPE for removal of bilirubin, with decreased rates of albumin loss. In this study of 60 patients with ACLF secondary to HBV, however, both therapies resulted in equivalent improvement in survival.[23] A subsequent retrospective analysis compared DPMAS with low-dose TPE in patients with hepatitis B virus (HBV)-ACLF. In this analysis, 28-day survival was improved in patient with more severe ACLF.[24] A RCT (NCT05030571) is currently underway for evaluation of DPMAS compared with SMT in ACLF.

BIOARTIFICIAL LIVER SUPPORT SYSTEMS

Although traditional modalities focus on extracorporeal filtration and absorption of toxins, advancing technologies have allowed for the development of several bioartificial liver devices. These are differentiated by their utilization of living mammalian cells to temporarily augment the functions of the failing liver externally and to supply growth factors essential for liver regeneration. In general, cellular components are deposited on an acellular inert extracellular matrix to allow gas and nutrient exchange by the cells. Several bioartificial systems have been developed, using cell lines, porcine, or human hepatocytes (eg, from discarded donor livers) as an artificial source of hepatocyte function. Hybrid approaches combining bioartificial cellular support with extracorporeal filtration and absorption are also being explored.

Extracorporeal Liver Assist Device

The extracorporeal liver assist device (ELAD) uses a C3A human hepatoblastoma cell line. This cell line has been selected for its anti-inflammatory, antiapoptotic, and antioxidative properties. Its upregulated CYP450 system allows for active cellular detoxification of circulating metabolites. In addition, the cell line expresses several growth factors crucial for hepatocyte regeneration, including vascular endothelial growth factor. Plasma from ultra-filtrated blood is passed through hollow-fiber cartridges containing C3A cells before being returned to the subject (**Fig. 2**).[25]

Several clinical studies have evaluated the efficacy of ELAD. In 2007, a Chinese study assessed ELAD + SMT with SMT alone for patients with ACLF. They observed a significant improvement in biochemical markers, transplant-free survival, and overall survival associated with longer length of treatment.[26] Unfortunately, these initial promising results have not been reinforced. A large open-label, a randomized-controlled clinical trial examining the use of ELAD in subjects with severe alcohol-associated hepatitis (sAH) detected no alteration in overall survival,[27] but subgroup analysis suggested some survival benefit in subjects with less severe disease (MELD < 28). Another trial assessing the device in alcohol-associated liver disease was terminated early due to safety concerns.[28] It is important to note that the initial study by Duan and colleagues primarily evaluated chronic HBV-related ACLF, raising the possibility that ELAD efficacy may be altered by the etiology of the liver disease. Additional homogenous trials are necessary before implementation of ELAD in ACLF.

HepatAssist

HepatAssist is a hybrid bioartificial liver support device, which uses porcine hepatocytes in combination with active charcoal filtration of the blood for detoxification. Patient's plasma is separated, passed through a charcoal filter and an oxygenator before

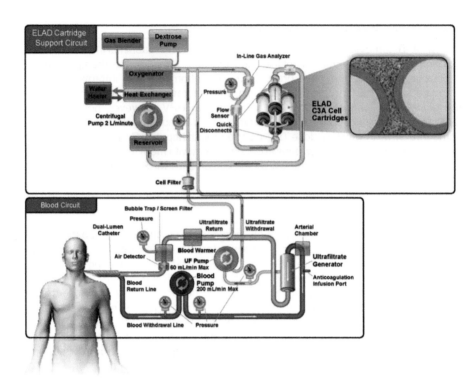

Fig. 2. The ELAD system is an extracorporeal human hepatic cell-based liver treatment. During ELAD treatment, blood is drawn from the subject via a dual-lumen catheter using an extracorporeal pumping unit and then is separated by a specifically designed ultrafiltration (UF) generator cartridge. The UF contains proteins the size of albumin and smaller but does not contain larger proteins such as antibodies. The UF is circulated at a high flow rate through the ELAD cartridges, which contain approximately 440 g of C3A cells. After circulation through the ELAD cartridges, the UF passes through a 0.2-mm pore size cell filter, is recombined with the cellular components of the subject's blood, and is then returned to the subject via the dual-lumen catheter. (*From* Thompson J, et al. Extracorporeal cellular therapy (ELAD) in severe alcoholic hepatitis: a multinational, prospective, controlled, randomized trial. Liver Transpl. 2018;24(3):380–93.)

passage over porcine hepatocytes deposited in a bioreactor (**Fig. 3**). A multicenter RCT of HepatAssist published in 2004 randomized 171 patients with ALF or post-OLT primary graft non-function to the HepatAssist device or SMT alone. There was no mortality difference at 30 days (71% vs 62%; $P = .26$) overall[29]; however, subgroup analysis of ALF demonstrated a reduction in mortality (relative risk [RR] 0.56, $P = .048$). Despite these findings, the device is not FDA-approved for use in the United States, and a phase III clinical trial would be required for wider application.

CELLULAR TRANSPLANTATION

Cellular transplantation (hepatocytes or stem cell) has been proposed as a potential bridge to transplant or liver recovery and as an alternative to liver transplant through the correction of isolated metabolic defects. Given the high regenerative capacity of the liver, the aim of cellular transplantation in ACLF is generally as a bridge to hepatocyte recovery through enhanced liver regeneration. Technically, cells may be

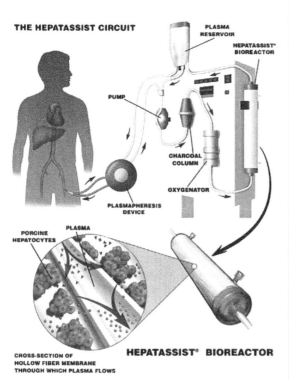

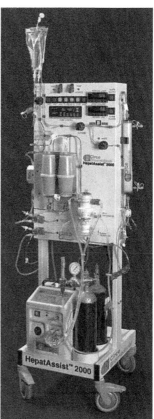

Fig. 3. The HepatAssist device.

deposited directly into the liver via portal vein injection, or hepatocytes may be trans-planted heterotopically into the spleen, peritoneum, or omentum. In cirrhotics, howev-er, altered parenchymal architecture might limit successful intrahepatic engraftment, making extrahepatic sites of engraftment more appealing. Although benefits include a decreased risk of surgical complications and lower financial cost than transplanta-tion, its clinical success to date has been somewhat limited. One of the barriers to suc-cessful hepatocyte transplantation (HT) has been difficulty with achieving long-term engraftment, most likely due to the robust allogeneic immune response elicited by he-patocytes in comparison to whole liver tissue.[30–32] As such, alternatives to primary he-patocytes, including less immunogenic stem cell-derived hepatocyte-like cells or encapsulated hepatocytes are being explored.

Hepatocyte Transplantation

Transplantation of exogenous allogenic mature hepatocytes has long been proposed as a potential therapeutic treatment of liver failure. HT was performed by Dr Najarian in Gunn rat model in 1976 for the treatment of isolated metabolic defects in uridine 5′-diphospho (UDP)-glucuronyl-transferase deficiency.[33] Human HT was pioneered in Japan in 1992 through the heterotopic implantation of human allogeneic hepatocytes into the spleen.[34] Since that time, numerous human hepatocyte transplant trials have been performed. More standardized techniques have emerged for isolation, culture, and preservation of hepatocytes; however, broad implementation has been limited due to a lack of long-term efficacy data. Most studies have focused on the utilization of hepatocyte transplant to correct inborn metabolic defects or a bridging therapy in ALF. In ALF, transplant hepatocytes may allow short-term promotion of host parenchymal regeneration, potentially promoting native liver spontaneous recovery, and orthotopic liver transplant remains a viable alternative if HT fails.

The hepatocytes may be harvested from discarded human livers for transplant or isolated hepatic lobes or segments. Cells may be infused immediately after isolation or cryopreserved for later use; however, the later risks some loss in cell viability due to the sensitivity of hepatocytes to in vitro conditions. The most preferred delivery method of HT is via intraportal injection to allow orthotopic implantation within the liver. This is achieved either through percutaneous transhepatic puncture of the portal vein or via inferior mesenteric vein catheterization. In newborns, access via the umbilical vein is also an option. During portal vein injection, care must be taken to monitor portal pressures and avoid portal hypertension. General estimates suggest that a total transplant volume equaling 5% to 15% of the liver mass is required to achieve physiological benefit.[35] Although cells may be administered in a single infusion, multiple infusions can also be performed, allowing for utilization of cells from multiple donors. One major barrier in HT is the lack of viable reporter proteins to monitor their fate following transplant; thus, graft monitoring is limited to identification on liver biopsies via human leukocyte antigens (HLA) or chromosomal differences. Animal models suggest a robust initiation of both cellular and humoral immune responses by hepatocytes,[31,32] but clinical correlation of this has been difficult due to the lack of monitoring.

In children, HT has primarily been evaluated as a treatment of inherited metabolic disorders such as Crigler-Najjar syndrome and Urea cycle defects. Multiple case reports demonstrate the improvement of serum bilirubin and ammonia levels in patients with inherited metabolic disorders and urea cycle, respectively[36]; however, HT only served to delay and not prevent the need to liver transplant. Liver transplant was required after 9 months secondary to a decline in cell function for unclear reasons, but rejection is a distinct possibility given the high immunogenicity in animal models. Worldwide more than 40 cases HT for drug or viral hepatitis-induced ALF have also been described. Short-term data demonstrate improvements in ammonia level, liver function, and hepatic encephalopathy, but, again, the majority ultimately required OLT. For treatment of ACLF, HT has been demonstrated to improve liver function and prolonged survival in a rat model of ACLF.[37] In humans, a small series of heterotopic HT into the spleen has been performed.[34] Of seven ACLF patients treated, three fully recovered, one ultimately received OLT, and three patients died between 2.5 and 12 months after HT.[38] Thus, HT may hold more promise as bridging or definitive therapy for ACLF.

Mesenchymal Stem Cell Transplantation

MSCs have emerged in recent decades as very promising treatments for a variety of diseases, including cirrhosis and ACLF. MSCs are pluripotent and can differentiate into multiple cell types, including hepatocytes[39] and MSC transplant in animal models demonstrated improved fibrosis and liver function.[40] The primary sources of MSCs are bone marrow MSCs (BM-MSCs) and umbilical cord MSCs (UC-MSCs), but peripheral blood and adipose tissue MSCs have also been evaluated. One benefit of the use of MSCs over allogeneic hepatocytes as cellular therapy is that cells may be derived from autologous sources, thus obviating the need to immunosuppression and the concerns for rejection. Alternatively, allogeneic sources may be used, and their early stage of differentiation may decrease their immunogenicity. Therapy with MSCs can be achieved through either single or multiple infusions via peripheral intravenous infusion or hepatic artery infusion. Barriers for use include optimization of cellular differentiation and the need for in vitro expansion to obtain sufficient sample volume for transplant.

Autologous BM-MSCs in clinical trials for chronic liver diseases have shown good safety data with short-term effectiveness but unsatisfactory long-term results.[41] Allogenic BM-MSCs, which are more readily accessible than autologous, BM-MSCs have also been proven safe in patients with cirrhosis and ACLF.[42–44] Numerous clinical trials have been reported regarding the clinical utility of MSCs in ACLF. Most of the trials have been performed in China, with a paucity of data from Europe or North America; thus, most of the cases have been performed in recipients with chronic HBV- induced cirrhosis and ACLF. A recent meta-analysis of 12 RCTs in MSC therapy for chronic liver disease and ACLF suggested improved liver function, MELD score, albumin levels, and coagulation profiles, as well as reduced rates of hepatic encephalopathy and gastrointestinal hemorrhage. Both MB-MSCs and UC-MSCs had similar efficacy. Fever as the only adverse event reported in 5/12 studies. Unfortunately, the analysis concluded that there was no discernible survival benefit with MSC therapy.[43] A second meta-analysis of 24 RTCs similarly reported good safety data for MSCs therapy, but they concluded that BM-MSCs are superior to UC-MSCs.[44] Overall, MSCs therapy seems to be safe overall, but data regarding long-term efficacy and sustained clinical benefit remain lacking. Furthermore, investigation of the efficacy in non-HBV-ACLF patients is warranted.

OTHER EMERGING MEDICAL THERAPIES
Granulocyte-Colony-Stimulating Factor

Systemic inflammation and inappropriate immune activation with resultant tissue damage and end-organ dysfunction are the hallmarks of ACLF pathophysiology. Granulocyte-colony-stimulating factor (G-CSF) stimulates the proliferation and differentiation of progenitor cells and mobilizes stem cells from the patient's bone marrow,[45] and it has been investigated as a potential therapeutic agent to augment immune injury in ACLF. G-CSF treatment seems to improve survival in RCTs for patients with severe alcohol-associated ACLF.[46–48] A meta-analysis of two of these RCTs demonstrates overall survival benefits for G-CSF + SMT treatment compared with SMT alone.[49] In contrast, the GRAFT trial, a multicenter RCT of 176 patients with ACLF defined by the EASL-CLIF classification, showed no significant mortality benefit or increase in transplant-free survival for patients treated with G-CSF + SMT compared with SMT alone.[50] Thus, there is currently insufficient evidence to recommend G-CSF routinely for the treatment of ACLF.

DUR-928

DUR-928 is an endogenous sulfated oxysterol molecule that influences hepatocyte regeneration and modulates inflammation. In an-open label RCT, DUR-928 treatment improved biochemical markers of liver dysfunction 89% of patients with sAH, with reduction of bilirubin and improvement in Lille score.[51] Currently, the recruitment is underway for phase two randomized, multicenter, placebo-controlled trial (NCT04563026) to evaluate the mortality benefits of DUR-928 in severe AH.

Albumin

Albumin infusion has multiple indications for use in decompensated cirrhotics and ACLF, including treatment of HRS, volume replacement after large volume paracentesis, and treatment of spontaneous bacteria peritonitis (SBP).[52] Owing to its antioxidative and immunomodulatory properties, several notable RCT studies have been evaluating the benefits of long-term albumin infusion in subjects with ACLF. The ANSWER trial evaluated the use of HA in decompensated cirrhotic in a multi-center, open-label design. After enrolling 431 subjects, the 18-month survival benefit was significantly higher in HA vs SMT group (77% vs 66%; P0.028).[53] Furthermore, there was a reduction in SBP, hepatic encephalopathy, and HRS for patients receiving HA. In contrast, the ATTIRE trial enrolled a large multicenter randomized cohort of 777 patients with acute decompensated cirrhosis. Treated patients were targeted to an albumin level above 3.0 g/dL, and there was ultimately no discernible survival benefit for albumin therapy compared with SMT (29.7% vs 30.2%; $P = .87$).[54] Finally, the INFECIR-2 study, which assessed the dose and frequency of albumin for the amelioration of inflammation, observed a reduction in cytokines and inflammatory markers in subjects who received HA with antibiotics compared to antibiotics alone.[55] An additional phase 3 multicenter RCT is currently underway to evaluate the efficacy of Albutein 20% in decompensated cirrhosis with or without ACLF (the PRECIOSA trial NCT03451292). Given the contradicting results of the available trial data, there is insufficient evidence to validate the benefits of HA in ACLF.

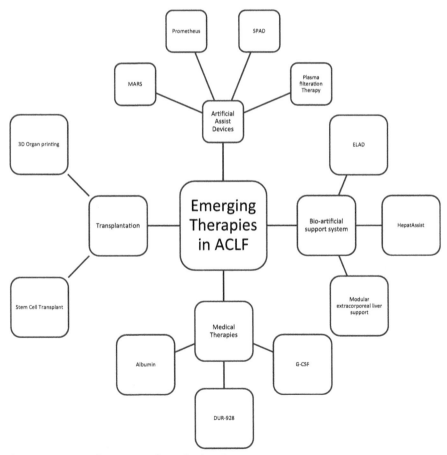

Fig. 4. Summary of emerging therapies in ACLF.

SUMMARY

ACLF has an exorbitantly high mortality, and although liver transplantation can be curative, patient access to transplant may be limited by organ availability, patient illness severity, underlying comorbidities, or psychosocial barriers. Thus, the development of alternative definitive and bridging therapies is crucial for improving patient outcomes from this disease. Although several therapeutic options have been developed and demonstrate some promise in improving metrics of disease severity, at least in the short term, none can yet substitute for liver transplantation (**Fig. 4**). Data highlight the need for further evaluation through RCTs as well as dedicated funding of further research and development to optimize therapeutic options for ACLF.

CLINICS CARE POINTS

- Liver transplantation remains the curative therapy for ACLF.
- Various artificial liver support devices exist but none have shown stronge survival benifits.
- Stems cell transplantation remains a potential future cure for ACLF patients whom liver tranplsnat is not avilable.

REFERENCE

1. Olson JC. Acute-on-chronic liver failure: management and prognosis. Curr Opin Crit Care 2019;25(2):165–70.
2. Sarin SK, Kedarisetty CK, Abbas Z, et al. Acute-on-chronic liver failure: consensus recommendations of the Asian Pacific Association for the Study of the Liver (APASL) 2014. Hepatol Int 2014;8(4):453–7.
3. Moreau R, Jalan R, Gines P, et al. Acute-on-chronic liver failure is a distinct syndrome that develops in patients with acute decompensation of cirrhosis. Gastroenterology 2013;144(7):1426–37.
4. Mahmud N, Kaplan DE, Taddei TH, et al. Incidence and mortality of acute-on-chronic liver failure using two definitions in patients with compensated cirrhosis. Hepatology 2019;69(5):2150–63.
5. Bajaj JS, O'Leary JG, Reddy KR, et al. Survival in infection-related acute-on-chronic liver failure is defined by extrahepatic organ failures. Hepatology 2014; 60(1):250–6.
6. Shen Y, Wang XL, Wang B, et al. Survival benefits with artificial liver support system for acute-on-chronic liver failure: a time series-based meta-analysis. Med (Baltim) 2016;95(3):e2506.
7. Kobashi-Margáin RA, Gavilanes-Espinar JG, Gutiérrez-Grobe Y, et al. Albumin dialysis with molecular adsorbent recirculating system (MARS) for the treatment of hepatic encephalopathy in liver failure. Ann Hepatol 2011;10:S70–6.
8. 510(k) Safety and effectiveness for the Molecular Adsorbent Recirculating System (MARS). 2012: FDA. Accessed 01 November, 2022.https://www.accessdata.fda.gov/cdrh_docs/pdf3/K033262.pdf.
9. Mitzner SR, Stange J, Klammt S, et al. Extracorporeal detoxification using the molecular adsorbent recirculating system for critically ill patients with liver failure. J Am Soc Nephrol 2001;12(Suppl17):S75–82.
10. Patel P, Okoronkwo N, Pyrsopoulos NT. Future approaches and therapeutic modalities for acute liver failure. Clin Liver Dis 2018;22(2):419–27.

11. Marangoni R, Bellati G, Castelli A, et al. Development of high-efficiency molecular adsorbent recirculating system: preliminary report. Artif Organs 2014;38:879–83.

12. Banares R, Nevens F, Larsen FS, et al. Extracorporeal albumin dialysis with the molecular adsorbent recirculating system in acute-on-chronic liver failure: the RE-LIEF trial. Hepatology 2013;57(3):1153–62.

13. Gerth HU, Pohlen M, Tholking G, et al. Molecular adsorbent recirculating system can reduce short-term mortality among patients with acute-on-chronic liver failure-a retrospective analysis. Crit Care Med 2017;45(10):1616–24.

14. Falkenhagen D, Strobl W, Vogt G, et al. Fractionated plasma separation and adsorption system: a novel system for blood purification to remove albumin bound substances. Artif Organs 1999;23(1):81–6.

15. Grodzicki M, Kotulski M, Leonowicz D, et al. Results of treatment of acute liver failure patients with use of the prometheus FPSA system. Transpl Proc 2009; 41(8):3079–81.

16. Rifai K, Das A, Rosenau J, et al. Changes in plasma amino acids during extracorporeal liver support by fractionated plasma separation and adsorption. Artif Organs 2010;34(2):166–70.

17. Rocen M, Kieslichova E, Merta D, et al. The effect of Prometheus device on laboratory markers of inflammation and tissue regeneration in acute liver failure management. Transpl Proc 2010;42(9):3606–11.

18. Kribben A, Gerken G, Haag S, et al. Effects of fractionated plasma separation and adsorption on survival in patients with acute-on-chronic liver failure. Gastroenterology 2012;142(4):782–9.

19. Sponholz C, Matthes K, Rupp D, et al. Molecular adsorbent recirculating system and single-pass albumin dialysis in liver failure–a prospective, randomised crossover study. Crit Care 2016;20:2.

20. Stenbøg P, Busk T, Larsen FS. Efficacy of liver assisting in patients with hepatic encephalopathy with special focus on plasma exchange. Metab Brain Dis 2013;28:333–5.

21. Larsen FS, Schmidt LE, Bernsmeier C, et al. High-volume plasma exchange in patients with acute liver failure: an open randomised controlled trial. J Hepatol 2016;64:69–78.

22. Swaroop S, Arora U, Biswas S, et al. Therapeutic plasma-exchange improves short-term, but not long-term, outcomes in patients with acute-on-chronic liver failure: a propensity score-matched analysis. J Clin Apher 2022.

23. Wan YM, Li YH, Xu ZY, et al. Therapeutic plasma exchange versus double plasma molecular absorption system in hepatitis B virus-infected acute-on-chronic liver failure treated by entercavir: a prospective study. J Clin Apher 2017;32(6): 453–61.

24. Yao J, Li S, Zhou L, et al. Therapeutic effect of double plasma molecular adsorption system and sequential half-dose plasma exchange in patients with HBV-related acute-on-chronic liver failure. J Clin Apher 2019;34(4):392–8.

25. Landeen LK, Van Allen J, Heredia N, et al. Expression of acute-phase proteins byELAD C3A Cells. Transplantation 2015;99:208, 21st Annual International Congress of the International-Liver-Transplant-Society (ILTS) July 08-11, 2015, Chicago, IL.

26. Dunn W, Jamil LH, Brown LS, et al. MELD accurately predicts mortality in patients with alcoholic hepatitis. Hepatology 2005;41:353–8.

27. Thompson J, Jones N, Al-Khafaji A, et al. Extracorporeal cellular therapy (ELAD) in severe alcoholic hepatitis: a multinational, prospective, controlled, randomized trial. Liver Transpl 2018;24(3):380–93.

28. Vital Therapies I. Assess safety and efficacy of ELAD (extracorporeal liver assist system) in subjects with alcohol-induced liver failure. 2015.

29. Demetriou AA, Brown RS Jr, Busuttil RW, et al. Prospective, randomized, multi-center, controlled trial of a bioartificial liver in treating acute liver failure. Ann Surg 2004;239(5):660–7, discussion 667-70.

30. Zimmerer JM, Horne PH, Fisher MG, et al. Unique CD8+ T cell-mediated immune responses primed in the liver. Transplantation 2016;100(9):1907–15.

31. Horne PH, Lunsford KE, Walker JP, et al. Recipient immune repertoire and engraftment site influence the immune pathway effecting acute hepatocellular allograft rejection. Cell Transplant 2008;17(7):829–44.

32. Lunsford KE, Horne PH, Koester MA, et al. Activation and maturation of alloreactive CD4-independent, CD8 cytolytic T cells. Am J Transplant 2006;6(10): 2268–81.

33. Matas AJ, Sutherland DER, Steffes MW, et al. Hepatocellular transplantation for metabolic deficiencies: decrease of plasma bilirubin in Gunn rats. Science 1976;192(4242):892–4.

34. Mito M, Kusano M, Kawaura Y. Hepatocyte transplantation in man. Transplant Proc 1992;24(6):3052–3.

35. Iansante V, Mitry RR, Filippi C, et al. Human hepatocyte transplantation for liver disease: current status and future perspectives. Pediatr Res 2018;83(1–2): 232–40.

36. Vimalesvaran S, Nulty J, Dhawan A. Cellular therapies in pediatric liver diseases. Cells 2022;11(16):2483.

37. Kobayashi N, Ito M, Nakamura J, et al. Hepatocyte transplantation improves liver function and prolongs survival in rats with decompensated liver cirrhosis. Transplant Proc 1999;31(1–2):428–9.

38. Wang F, Zhou L, Ma X, et al. Monitoring of intrasplenic hepatocyte transplantation for acute-on-chronic liver failure: a prospective five-year follow-up study. Transplant Proc 2014;46(1).

39. Snykers S, Henkens T, De Rop E, et al. Role of epigenetics in liver-specific gene transcription, hepatocyte differentiation and stem cell reprogrammation. J Hepatol 2009;51(1):187–211.

40. Jang YO, Cho M, Yun C, et al. Effect of function-enhanced mesenchymal stem cells infected with decorin-expressing adenovirus on hepatic fibrosis. Stem Cells Transl Med 2016;5(9):1247–56.

41. Peng L, Xie D-Y, Lin B-L, et al. Autologous bone marrow mesenchymal stem cell transplantation in liver failure patients caused by hepatitis B: short-term and long-term outcomes. Hepatology 2011;54(3):820–8.

42. Lin B-L, Chen J-F, Qiu W-H, et al. Allogeneic Bone Marrow-Derived Mesenchymal Stromal Cells for Hepatitis B Virus-Related Acute-on-Chronic Liver Failure: a Randomized Controlled Trial American Association for the Study of Liver Diseases. Hepatology 2017;66(1):209–19. https://doi.org/10.1002/hep.29189/suppinfo.

43. Liu Y, Dong Y, Wu X, et al. The assessment of mesenchymal stem cells therapy in acute on chronic liver failure and chronic liver disease: a systematic review and meta-analysis of randomized controlled clinical trials. Stem Cell Res Ther 2021; 13(1):204.

44. Zhou GP, Jiang YZ, Sun LY, et al. Therapeutic effect and safety of stem cell therapy for chronic liver disease: a systematic review and meta-analysis of randomized controlled trials. Stem Cell Res Ther 2020;11(1):1–19.

45. Theocharis SE, Papadimitriou LJ, Retsou ZP, et al. Granulocyte colony stimulating factor administration ameliorates liver regeneration in animal model of fulminant hepatic failure and encephalopathy. Dig Dis Sci 2003;48(9):1797–803.

46. Singh V, Sharma AK, Narasimhan RL, et al. Granulocyte colony-stimulating factor in severe alcoholic hepatitis: a randomized pilot study. Am J Gastroenterol 2014; 109(9):1417–23.

47. Singh V, Keisham A, Bhalla A, et al. Efficacy of granulocyte colony-stimulating factor and N-acetylcysteine therapies in patients with severe alcoholic hepatitis. Clin Gastroenterol Hepatol 2018;16(10):1650–6. E2.

48. Shasthry SM, Sharma MK, Shasthry V, et al. Efficacy of granulocyte colony-stimulating factor in the management of steroid-nonresponsive severe alcoholic hepatitis: a double-blind randomized controlled trial. Hepatology 2019;70(3):802–11.

49. Chavez-Tapia NC, Mendiola-Pastrana I, Ornelas-Arroyo VJ, et al. Granulocyte-colony stimulating factor for acute-on-chronic liver failure: systematic review and meta-analysis. Ann Hepatol 2015;14(5):631–41.

50. Engelmann C, Herber A, Franke A, et al. Granulocyte-colony stimulating factor (G-CSF) to treat acute-on-chronic liver failure: a multicenter randomized trial (GRAFT study). J Hepatol 2021;75(6):1346–54.

51. Hassanein T, Stein LL, Flamm S, et al. Safety and efficacy of DUR-928: a potential new therapy for acute alcoholic hepatitis. Hepatology 2019;70:1483A–4A.

52. EASL clinical practice guidelines for the management of patients with decompensated cirrhosis. J Hepatol 2018;69(2):406–60.

53. Di Pascoli M, Fasolato S, Piano S, et al. Long-term administration of human albumin improves survival in patients with cirrhosis and refractory ascites. Liver Int Off J Int Assoc Study Liver 2019;39:98–105.

54. China L, Freemantle N, Forrest E, et al. A randomized trial of albumin infusions in hospitalized patients with cirrhosis. N Engl J Med 2021;384(9):808–17.

55. Fernández J, Clària J, Amorós A, et al. Effects of albumin treatment on systemic and portal hemodynamics and systemic inflammation in patients with decompensated cirrhosis. Gastroenterology 2019;157(1):149–62.

Moving?

Make sure your subscription moves with you!

To notify us of your new address, find your **Clinics Account Number** (located on your mailing label above your name), and contact customer service at:

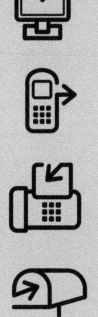

Email: journalscustomerservice-usa@elsevier.com

800-654-2452 (subscribers in the U.S. & Canada)
314-447-8871 (subscribers outside of the U.S. & Canada)

Fax number: 314-447-8029

Elsevier Health Sciences Division
Subscription Customer Service
3251 Riverport Lane
Maryland Heights, MO 63043

*To ensure uninterrupted delivery of your subscription, please notify us at least 4 weeks in advance of move.

Printed and bound by CPI Group (UK) Ltd, Croydon, CR0 4YY

03/10/2024

01040469-0006